Emergent Neuroimaging: A Patient Focused Approach

Editor

DIEGO B. NUNEZ

NEUROIMAGING CLINICS OF NORTH AMERICA

www.neuroimaging.theclinics.com

Consulting Editor
SURESH K. MUKHERJI

August 2018 • Volume 28 • Number 3

ELSEVIER

1600 John F. Kennedy Boulevard • Suite 1800 • Philadelphia, Pennsylvania, 19103-2899

http://www.neuroimaging.theclinics.com

NEUROIMAGING CLINICS OF NORTH AMERICA Volume 28, Number 3
August 2018 ISSN 1052-5149, ISBN 13: 978-0-323-61400-9

Editor: John Vassallo (j.vassallo@elsevier.com)
Developmental Editor: Casey Potter

Neuroimaging Clinics of North America (ISSN 1052-5149) is published quarterly by Elsevier Inc., 360 Park Avenue South, New York, NY 10010-1710. Months of issue are February, May, August, and November. Business and editorial offices: 1600 John F. Kennedy Blvd., Suite 1800, Philadelphia, PA 19103-2899. Business and editorial offices: 6277 Sea Harbor Drive, Orlando, FL 32887-4800. Periodicals postage paid at New York, NY, and additional mailing offices. Subscription prices are USD 387 per year for US individuals, USD 622 per year for US institutions, USD 100 per year for US students and residents, USD 440 per year for Canadian individuals, USD 791 per year for Canadian institutions, USD 525 per year for international individuals, USD 791 per year for international institutions and USD 260 per year for Canadian and foreign students and residents. To receive student/resident rate, orders must be accompanied by name of affiliated institution, date of term, and the *signature* of program/residency coordinator on institution letterhead. Orders will be billed at individual rate until proof of status is received. Foreign air speed delivery is included in all *Clinics* subscription prices. All prices are subject to change without notice. POSTMASTER: Send address changes to *Neuroimaging Clinics of North America*, Elsevier Health Sciences Division, Subscription **Customer Service, 3251 Riverport Lane, Maryland Heights, MO 63043. Telephone: 1-800-654-2452 (U.S. and Canada); 314-447-8871 (outside U.S. and Canada). Fax: 314-447-8029. E-mail: journalscustomer service-usa@elsevier.com (for print support); journalsonlinesupport-usa@elsevier.com (for online support).**

Reprints. For copies of 100 or more of articles in this publication, please contact the Commercial Reprints Department, Elsevier Inc., 360 Park Avenue South, New York, NY 10010-1710. Tel.: 212-633-3874; Fax: 212-633-3820; E-mail: reprints@elsevier.com.

Neuroimaging Clinics of North America is covered by *Excerpta Medical/EMBASE,* the RSNA Index of Imaging Literature, *MEDLINE/PubMed (Index Medicus),* MEDLINE/MEDLARS, SciSearch, Research Alert, and Neuroscience Citation Index.

Printed in the United States of America.

PROGRAM OBJECTIVE

The goal of *Neuroimaging Clinics of North America* is to keep practicing radiologists and radiology residents up to date with current clinical practice in radiology by providing timely articles reviewing the state of the art in patient care.

TARGET AUDIENCE

Practicing radiologists, radiology residents, and other healthcare professionals who utilize neuroimaging findings to provide patient care.

LEARNING OBJECTIVES

Upon completion of this activity, participants will be able to:
1. Review special considerations in elderly patients head and neck injuries.
2. Discuss emergent neuroimaging during pregnancy and the post-partum period, as well as in the oncologic and immunosuppressed patient.
3. Recognize current challenges in the use of CT and MRI in suspected cervical spine trauma.

ACCREDITATION

The Elsevier Office of Continuing Medical Education (EOCME) is accredited by the Accreditation Council for Continuing Medical Education (ACCME) to provide continuing medical education for physicians.

The EOCME designates this enduring material for a maximum of 15 *AMA PRA Category 1 Credit*(s)™. Physicians should claim only the credit commensurate with the extent of their participation in the activity.

All other healthcare professionals requesting continuing education credit for this enduring material will be issued a certificate of participation.

DISCLOSURE OF CONFLICTS OF INTEREST

The EOCME assesses conflict of interest with its instructors, faculty, planners, and other individuals who are in a position to control the content of CME activities. All relevant conflicts of interest that are identified are thoroughly vetted by EOCME for fair balance, scientific objectivity, and patient care recommendations. EOCME is committed to providing its learners with CME activities that promote improvements or quality in healthcare and not a specific proprietary business or a commercial interest.

Mohamad Abdalkader, MD; Timothy J. Amrhein, MD; Mark P. Bernstein, MD, FASER; Anthony M. Durso, MD; Nisreen S. Ezuddin, MD; Chad Farris, MD; Dheeraj Gandhi, MD; Guangzu Gao, MD; Liangge Hsu, MD; Shahmir Kamalian, MD; Alison Kemp; Peter G. Kranz, MD; Pradeep Kuttysankaran; Catalina Restrepo Lopera, MD; Ajay Malhotra, MD, MMM; Michael D. Malinzak, MD, PhD; Kushal Y. Mehta, MD; Ali Y. Mian, MD; Asim Mian, MD; Frank J. Minja, MD; Suresh K. Mukherji, MD, MBA, FACR; Felipe Munera, MD; Thanh B. Nguyen, MD, FRCPC; Diego B. Nunez, MD, MPH, FACR; Casey Potter; Christopher A. Potter, MD; Gaurav Saigal, MD; Claire K. Sandstrom, MD; Pina Sanelli, MD, MPH, FACR; Edward K. Sung, MD; Sean Symons, BASc, MPH, MD, FRCPC, DABR, MBA; Carlos Torres, MD, FRCPC; Gabriela de la Vega, MD; John Vassallo; Walter F. Wiggins, MD, PhD; Aaron Winn, MD; Xiao Wu, BS; Nader Zakhari, MD, FRCPC; Rebecca L. Zucconi, MD, FACOG; William B. Zucconi, DO.

The planning committee, staff, authors and editors listed below have identified no financial relationships or relationships to products or devices they or their spouse/life partner have with commercial interest related to the content of this CME activity:
Michael H. Lev, MD, FAHA, FACR: *has participated in a speaker's bureau and acted as a consultant and/or advisor for the General Electric Company and Takeda Pharmaceutical Company Limited. He has also participated in a speaker's bureau and received research support from Siemens Medical Solutions, USA.*
Aaron D. Sodickson, MD, PhD: *has acted as a consultant and/or advisor for General Electric Company, Bayer AG and has been a consultant and/or advisor and received research support from Siemens Medical Solutions USA, Inc.*

UNAPPROVED/OFF-LABEL USE DISCLOSURE

The EOCME requires CME faculty to disclose to the participants:
1. When products or procedures being discussed are off-label, unlabelled, experimental, and/or investigational (not US Food and Drug Administration [FDA] approved); and
2. Any limitations on the information presented, such as data that are preliminary or that represent ongoing research, interim analyses, and/or unsupported opinions. Faculty may discuss information about pharmaceutical agents that is outside of FDA-approved labelling. This information is intended solely for CME and is not intended to promote off-label use of these medications. If you have any questions, contact the medical affairs department of the manufacturer for the most recent prescribing information.

TO ENROLL

To enroll in the *Neuroimaging Clinics of North America* Continuing Medical Education program, call customer service at 1-800-654-2452 or sign up online at http://www.theclinics.com/home/cme. The CME program is available to subscribers for an additional annual fee of USD 244.40.

METHOD OF PARTICIPATION

In order to claim credit, participants must complete the following:

1. Complete enrolment as indicated above.
2. Read the activity.
3. Complete the CME Test and Evaluation. Participants must achieve a score of 70% on the test. All CME Tests and Evaluations must be completed online.

CME INQUIRIES/SPECIAL NEEDS

For all CME inquiries or special needs, please contact elsevierCME@elsevier.com.

NEUROIMAGING CLINICS OF NORTH AMERICA

THE CLINICS ARE AVAILABLE ONLINE!
Access your subscription at:
www.theclinics.com

Contributors

CONSULTING EDITOR

SURESH K. MUKHERJI, MD, MBA, FACR
Professor and Chairman, Walter F. Patenge
Endowed Chair, Department of Radiology,
Michigan State University, Chief Medical
Officer and Director of Health Care Delivery,
Michigan State University Health Team,
East Lansing, Michigan, USA

EDITOR

DIEGO B. NUNEZ, MD, MPH, FACR
Chief, Division of Neuroradiology, Director,
Emergency Neuroradiology, Department of
Radiology, Brigham and Women's Hospital,
Senior Lecturer, Harvard Medical School,
Boston, Massachusetts, USA

AUTHORS

MOHAMAD ABDALKADER, MD
Neurointerventional Radiology Fellow,
Department of Radiology, Boston University
Medical Center, Boston, Massachusetts,
USA

TIMOTHY J. AMRHEIN, MD
Assistant Professor, Department of Radiology,
Duke University Medical Center, Durham,
North Carolina, USA

MARK P. BERNSTEIN, MD, FASER
Clinical Associate Professor, Department of
Radiology, NYU Langone Health, Bellevue
Hospital and Trauma Center, New York,
New York, USA

ANTHONY M. DURSO, MD
Assistant Professor, Department of Radiology,
University of Miami Miller School of Medicine,
Ryder Trauma Center, Jackson Memorial
Hospital, Miami, Florida, USA

NISREEN S. EZUDDIN, MD
Department of Radiology, University of Miami
Miller School of Medicine, Jackson Memorial
Hospital, Miami, Florida, USA

CHAD FARRIS, MD
Resident in Training, Department of Radiology,
Boston University Medical Center, Boston,
Massachusetts, USA

DHEERAJ GANDHI, MD
Professor and Director, Interventional
Neuroradiology, Professor of Radiology,
Nuclear Medicine, Neurology and
Neurosurgery, University of Maryland School
of Medicine, Baltimore, Maryland, USA

GUANGZU GAO, MD
Chief Resident, Department of Radiology
and Biomedical Imaging, Yale Diagnostic
Radiology, Yale School of Medicine,
New Haven, Connecticut, USA

LIANGGE HSU, MD
Division of Neuroradiology, Department of Radiology, Brigham and Women's Hospital, Boston, Massachusetts, USA

SHAHMIR KAMALIAN, MD
Director, Emergency Radiology CT, Massachusetts General Hospital, Instructor, Department of Radiology, Harvard Medical School, Boston, Massachusetts, USA

PETER G. KRANZ, MD
Director of Spine Intervention, Associate Professor, Department of Radiology, Duke University Medical Center, Durham, North Carolina, USA

MICHAEL H. LEV, MD, FAHA, FACR
Division Chief, Emergency Radiology, Massachusetts General Hospital, Professor, Department of Radiology, Harvard Medical School, Boston, Massachusetts, USA

CATALINA RESTREPO LOPERA, MD
Radiology Resident, CES University, Medellin, Antioquia, Colombia

AJAY MALHOTRA, MD, MMM
Department of Radiology and Biomedical Imaging, Yale School of Medicine, The Imaging Clinical Effectiveness and Outcomes Research, Northwell Health, New Haven, Connecticut, USA

MICHAEL D. MALINZAK, MD, PhD
Medical Instructor, Department of Radiology, Duke University Medical Center, Durham, North Carolina, USA

KUSHAL Y. MEHTA, MD
Neuroradiology Fellow, Department of Radiology and Biomedical Imaging, Yale School of Medicine, New Haven, Connecticut, USA

ALI Y. MIAN, MD
Neuroradiology Fellow, Department of Radiology and Biomedical Imaging, Yale School of Medicine, New Haven, Connecticut, USA

ASIM MIAN, MD
Assistant Professor, Department of Radiology, Program Director of Radiology Residency, Boston University Medical Center, Boston, Massachusetts, USA

FRANK J. MINJA, MD
Assistant Professor Neuroradiology, Department of Radiology and Biomedical Imaging, Yale School of Medicine, New Haven, Connecticut, USA

FELIPE MUNERA, MD
Professor and Vice Chair for Clinical Operations, Department of Radiology, University of Miami Miller School of Medicine, Ryder Trauma Center, Jackson Memorial Hospital, Service Chief, University of Miami Hospital, Miami, Florida, USA

THANH B. NGUYEN, MD, FRCPC
Associate Professor, Department of Radiology, University of Ottawa, The Ottawa Hospital, Civic and General Campus, Ottawa, Ontario, Canada

DIEGO B. NUNEZ, MD, MPH, FACR
Chief, Division of Neuroradiology, Director, Emergency Neuroradiology, Department of Radiology, Brigham and Women's Hospital, Senior Lecturer, Harvard Medical School, Boston, Massachusetts, USA

CHRISTOPHER A. POTTER, MD
Emergency and Neuroradiology Divisions, Department of Radiology, Brigham and Women's Hospital, Boston, Massachusetts, USA

GAURAV SAIGAL, MD
Department of Radiology, University of Miami Miller School of Medicine, Jackson Memorial Hospital, Miami, Florida, USA

CLAIRE K. SANDSTROM, MD
Section of Emergency and Trauma Radiology, Department of Radiology, Harborview Medical Center, Seattle, Washington, USA

PINA SANELLI, MD, MPH, FACR
Vice Chairman of Research, Professor, Department of Radiology, The Imaging Clinical Effectiveness and Outcomes Research, Northwell Health, North Shore University Hospital, Manhasset, New York, USA

AARON D. SODICKSON, MD, PhD
Division Chief of Emergency Radiology and Medical Director of CT, Department of Radiology, Brigham and Women's Hospital, Associate Professor of Radiology, Harvard Medical School, Boston, Massachusetts, USA

EDWARD K. SUNG, MD
Assistant Professor, Department of Radiology, Boston University Medical Center, Boston, Massachusetts, USA

SEAN SYMONS, BASc, MPH, MD, FRCPC, DABR, MBA
Associate Professor of Radiology, Division Head, Neuroradiology, Department of Medical Imaging, University of Toronto, Sunnybrook Health Sciences Centre, Toronto, Ontario, Canada

CARLOS TORRES, MD, FRCPC
Associate Professor, Department of Radiology, University of Ottawa, Neuroradiologist, Department of Medical Imaging, The Ottawa Hospital, Civic Campus, Clinical Investigator, Ottawa Hospital Research Institute, Ottawa, Ontario, Canada

GABRIELA DE LA VEGA, MD
Department of Radiology, University of Miami Miller School of Medicine, Jackson Memorial Hospital, Miami, Florida, USA

WALTER F. WIGGINS, MD, PhD
Resident, Department of Radiology, Brigham and Women's Hospital, Clinical Fellow in Radiology, Harvard Medical School, Boston, Massachusetts, USA

AARON WINN, MD
Senior Resident, Department of Radiology, University of Miami Miller School of Medicine, Ryder Trauma Center, Jackson Memorial Hospital, Miami, Florida, USA

XIAO WU, BS
Department of Radiology and Biomedical Imaging, Yale School of Medicine, New Haven, Connecticut, USA

NADER ZAKHARI, MD, FRCPC
Assistant Professor, Department of Radiology, University of Ottawa, The Ottawa Hospital, Civic and General Campus, Ottawa, Ontario, Canada

REBECCA L. ZUCCONI, MD, FACOG
Assistant Professor, Department of Medical Sciences, Frank H Netter MD School of Medicine, Quinnipiac University, Hamden, Connecticut, USA

WILLIAM B. ZUCCONI, DO
Assistant Professor, Neuroradiology Fellowship Director, Associate Residency Program Director, Department of Radiology and Biomedical Imaging, Yale Diagnostic Radiology, Yale School of Medicine, New Haven, Connecticut, USA

Contents

Stroke is the clinical syndrome of abrupt onset of acute neurologic deficit owing to decreased oxygen delivery to the brain, resulting in ischemia or infarction. Approximately 87% of strokes are ischemic and 13% are hemorrhagic. Improved awareness of the neuroimaging findings highlighted in recent stroke clinical trials, as well as of their role in patient selection for novel treatment options, including "late window" (8–24 hours post ictus) intraarterial thrombectomy, has become increasingly important. This article focuses on the role of neuroimaging in the assessment and management of patients with acute ischemic stroke.

Thunderclap headache is a common presentation in the emergency department, and, although multiple causes have been described, subarachnoid hemorrhage (SAH) is the primary concern and early diagnosis is critical. Computed tomography (CT) is highly sensitive if performed within 6 hours of onset. Patients with aneurysmal or perimesencephalic SAH should be evaluated with CT angiography. Further workup should be guided by the pattern of blood. Patients with negative CT angiography may be further evaluated with MR imaging, especially patients with peripheral convexity SAH.

Spontaneous intracranial hemorrhage (ICH) is a commonly encountered neurologic emergency. Imaging plays important roles in both guiding the emergent stabilization of patients with ICH and elucidating the cause of the hemorrhage to prevent rebleeding. A thorough understanding of the factors that have an impact on immediate management, the causes of hemorrhage, and the strengths of various imaging techniques in addressing these 2 concerns is vital to crafting a patient-centered approach to this condition.

MR imaging with diffusion-weighted imaging has been essential in the evaluation of acute stroke but is also crucial for the diagnosis, treatment, and follow-up in patients with various nonischemic disorders, including infectious processes, trauma, toxic/metabolic disorders, and other abnormalities. This article reviews various disorders with diffusion abnormality that can be commonly seen in the emergency setting.

Neuroimaging in the emergency department increasingly involves patients at increased risk for acute neurologic complications from malignancy and immunosuppression, including patients with organ transplantation, diabetes mellitus, treatment of chronic disease, and human immunodeficiency virus positivity. These patients are susceptible to the same infections and emergencies as immunocompetent patients but may present differently with common illnesses and are susceptible to a variety of other diseases. This article reviews important patient risk factors, emergent central nervous system abnormalities, and their imaging findings. Detailed knowledge of risk factors and specific complications in these complex patients is essential for optimal image acquisition, interpretation, diagnosis, and treatment.

Acute neurologic emergencies in pregnancy often require neuroimaging to guide diagnosis and treatment. Implementation of a patient-centered care model in radiology can alleviate a patient's stress, reinforce appropriate imaging workup, improve patient satisfaction, and lead to improved outcomes. The authors present the evaluation, differential diagnosis, and recommended imaging protocols for the three most common acute neurologic symptoms in pregnancy and the postpartum period: headache, seizure, and focal neurologic deficits. With the patient's symptoms as a reference point, the referring physician in consultation with the radiologist can effectively implement the optimal imaging procedures.

Unconsciousness may be due to severe brain damage or to potentially reversible causes. Noncontrast head computed tomography (CT) helps identify acute ischemic and hemorrhagic lesions as well as certain patterns of toxic encephalopathy. MR imaging plays an important role in the assessment of acutely encephalopathic patients who may show no significant abnormality on CT. This article describes some of the common and infrequent entities that can lead to unconsciousness, including epilepsy and vascular, traumatic, metabolic, and toxic disorders.

This article summarizes common neurologic emergencies presenting in pediatric patients. Imaging techniques and appearances of specific conditions are detailed, including pearls and pitfalls for each presentation. Specific attention is given to differential diagnoses that can serve as mimickers of pediatric neurologic emergencies.

Traumatic injuries to the head and neck are common in the elderly, which is a rapidly growing sector of the American population. Most injuries result from low-energy falls and therefore might be at risk for delayed presentation and undertriage. Imaging, particularly with computed tomography, plays a vital role in the evaluation of traumatic head and neck injuries in geriatric patients. A thorough understanding of the differing patterns of trauma in the elderly patient and the factors that are associated with poorer outcomes is essential.

Current Challenges in the Use of Computed Tomography and MR Imaging in Suspected Cervical Spine Trauma

Frank J. Minja, Kushal Y. Mehta, and Ali Y. Mian

There is controversy regarding the optimal imaging strategy in adult patients with blunt trauma for suspected cervical spine trauma. Some investigators recommend negative computed tomography (CT) alone to clear the cervical spine in adult patients with blunt trauma, whereas others insist that MR imaging is necessary, especially among obtunded adult patients with blunt trauma. CT is an excellent imaging modality for bony cervical spine injury; however, there is a nonzero rate of clinically significant cervical spine injuries missed on CT. MR imaging has high sensitivity for soft tissue cervical spine injuries but low specificity for the rare isolated unstable ligamentous cervical spine injury.

Blunt Craniocervical Trauma: Does the Patient Have a Cerebral Vascular Injury?

Aaron Winn, Anthony M. Durso, Catalina Restrepo Lopera, and Felipe Munera

Blunt cerebrovascular injury involves injury to the carotid and/or vertebral arteries sustained via generalized multitrauma or directed blunt craniocervical trauma. Stroke remains the most consequential outcome. Timely diagnosis and initiation of treatment before the development of neurologic complications have a well-established role in decreasing morbidity and mortality. This article presents evidence and controversies surrounding the optimization of diagnostic imaging for suspected blunt cerebrovascular injury. Discussion centers on the increasing reliance on multidetector computed tomography angiography for screening, considering relevant clinical criteria for determining screening. Imaging protocols, imaging findings, injury grading, pearls, and pitfalls are discussed.

The Imaging of Maxillofacial Trauma 2017

Mark P. Bernstein

Maxillofacial injuries account for a large portion of emergency department visits and often result in surgical consultation. Although many of the principles of fracture detection and repair are basic, the evolution of technology and therapeutic strategies has led to improved patient outcomes. This article provides a clinical review of imaging aspects involved in maxillofacial trauma and delineates its relevance to patient management.

Radiation Dose Considerations in Emergent Neuroimaging

Walter F. Wiggins and Aaron D. Sodickson

Computed tomography is often the first-line diagnostic imaging modality in the evaluation of patients with neurologic emergencies. A patient-centered approach to radiation dose management in emergent neuroimaging thus revolves around the appropriate use of computed tomography, including clinical decision support for ordering providers, thoughtful protocol design, the use of available technological advances in computed tomography, and radiation exposure monitoring at a population level. A multifaceted approach can help to minimize radiation exposure to individual patients while preserving diagnostic quality imaging.

Foreword
Emergent Neuroimaging: A Patient-Focused Approach

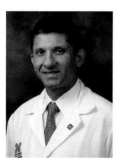

Suresh K. Mukherji, MD, MBA, FACR
Consulting Editor

Two of the largest growth areas in medicine are neuroimaging and emergency care, and I am thrilled that this issue of *Neuroimaging Clinics* is dedicated to emergency neuroimaging. This very practical issue addresses both traumatic and nontraumatic neurologic conditions that will be present in the "middle of the night." The breadth of topics is expansive and includes brain, spine, and head and neck. I especially appreciate the focus on clinical presentations and articles dedicated to pediatric neurologic emergencies, pregnancy, and radiation dose. This is a unique approach!

I want to thank Dr Nunez for his willingness to accept such a challenging topic. I have known Diego for many years and have always been impressed by his expertise, but more importantly, by his humbleness and humanity. He is the definition of a "gentleman," and I am honored to refer to him as a friend and colleague.

The articles are authored by recognized authorities in their field of expertise. I want to express my sincerest gratitude to all of the article contributors for their efforts in creating such outstanding content. The information is timely and relevant and will immediately benefit the daily clinical practice of all physicians involved in acute neurological care.

Suresh K. Mukherji, MD, MBA, FACR
Department of Radiology
Michigan State University
Michigan State University Health Team
846 Service Road
East Lansing, MI 48824, USA

E-mail address:
mukherji@rad.msu.edu

Neuroimag Clin N Am 28 (2018) xv
https://doi.org/10.1016/j.nic.2018.05.002
1052-5149/18/© 2018 Published by Elsevier Inc.

Preface
Emergent Neuroimaging: A Patient-Focused Approach

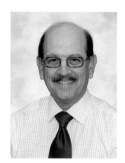

Diego B. Nunez, MD, MPH
Editor

With the progressive shift of health care delivery toward a patient-centered approach, we have seen extension of these initiatives to radiology practices that are now focusing on opportunities to improve patient satisfaction, quality, and safety. These include effective communication with patients while developing system changes and creating the appropriate physical environment for access to appropriate imaging.

In the emergency setting, it is inherently difficult for radiologists to have patient facing time as a way to contribute to customized care. Notwithstanding, we have a great opportunity to positively affect patient management and outcomes by ensuring that they get the imaging they need and that they promptly get the right imaging in the emergency department.

To that end, we need to be proactive participants of the health care managing team in emergency departments by developing and tailoring the imaging strategies that more effectively address specific clinical problems in targeted subset of patients.

In this issue of the *Neuroimaging Clinics*, a mix of traumatic and nontraumatic conditions is covered to address best practices for different patient demographics. "Stroke" articles include imaging updates for patients with acute neurologic deficit, with thunderclap headache and with impaired level of consciousness. Imaging protocols adapted to clinical issues affecting children and elderly patients as well as specific factors that alter physiological stages, such as pregnancy and compromise of the immune system, are all addressed with a patient-focused approach. We also covered the scope of emergent MR applications beyond the usual stroke suspects, and importantly, an article is dedicated to radiation considerations when imaging patients with neurological emergencies. The current evidence supporting imaging strategies for the traumatized patient with suspected cervical spine and cerebrovascular injuries is also highlighted.

I am indebted to the extraordinary group of colleagues who contributed their time and expertise to cover such a variety of subjects. They all represent major academic radiology practices across the United States. I hope the radiology readership finds this issue informative and helpful in clinical practice. The topics of the articles could also benefit physicians in other disciplines, in particular, our emergency medicine colleagues. To that end, and from our own experience during the best part of the last three decades practicing emergency neuroradiology, it remains uncontested that to achieve better patient experience and outcomes we need a genuine partnership with our emergency radiology colleagues.

Diego B. Nunez, MD, MPH
Department of Radiology
Brigham and Women's Hospital
75 Francis Street
Boston, MA 02115, USA

E-mail address:
dnunez@bwh.harvard.edu

Neuroimag Clin N Am 28 (2018) xvii
https://doi.org/10.1016/j.nic.2018.05.001
1052-5149/18/© 2018 Published by Elsevier Inc.

neuroimaging.theclinics.com

The Adult Patient with Acute Neurologic Deficit
An Update on Imaging Trends

Shahmir Kamalian, MD*, Michael H. Lev, MD, FAHA, FACR

KEYWORDS

- Stroke • CT • CT angiography • MR imaging • Intravenous thrombolysis
- Intraarterial thrombectomy • Endovascular thrombectemy

KEY POINTS

- Abrupt onset of a focal neurologic deficit typically defines the clinical syndrome of stroke.
- Neuroimaging has an essential role in differentiating ischemic from hemorrhagic stroke and guiding patient selection for intravenous thrombolysis (IVT) and intra-arterial thrombectomy (IAT).
- Obtaining advanced imaging (CTA, DWI) for patient selection for IAT should never delay the administration of IVT when the patient is otherwise eligible, up to 4.5 hours post-ictus.
- The recent DAWN and DEFUSE 3 trial results showed a strong benefit of IAT when administered within 24-hours post-ictus, in appropriately selected patients using advanced imaging.

INTRODUCTION

Abrupt onset of a focal neurologic deficit typically defines the clinical syndrome of stroke, although stroke mimics—which include but are not limited to seizure (20%), syncope (10%–20%), sepsis or hypo/hyperglycemia (14%), subdural hematoma or tumor (10%–12%), somatization/anxiety and hyperventilation (5%–10%), transient global amnesia, and complex migraine (30%–35%)—have been estimated to occur as often as 10 times more frequently as ischemic or hemorrhagic stroke.[1] Stroke reflects neuronal dysfunction secondary to hypo-oxygenation and can be associated with temporary (transient ischemic attack) or permanent (infarction) neuronal injury. Because only a small number (<5%) of patients with signs & symptoms of acute stroke present to an emergency department within the 3 to 4.5-hour time window for treatment by intravenous "clot busting" tissue plasminogen activator (IV-rPA), timely advanced imaging with CT, CT angiography (CTA), and, whenever possible, diffusion-weighted MR imaging (DWI-MR) remains essential to patient assessment - even in patients with transient ischemic attack or rapid clinical improvement (ie, "too good to treat"), to identify treatable causes of ischemia and prevent a stroke (eg, severe internal carotid artery stenosis or dissection). Unenhanced CT (noncontrast CT) is required for all stroke patients to exclude hemorrhage. Advanced imaging requires, at minimum, CT angiography (CTA), to both identify a proximal large vessel occlusion (LVO) and to access collaterals. To the greatest extent possible, diffusion-weighted MR imaging (DWI) should be performed as the most accurate modality for determining irreversibly infarcted tissue core; additional CT or MR perfusion imaging (MRP) is increasingly obtained at many centers. Recent prospective clinical trials published in *The New England Journal of Medicine* (*NEJM*) and other high-impact journals, have not only helped define the central role of advanced neuroimaging modalities—CTA, CTA collaterals,

Conflicts of Interest: None (S. Kamalian). Consultant for Takeda Pharm, GE Healthcare, MedyMatch, and D-Pharm (M.H. Lev).

Division of Emergency Radiology, Department of Radiology, Massachusetts General Hospital, Harvard Medical School, 55 Fruit Street, Blake SB Room 29A, Boston, MA 02114, USA

* Corresponding author.

E-mail address: skamalian@mgh.harvard.edu

neuroimaging.theclinics.com

CT perfusion (CTP), MR imaging–DWI, MR imaging–fluid-attenuated inversion recovery (FLAIR), and magnetic resonance angiography (MRA)—in patient selection for intra-arterial thrombectomy (IAT) treatment but also helped make possible extending the time window for this treatment up to 24 hours post-ictus, as recently demonstrated in the DAWN and DEFUSE 3 trials.[2,3]

Core is brain tissue that has been irreversibly infarcted at presentation; *penumbra* is markedly hypoperfused at-risk tissue that has a high probability of infarction in the absence of timely reperfusion. Most true stroke syndromes are ischemic, with a majority due to an intracranial, circle of Willis LVO from an embolus (approximately 85%) and with only a small percentage attributable to global cerebral hypoperfusion (so called low-flow or border-zone strokes); global anoxic injury, from near-drowning, carbon monoxide poisoning, or other causes of suffocation, is also less common. Approximately 10% of strokes are hemorrhagic due to intracerebral hemorrhage, with 3% due to subarachnoid hemorrhage.[4,5]

It is estimated that 795,000 persons have a stroke each year in the United States, causing 140,000 deaths.[4,5] That said, stroke has moved from the third leading cause of death in 2007 to the fifth in 2017.[4–6] Although major recent advances in neuroimaging and stroke treatment have contributed to a decrease in mortality, stroke remains the leading cause of serious long-term disability in the United States and costs the health care system an estimated $34 billion each year.[4]

Neuroimaging has a central role in the differential diagnosis of patients with suspected stroke, by differentiating ischemic from hemorrhagic stroke, identifying other causes of acute neurologic deficit (ie, stroke mimics), and helping in patient selection for IAT. An estimated 9% to 30% of patients with suspected stroke—and 3% to 17% of patients treated with IV-tPA—have stroke mimics.[7–16] Current treatment options for acute embolic stroke include IV-tPA, IAT, or a combination of both. Therapeutic options for intracerebral hemorrhage, subarachnoid hemorrhage, and stroke mimics vary by the etiology.

ETIOLOGY AND TIMELINE OF ISCHEMIC STROKE

Ischemic strokes are divided into 5 subtypes based on etiology: large-artery atherosclerosis (most commonly from the cervical carotid arteries), cardioembolism (secondary to clot formation in the heart), small-vessel occlusion (lacunar infarct, which is <20 mm diameter), stroke of other determined etiology (such as dissection, nonatherosclerotic vasculopathies, or global hypoperfusion), and stroke of undetermined etiology.[17]

The most common causes of the stroke vary in different age groups. Carotid disease (large artery) and atrial fibrillation (cardioembolism) are the most common causes of acute ischemic stroke in patients over age 40. Hypertensive and coronary heart diseases are the most common underlying disorders in patients with atrial fibrillation. Atrial fibrillation is highly associated with left atrium enlargement with 39% increase in risk per 5-mm increment.[18] Therefore, in an older patient with an enlarged left atrium, the stroke may be due to atrial fibrillation. The most common causes of ischemic stroke in patients below age 40 include dissection, nonatherosclerotic vasculopathies, and paradoxic stroke in conditions, such as a patent foramen ovale and arteriovenous shunts in the lungs.

Clinical history can provide important clues in determining the cause of stroke. For example, dissection should be considered in young patients (typically age <40) after yoga, weight lifting, or chiropractic manipulation, whereas paradoxic embolus from deep vein thrombosis through a patent foramen ovale is at the top of the differential diagnosis list as the cause of acute ischemic stroke in a pilot or a long-distance traveler presenting with abrupt onset of new neurologic deficit.[19,20]

Ischemic stroke is loosely classified as hyperacute, acute, subacute, and chronic, based on the symptom onset time. Typically, the hyperacute phase is within 6 hours to 8 hours of stroke onset, when patients are potentially eligible for various well-established reperfusion treatments (ie, IV-tPA and/or IAT). Acute stroke is considered stroke of less than 24 hours' duration, with the subacute and chronic stages ranging from 1 day to 1 month and greater than 1 month, respectively. Part of the problem with these loose definitions, however, is that stroke progression and infarct growth vary widely from patient to patient, largely attributable to the quality of the intracranial collateral blood flow around a site of proximal LVO. One of the overarching goals of patient selection using advanced imaging is to replace the concept of making treatment decisions based on an arbitrary clock time with the concept of making treatment decisions based on stroke physiology, as determined by the concurrent neuroimaging findings at the time of triage.

ROLE OF NEUROIMAGING IN DIAGNOSIS AND MANAGEMENT OF PATIENTS WITH ACUTE ISCHEMIC STROKE

Neuroimaging has 4 critical roles in the assessment of patients with an acute ischemic stroke: (1) exclusion of an acute intracranial hemorrhage, (2) identification of a proximal LVO as a target for IAT, (3) determining the volume of already irreversibly dead brain at presentation (infarction core), and (4) estimating the volume of potentially salvageable ischemic tissue that is a target for treatment, which is likely to undergo irreversible injury in the absence of timely reperfusion (ischemic penumbra).

Presence of an acute intracranial hemorrhage is an absolute contraindication to IV-tPA therapy. Large artery proximal occlusions of the middle cerebral artery (MCA) or other proximal circle of Willis vessels typically account for most of the morbidity and mortality of stroke; clot dissolution or retrieval to restore normal brain perfusion is therefore the goal of IV and/or intra-arterial thrombolysis. Determining the infarct core volume is important because patients with large cores—many studies have established 70 mL as a threshold beyond which a good clinical outcome is unlikely—are at higher risk for intraparenchymal hemorrhage after successful reperfusion.[21,22] Finally, in the absence

of a substantial volume of potentially salvageable ischemic target tissue (ie, penumbra), the risks of attempting reperfusion therapies may outweigh the benefits.

IMAGING FINDINGS IN ACUTE ISCHEMIC STROKE
Noncontrast CT

Noncontrast CT is a specific but relatively insensitive modality for the detection of early ischemic changes. It has a pivotal role, however, in addressing the first critical question in treating acute stroke—Is there an acute intracranial hemorrhage that is an absolute contraindication for IV-tPA or IAT therapy? Signs of early infarct on noncontrast head CT include loss of the gray matter–white matter differentiation along the cortical ribbon (especially in the insula) or lentiform nucleus, hyperdense vessel sign (which indicates an embolus in the vessel), and sulcal effacement from edema (**Fig. 1**A, B).[23] Presence of an obvious, well-established large hypodense infarct (>1/3 of MCA territory or 100 mL) is also

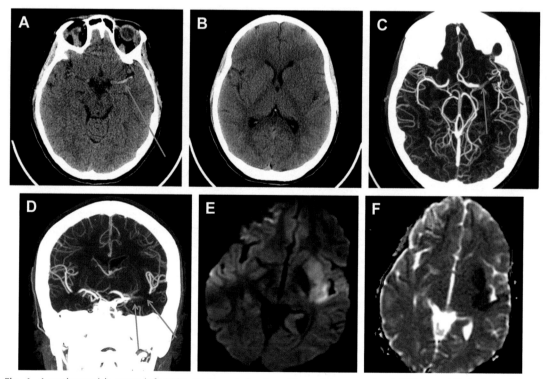

Fig. 1. A patient with acute left MCA territory infarction. The axial noncontrast CT image (*A*) depicts a hyperdense vessel sign (*arrow*). At the level of insula, the CT (*B*) shows loss of gray matter–white matter differentiation in the posterior insula and lentiform nucleus and mild edema, which is evident by asymmetric effacement of the left sylvian fissure compared with the right side. The axial (*C*) and coronal (*D*) MIP CTA images depict an occlusive thrombus in the M1 segment of the left MCA (*arrows*). The MR images (DWI [*E*] and ADC [*F*]) show the posterior insula and lentiform nucleus, with restricted diffusion, consistent with acute infarct.

typically considered a contraindication to IV-tPA therapy. Noncontrast CT can also help identify a proximal thrombus and assessment clot burden, through the presence of a hyperdense vessel sign, a specific but not sensitive marker for intravascular clot in the clinical setting of an abrupt-onset new neurologic deficit.

CT Angiography

CTA is a quick and accurate method for addressing the second critical question in the imaging assessment of patients with acute ischemic stroke—Is there a proximal circle of Willis LVO, which might be a target for IAT treatment?

Maximum intensity projection (MIP) images are helpful for rapid identification of more distal vascular stenosis or occlusions (eg, at the secondary [M2] or tertiary [M3] branch vessels) as well as for assessment of clot burden (ie, clot length) and leptomeningeal collateral status (Fig. 1C, D)[24,25] For optimal MIP image review and interpretation, the reformatting—which can be rapidly performed, typically in under a minute, by the CT technologists at the scanner console—should be obtained as thick slab/thin overlapping intervals (3-cm thick at 5-mm overlapping intervals at the authors' institution). Moreover, to be certain that the observed collateral pattern reflects the true collateral status— and is not an artifact of a delayed circulation time of contrast taking longer to reach the pial collateral circulation through a more circuitous pathway bypassing a proximal LVO—it is essential that delayed-phase CTA images be obtained routinely in acute stroke patients who are potential IAT candidates; some institutions use a multiphase CTA protocol for collateral assessment.[26]

Clot burden is an important marker that predicts response to IV-tPA.[24] Patients with LVO and a clot length of more than 8 mm have a low likelihood of successful recanalization by IV-tPA alone and hence may be good candidates for IAT treatment.[24,27]

The quality of the leptomeningeal collateral vasculature on CTA can also help distinguish patients most likely to benefit from IAT from those least likely to benefit.[28] Poor leptomeningeal collateralization has been associated with higher incidence and larger size of hemorrhage.[25,29,30] Patients with a proximal occlusion and good collateral vasculature usually have a small infarction core and a large potentially salvageable ischemic tissue (Fig. 2).[25] Likewise, patients with a proximal occlusion and poor collateral vasculature usually have a large

infarction core and a small potentially salvageable ischemic penumbra (Fig. 3).[25] Hence, when DWI MR imaging is unavailable or contraindicated as the modality to most accurately determine infarct core volume, the stratification of leptomeningeal CTA collaterals into robust (ie, symmetric), poor (absent in >30%–50% of the territory at risk), or intermediate categories can help in estimating the potential benefits versus risks of attempting IAT in any given individual patient (Fig. 4). Although patients with robust collaterals have higher odds of good clinical outcome after reperfusion than patients with poor collaterals, in the absence of robust complete or near-complete recanalization, the outcome of patients is similar, regardless of collateral status.[31]

CT Perfusion

CTP can visually depict and potentially measure several perfusion parameters at the microvascular level, such as cerebral blood flow (CBF), cerebral blood volume (CBV), and mean transit time (MTT). CTP has been the focus of many imaging research studies for identification of infarct core and ischemic penumbra. CBF and CBV maps can be used for infarct core measurement and CBF and MTT maps for ischemic penumbra measurement (see Fig. 4C).[32–35]

Although CTP findings may be useful for stroke differential diagnosis, clinical management (notably for titration of antihypertensive medications), and disposition decisions/prognostication in acute ischemic stroke patients,[36] its specific role in the selection of patients for IV or intra-arterial reperfusion therapies remains highly controversial and hotly debated. Compared with a DWI reference standard, CTP may be insufficiently accurate for assessing core infarct volume in any given individual patient who is a potential IAT candidate; this is largely due to both image noise and lack of standardization—leading not only to potential inaccuracy but also to marked interscan variability in the quantification of perfusion parameter values as well as large measurement error in the estimation of infarct core volumes.[32,33,37–39] Moreover, using CTP to estimate penumbral volume may be unnecessary, in that patients who present within the time window for reperfusion therapy with a proximal LVO and a small infarct core almost always have a sufficiently large ischemic penumbra to warrant IAT if otherwise eligible.[40] Thus, using CTP might not only be unneeded for triage of patients to appropriate IV or intra-arterial reperfusion therapies but also inappropriately exclude patients who might

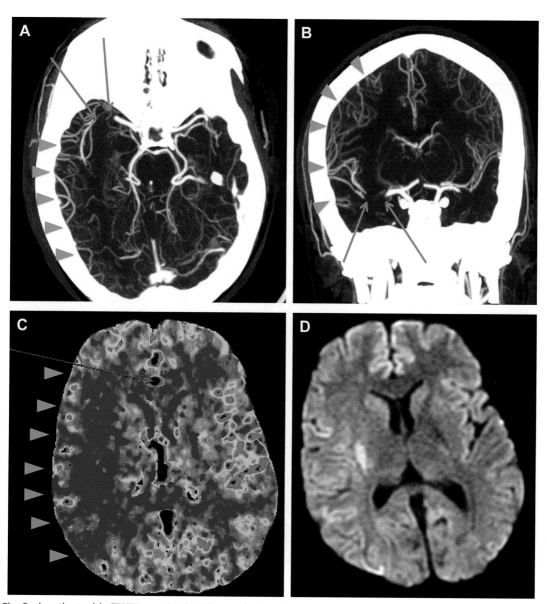

Fig. 2. A patient with CT/CTA acquired 1.5 hours after stroke onset: the axial (*A*) and coronal (*B*) MIP CTA images depict a thrombus in the M1 segment of the right MCA (*arrows*), with good (symmetric) pial collateral vessels (*arrowheads*). Although the CBF map from the CPT data set (*C*) demonstrated a large area perfusion defect (*arrowheads*), the DWI (*D*) showed a small infarct core, with an associated large area of at-risk tissue (penumbra). This combination of proximal LVO, small core, large penumbra defines a cohort of patients most likely to benefit from IAT.

otherwise benefit from such therapies by overestimating the infarct core or, at the other extreme, put patients at increased risk of hemorrhagic complications by underestimating the infarct core size. Hence, at several institutions, CTP is not considered essential for the selection of patients for available revascularization therapies when MR imaging is contraindicated or unavailable, but rather both the presence of a proximal LVO and the quality of the pial CTA-collateral flow (robust, intermediate, or poor) are considered when making IAT decisions.

It should again be underscored, however, that perfusion imaging has other important potential applications in acute stroke management when MR imaging is unavailable or contraindicated, including (but not limited to) differential diagnosis (especially identifying distal branch occlusions

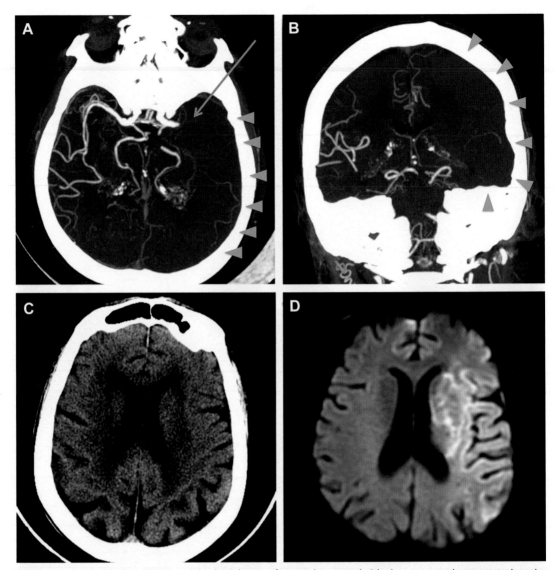

Fig. 3. A patient with the CT/CTA acquired 1.5 hours after stroke onset (with the same stroke onset to imaging time interval as the patient shown in **Fig. 2**). The axial (A) and coronal (B) MIP CTA images depict a thrombus in the M1 segment of the left MCA (*arrow*), with almost complete absence of collateral flow (*arrowheads*); a poor (or in this case, malignant collateral pattern). Although the noncontrast CT examination (C) shows no obvious hypodensity to suggest acute infarction, the DWI (D) depicts a large infarct core, involving almost the entire left MCA territory.

that may not be evident on CTA thick-slab MIPs), hypertensive management, and disposition/prognosis.[41]

MR Imaging

As with unenhanced CT, standard MR imaging sequences (T1-weighted, T2-weighted, and FLAIR) can be relatively insensitive for the detection of ischemia/infarction in the first few hours post-ictus.[23] Rather, the greatest value of MR imaging lies in the early detection and delineation of infarct core using DWI (**Fig. 1E, F**). DWI is highly sensitive (88%–100%), specific (95%–100%), and accurate (95%) for detecting and delineating ischemic brain tissue likely to be irreversibly infarcted despite early, robust reperfusion. DWI can often detect ischemia even within minutes of onset; ischemia causes restricted free water diffusion in brain tissue, which results in marked hyperintense (bright) signal on DWI sequences. The DWI signal intensity is an exponential

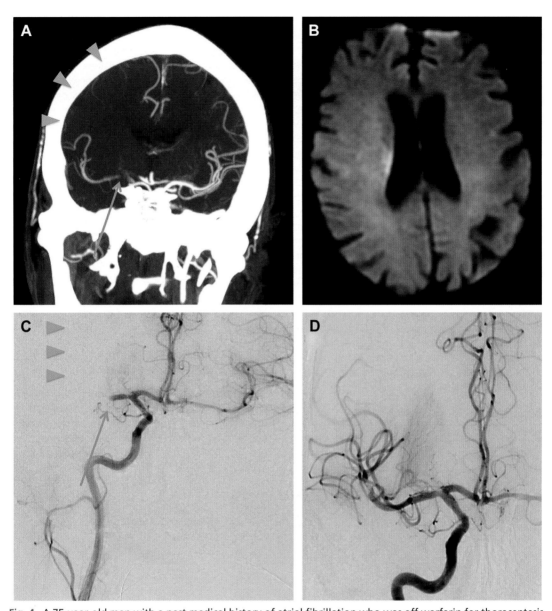

Fig. 4. A 75-year-old man with a past medical history of atrial fibrillation who was off warfarin for thoracentesis. The patient presented 25 minutes after stroke onset. Despite an occlusive M1 thrombus in the right MCA (*arrow*) and poor collateral pattern (*arrowheads*), as depicted by the coronal MIP CTA (*A*), the patient had a small infarct core (DWI [*B*]) in the right posterior caudate body. The patient underwent immediate IAT. The catheter angiogram (*C*) confirms the presence of a complete right M1-MCA occlusion (*arrow*) with poor collaterals (*arrowheads*). After a single pass of a penumbra suction device, the patient had successful, complete recanalization (*D*). The follow-up noncontrast CTP 24 hours later (not shown) was without significant abnormality in the right MCA territory.

function of the random Brownian motion of water molecules within a voxel of tissue, with a linear component based on T2-weighted signal intensity, and with brighter signal reflecting lesser (ie, more restricted) diffusibility. The gray scale on the apparent diffusion coefficient (ADC) maps reflect a linear function of diffusibility, without the T2 component, and with brighter signal reflecting greater diffusibility (eg, cerebrospinal fluid appears bright because the hydrogen atoms in water are more freely mobile). The ADC maps can, therefore, help distinguish a DWI-bright lesion as true restricted diffusion (ie, DWI bright, T2 bright, and ADC dark) from T2 shine-through (DWI bright, T2 bright, and ADC bright).[23]

Infarct core size is a well-established and important marker for the likelihood of good outcome in MCA occlusive stroke. Infarct core volume on MR-DWI can be estimated with an acceptable level of accuracy by multiplying the largest cross-sectional dimensions on axial, sagittal, and coronal reconstructed images and dividing the product by 2 (Length × Width × Height/2). Patients with small infarct core volumes (<70 mL) at presentation, in the setting of acute MCA occlusion, have the potential to derive the greatest benefit after successful reperfusion; conversely, those with initial large infarct core volumes (>100 mL) are at increased risk of hemorrhage after reperfusion and are unlikely to benefit from IAT.[42,43] Infarcts between 70 mL and 100 mL at presentation are uncertain to benefit from IAT.

In the posterior circulation, the correlation between initial infarct size and clinical outcome is poor, because even a tiny ischemic focus in a critical location in the brainstem can result in a devastating neurologic deficit.[24]

MR Angiography

Although CTA is considered the first-line imaging modality to rule in an LVO in setting of acute stroke, MRA provides a useful screening test to detect proximal LVO in patients who cannot receive iodinated CT IV contrast material due to allergy or acute renal failure.[44] The main limitations of MRA are overestimating the degree of stenosis and inaccuracy in detection of distal occlusions, owing to the fact that MRA images are flow-dependent rather than reflecting true intraluminal anatomy as does CTA.[23]

MR Perfusion

MRP can produce perfusion maps, including CBF, CBV, MTT and time to peak/time to maximum. The role of MRP in the selection of patients for IV thrombolytic or IAT therapies is controversial and debated, as is the role of CTP. Arterial spin-labeled MRP is a method of estimating tissue-level perfusion in the brain without the need for IV gadolinium contrast; however it, too, has several limitations; MRP methods are also notable for not requiring ionizing radiation.[23]

THE MASSACHUSETTS GENERAL HOSPITAL STROKE IMAGING ALGORITHM

The Massachusetts General Hospital stroke imaging algorithm is an evidence-based tool to identify patients with severe ischemic strokes caused by anterior circulation occlusions, who are candidates for IAT stroke therapy (Fig. 5).

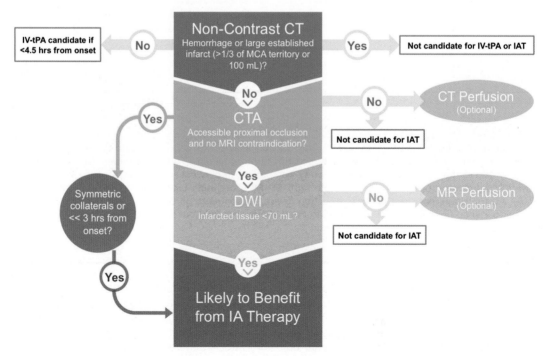

Fig. 5. Massachusetts General Hospital acute stroke imaging algorithm.

Table 1
Causes of restricted diffusion

Na$^+$/K$^+$-ATPase pump failure (ischemic and/or excitotoxic injury)	Seizures, hypoglycemia, hyperglycemia, ketosis, transient global amnesia, drug-induced encephalopathies like metronidazole or methotrexate, necrotizing infections like HSV, Wernicke encephalopathy
Tissue vacuolization or spongiform changes	Creutzfeldt-Jakob disease, heroin leukoencephalopathy, demyelination, diffuse axonal injury
High protein concentration or increased viscosity	Pyogenic infection, hemorrhage
Dense cell packing	High-grade glioma, lymphoma, small-blue-round-cell metastases, such as small cell lung cancer

First, noncontrast CT is performed—with an expected door-to-CT time of less than 25 minutes per national Get With The Guidelines criteria—to evaluate for hemorrhage (an absolute contraindication to IV-tPA or IAT) or a large well-established hypodensity (>1/3 MCA territory; a relative contraindication to IV thrombolysis [IVT] or IAT). If neither is present and the patient is IV-tPA eligible, CTA is next performed and postprocessed during the 5 minutes to 10 minutes it takes to prepare the tPA for IV administration; obtaining advanced imaging, however, should never slow the administration of definitive thrombolytic treatment in patients who are otherwise eligible. Next, in the setting of a proximal LVO (intracranial ICA or MCA) —and if there are no contraindications to MR imaging—DWI is acquired. If DWI depicts a small (<70 mL) infarct, the patient is considered likely to benefit from IAT (assuming other criteria have been met) and immediately triaged to the interventional suite. If MR imaging is unavailable

and the patient is not a candidate for IAT, CTP can be considered to help exclude stroke mimics or to help guide management decisions, such as the need for hypertensive therapy.[45]

In addition to detection of LVO, CTA is also useful for assessment of pial collateral flow. In the setting of a proximal LVO, a malignant collateral flow pattern (no contrast filling in >50% of the territory at risk on delayed CTA images) strongly correlates with DWI infarct volume greater than 70 mL to 100 mL.[46] Conversely, robust (ie, symmetric) collaterals—although they do not necessarily guarantee a DWI infarct volume less than 70 mL—mean that a final infarct volume less than 70 mL is more likely in the setting of early, complete recanalization. Hence, patients with a poor collateral pattern are likely to have a poor clinical outcome, despite successful recanalization, whereas patients with robust (ie, symmetric) collaterals have the potential to benefit from IAT.[31,47] In the absence of recanalization, the

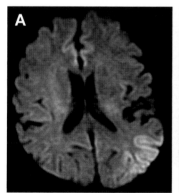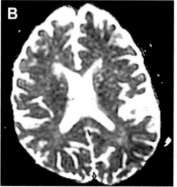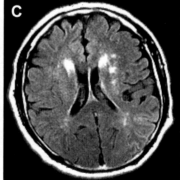

Fig. 6. A 66-year-old patient with altered mental status and acute onset aphasia and right gaze deviation. The patient received IV-tPA for presumed stroke but was later found to have had a seizure. Admission MR imaging showed gyriform restricted diffusion (DWI [A], ADC map [B]) in the left parieto-occipital cortex, with cortical and subcortical white matter swelling (FLAIR [C]). The imaging findings completely resolved by the time of discharge (not shown).

outcome of patients with good versus collateral vasculature does not differ significantly.[31]

ACUTE ISCHEMIC STROKE DIFFERENTIAL DIAGNOSIS (STROKE MIMICS)

It is estimated that 9% to 30% of patients suspected for stroke and 2.8% to 17% of patients treated with IV-tPA have stroke mimics.[7–16] Although several diverse entities can mimic stroke, most mimics are due to seizures, migraines, tumors, or toxic-metabolic disturbances. Imaging usually facilitates diagnosis, because true ischemic stroke typically has the imaging features previously described, although some of these features—even restricted diffusion (**Table 1**)—are not

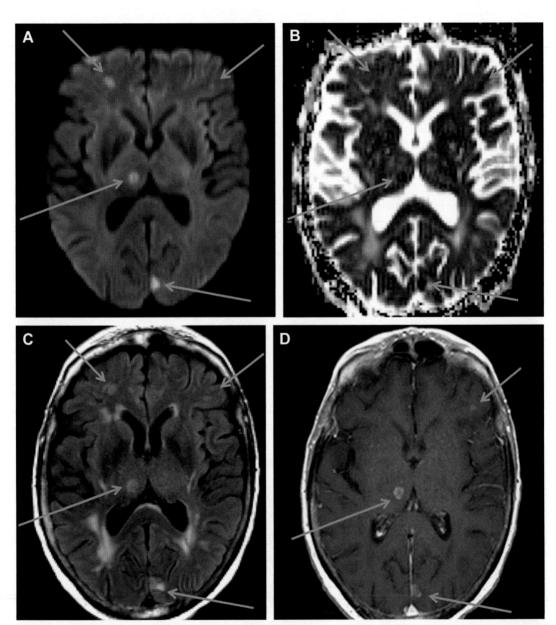

Fig. 7. A 69 year old with small cell lung carcinoma presented with sudden onset of visual changes and gait imbalance. MR imaging depicted multiple foci of restricted diffusion (*arrows*) in the left occipital lobe, right thalamus, and bilateral frontal lobes (DWI [*A*] and ADC map [*B*]). All the lesions (*arrows*) demonstrate associated T2/FLAIR hyperintensity (*C*) and contrast enhancement on the postcontrast T1-weighted images (*D*). The lesion in the right frontal lobe is not included on the representative axial postcontrast T1-weighted image due to the patient movement between the sequences.

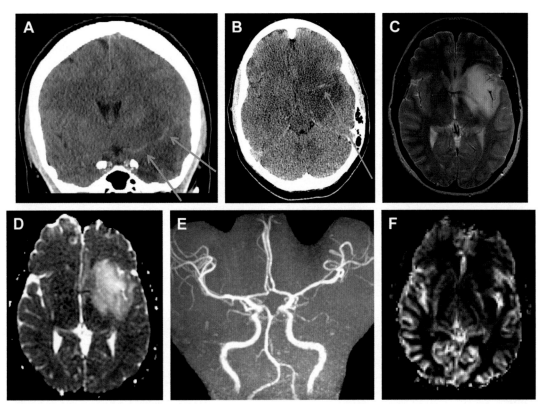

Fig. 8. A 49 year old with sudden-onset aphasia. The initial noncontrast CT (*A, B*) was interpreted as a left MCA infarction with a hyperdense left MCA sign (*arrows*). MR imaging showed a T2 hyperintense expansile lesion (T2-weighted imaging [*C*]) with elevated diffusion (ADC map [*D*]). The MRA showed patency of the left MCA (*E*), and the MRP (CBF [*F*]) showed no areas of decreased CBF. The patient underwent biopsy, which subsequently showed an anaplastic oligoastrocytoma.

unique to stroke and can be associated with other entitites.[48] The topographic pattern of the DWI lesion, in combination with vascular imaging and CT or MRP findings, often helps diagnose these other entities (**Figs. 6–8**).

TREATMENT OF PATIENTS WITH ACUTE ISCHEMIC STROKE

The management of acute ischemic stroke (within the first few hours) differs from long-term management. The immediate goal of treatment is minimizing brain injury and preventing complications. Treatment of stroke requires stabilization of airway, breathing, and circulation; control of blood pressure; fluid management; treatment of hypoglycemia or hyperglycemia; and swallowing assessment, in addition to IV-tPA and IA therapy.[49,50] The IV and intra-arterial treatment is discussed.

Intravenous Thrombolysis

The goal of IV-tPA thrombolysis is timely restoration of blood flow and salvaging the ischemic brain tissue not already infarcted. In 1995, the National Institute of Neurological Disorders and Stroke stroke trial showed the benefit of IV thrombolytic therapy given during the first 3 hours after stroke onset.[51] Later in 2008, the European Cooperative Acute Stroke Study III—a double-blinded, parallel-group, and randomized trial—showed that the benefit of IV-tPA thrombolysis extends up to 4.5 hours after stroke onset.[52]

All data suggest that the sooner IV-tPA therapy is initiated, the more likely it is to be beneficial and that this benefit extends up to 4.5 hours after stroke onset. Therefore, all eligible patients (**Table 2**) should be treated with IV-tPA as soon as possible, even if IAT is considered.

As discussed previously, if hyperdense vessel clot length is greater than 8 mm, the likelihood that IV-tPA alone will result in complete recanalization approaches zero, and these patients should be considered for IAT if possible.[24,53]

Intra-arterial Thrombolysis

In 2015, 5 multicenter randomized clinical trials (MR CLEAN, ESCAPE, REVASCAT, EXTEND-IA,

Table 2
Eligibility criteria for intravenous tissue plasminogen activator administration

Inclusion criteria

- Clinical diagnosis of ischemic stroke
- Symptom onset <4.5 h before start of treatment
- Age ≥18 y

Absolute exclusion criteria

Historical	• Stroke or head trauma in the last 3 mo • Previous intracranial hemorrhage • Intracranial neoplasm, arteriovenous malformation, or aneurysm • Recent intracranial or intraspinal surgery • Arterial puncture at a noncompressible site in the previous 7 d
Clinical	• Symptoms suggestive of subarachnoid hemorrhage • Persistent hypertension (systolic ≥185 or diastolic ≥110 mm Hg) • Serum glucose <50 mg/dL (<2.8 mmol/L) • Active internal bleeding • Acute bleeding diathesis, including but not limited to conditions defined in Hematologic section
Hematologic	• Platelet count <100,000/mm^{3a} • Current anticoagulant use with an INR >1.7 or PT >15 s[a] • Heparin use within 48 h and an abnormally elevated aPTT[a] • Current use of a direct thrombin inhibitor or direct factor Xa inhibitor with evidence of anticoagulant effect by laboratory tests
Head CT	• Evidence of hemorrhage • Extensive well-established hypodensity (>1/3 of MCA territory)

Relative exclusion criteria

- Minor and isolated neurologic signs or rapidly improving stroke symptoms
- Seizure at the onset of stroke with postictal neurologic impairments
- Major surgery or serious trauma in the previous 14 d
- Gastrointestinal or urinary tract bleeding in the previous 21 d
- Myocardial infarction in the previous 3 mo
- Pregnancy

Additional, relative exclusion criteria for treatment 3–4.5 h post-ictus

- Age >80 y
- Severe stroke (NIHSS score >25)
- Combination of both previous ischemic stroke and diabetes mellitus

Abbreviations: aPTT, activated partial thromboplastin time; INR, international normalized ratio; NIHSS, National Institutes of Health Stroke Scale; PT, prothrombin time.

  [a] It is desirable to have the results of these tests, but thrombolytic therapy should not be delayed for the test results unless (1) there is clinical suspicion of a bleeding abnormality or thrombocytopenia or (2) the patient is currently on or has recently received anticoagulants.

and SWIFT PRIME) were published *NEJM*, all of which showed the benefit of IAT treatment after IV-tPA compared with IV-tPA alone, in patients with acute ischemic stroke (**Table 3**).[26,54–57]

Despite the success of these recent IAT trials, several prior studies from 2013 failed to show a benefit of IAT. The success of these more recent studies can be attributed both to the availability of more effective current-generation clot retriever devices (stent retriever and penumbra devices versus older-generation concentric MERCI retriever device) and to the use of advanced imaging (CTA plus some measure of infarct core) for patient selection.[58,59]

In patients with anterior circulation occlusion stroke and contraindications to IV-tPA, endovascular therapy with stent retriever devices within 6 hours of stroke onset is a reasonable option.[50] Most recently, the DAWN and DEFUSE 3 trials—published in NEJM in November 2017 and February 2018, respectively—has shown that, with advanced imaging selection, patients can be safely treated with IAT up to 24 hours post-ictus.[2,3] DAWN patients achieved 49% functional

Table 3
Summary of 5 *The New England Journal of Medicine* 2015 randomized clinical trials showing efficacy of intra-arterial thrombectomy plus intravenous thrombolysis over that of intravenous thrombolysis alone in patients with acute ischemic stroke secondary to proximal large vessel occlusion

	MR CLEAN	ESCAPE	REVASCAT	SWIFT PRIME	EXTEND-IA
Subjects	PIACO	PIACO	PIACO	PIACO	PIACO + salvageable tissue on CTP
Number of patients	500	315	206	196	70
Imaging	CT, CTA	CT, CTA	CT, CTA/MRA	CT, CTA, CTP/MRP	CT, CTA, CTP
Intervention group	Any IA method	Any IA method	IA treatment with a stent retriever device	IA treatment with a stent retriever device	IA treatment with a stent retriever device
Control group	Medical treatment (± IV-tPA)	Medical treatment (± IV-tPA)	IV-tPA	IV-tPA	IV-tPA
Time to intervention	<6 h	<12 h	<8 h	<6 h	<4.5 h
Median time to groin puncture	260 min	241 min	269 min	224 min	210 min
90-d modified Rankin scale improvement	I: 32.6%[a] C: 22.1%	I: 53%[a] C: 29.3%	I: 43.7%[a] C: 28.2%	I: 60.2%[a] C: 35.5%	I: 71.4%[a] C: 40%
90-d mortality reduction	I: 21% C: 22.1%	I: 10.4%[a] C: 19%	I: 21% C: 22.1%	I: 9.2% C: 12.4%	I: 18.4% C: 15.5%
Conclusion	IA therapy within 6 h of stroke onset is effective and safe.	Rapid IA therapy in patients with small infarct and moderate-to-good collaterals improves functional outcome and mortality.	IA therapy with a stent retriever improves functional outcome.	IA therapy with a stent retriever within 6 h improves functional outcomes.	Early IA therapy with a stent retriever compared with IV-tPA alone improves reperfusion, early neurologic recovery, and functional outcome.

Abbreviations: C, control group; I, interventional group; IA, intra-arterial; PIACO, proximal intracranial anterior circulation occlusion.
a Statistically significant.

independence at 90 days versus 13% in controls; for every 2.8 treated patients, 1 additional patient was functionally independent at 90 days.

SUMMARY

Abrupt onset of a focal neurologic deficit typically defines the clinical syndrome of stroke. Neuroimaging has an essential role in the assessment of patients with suspected stroke, by differentiating ischemic from hemorrhagic stroke, identifying stroke mimics, and guiding patient selection for available therapies. Improved awareness of the neuroimaging findings highlighted in recent stroke clinical trials as well as of their role in patient selection for novel treatment options—including late window (8–24 hours post-ictus) IAT—has become increasingly important as advanced neuroimaging methods (ie, head and neck CTA, MRA, and perfusion and diffusion techniques) are gaining widespread acceptance for acute stroke evaluation.

REFERENCES

1. Kidwell CS, Saver JL, Schubert GB, et al. Design and retrospective analysis of the los angeles prehospital stroke screen (lapss). Prehosp Emerg Care 1998;2:267–73.
2. Jovin TG, Saver JL, Ribo M, et al. Diffusion-weighted imaging or computerized tomography perfusion assessment with clinical mismatch in the triage of wake up and late presenting strokes undergoing neurointervention with trevo (DAWN) trial methods. Int J Stroke 2017;12:641–52.
3. Albers GW, Marks MP, Kemp S, et al. Thrombectomy for stroke at 6 to 16 hours with selection by perfusion imaging. N Engl J Med 2018;378(8):708–18.
4. Benjamin EJ, Blaha MJ, Chiuve SE, et al. Heart disease and stroke statistics-2017 update: a report from the american heart association. Circulation 2017;135:e146–603.
5. Xu J, Murphy SL, Kochanek KD, et al. Mortality in the united states, 2015. NCHS Data Brief 2016;(267):1–8.
6. Xu J, Kochanek KD, Murphy SL, et al. Deaths: final data for 2007. Natl Vital Stat Rep 2010;58:1–19.
7. Hand PJ, Kwan J, Lindley RI, et al. Distinguishing between stroke and mimic at the bedside: the brain attack study. Stroke 2006;37:769–75.
8. Hemmen TM, Meyer BC, McClean TL, et al. Identification of nonischemic stroke mimics among 411 code strokes at the university of california, san diego, stroke center. J Stroke Cerebrovasc Dis 2008;17:23–5.
9. Allder SJ, Moody AR, Martel AL, et al. Limitations of clinical diagnosis in acute stroke. Lancet 1999;354:1523.
10. Moritani T, Smoker WR, Sato Y, et al. Diffusion-weighted imaging of acute excitotoxic brain injury. AJNR Am J Neuroradiol 2005;26:216–28.
11. Libman RB, Wirkowski E, Alvir J, et al. Conditions that mimic stroke in the emergency department. Implications for acute stroke trials. Arch Neurol 1995;52:1119–22.
12. Merino JG, Luby M, Benson RT, et al. Predictors of acute stroke mimics in 8187 patients referred to a stroke service. J Stroke Cerebrovasc Dis 2013;22:e397–403.
13. Chernyshev OY, Martin-Schild S, Albright KC, et al. Safety of tpa in stroke mimics and neuroimaging-negative cerebral ischemia. Neurology 2010;74:1340–5.
14. Multicenter Acute Stroke Trial–Europe Study Group, Hommel M, Cornu C, Boutitie F, et al. Thrombolytic therapy with streptokinase in acute ischemic stroke. N Engl J Med 1996;335:145–50.
15. Winkler DT, Fluri F, Fuhr P, et al. Thrombolysis in stroke mimics: Frequency, clinical characteristics, and outcome. Stroke 2009;40:1522–5.
16. Guillan M, Alonso-Canovas A, Gonzalez-Valcarcel J, et al. Stroke mimics treated with thrombolysis: further evidence on safety and distinctive clinical features. Cerebrovasc Dis 2012;34:115–20.
17. Adams HP Jr, Bendixen BH, Kappelle LJ, et al. Classification of subtype of acute ischemic stroke. Definitions for use in a multicenter clinical trial. Toast. Trial of org 10172 in acute stroke treatment. Stroke 1993;24:35–41.
18. Kannel WB, Wolf PA, Benjamin EJ, et al. Prevalence, incidence, prognosis, and predisposing conditions for atrial fibrillation: population-based estimates. Am J Cardiol 1998;82:2N–9N.
19. Miley ML, Wellik KE, Wingerchuk DM, et al. Does cervical manipulative therapy cause vertebral artery dissection and stroke? Neurologist 2008;14:66–73.
20. Biller J, Sacco RL, Albuquerque FC, et al. Cervical arterial dissections and association with cervical manipulative therapy: a statement for healthcare professionals from the American Heart Association/American Stroke Association. Stroke 2014;45:3155–74.
21. Sanak D, Nosal V, Horak D, et al. Impact of diffusion-weighted MRI-measured initial cerebral infarction volume on clinical outcome in acute stroke patients with middle cerebral artery occlusion treated by thrombolysis. Neuroradiology 2006;48:632–9.
22. Yoo AJ, Verduzco LA, Schaefer PW, et al. MRI-based selection for intra-arterial stroke therapy: value of pretreatment diffusion-weighted imaging lesion volume in selecting patients with acute stroke

who will benefit from early recanalization. Stroke 2009;40:2046–54.

23. Kidwell CS, Hsia AW. Imaging of the brain and cerebral vasculature in patients with suspected stroke: advantages and disadvantages of CT and MRI. Curr Neurol Neurosci Rep 2006;6:9–16.

24. Kamalian S, Morais LT, Pomerantz SR, et al. Clot length distribution and predictors in anterior circulation stroke: implications for intra-arterial therapy. Stroke 2013;44:3553–6.

25. Berkhemer OA, Jansen IG, Beumer D, et al. Collateral status on baseline computed tomographic angiography and intra-arterial treatment effect in patients with proximal anterior circulation stroke. Stroke 2016;47:768–76.

26. Goyal M, Demchuk AM, Menon BK, et al. Randomized assessment of rapid endovascular treatment of ischemic stroke. N Engl J Med 2015;372:1019–30.

27. Meyne JK, Zimmermann PR, Rohr A, et al. Thrombectomy vs. Systemic thrombolysis in acute embolic stroke with high clot burden: a retrospective analysis. Rofo 2015;187:555–60.

28. Tan IY, Demchuk AM, Hopyan J, et al. CT angiography clot burden score and collateral score: correlation with clinical and radiologic outcomes in acute middle cerebral artery infarct. AJNR Am J Neuroradiol 2009;30:525–31.

29. Puetz V, Dzialowski I, Hill MD, et al. Intracranial thrombus extent predicts clinical outcome, final infarct size and hemorrhagic transformation in ischemic stroke: the clot burden score. Int J Stroke 2008;3:230–6.

30. Puetz V, Dzialowski I, Hill MD, et al. Malignant profile detected by CT angiographic information predicts poor prognosis despite thrombolysis within three hours from symptom onset. Cerebrovasc Dis 2010; 29:584–91.

31. Tong E, Patrie J, Tong S, et al. Time-resolved CT assessment of collaterals as imaging biomarkers to predict clinical outcomes in acute ischemic stroke. Neuroradiology 2017;59(11):1101–9.

32. Kamalian S, Kamalian S, Konstas AA, et al. CT perfusion mean transit time maps optimally distinguish benign oligemia from true "at-risk" ischemic penumbra, but thresholds vary by postprocessing technique. AJNR Am J Neuroradiol 2012;33:545–9.

33. Kamalian S, Kamalian S, Maas MB, et al. CT cerebral blood flow maps optimally correlate with admission diffusion-weighted imaging in acute stroke but thresholds vary by postprocessing platform. Stroke 2011;42:1923–8.

34. Campbell BC, Christensen S, Levi CR, et al. Cerebral blood flow is the optimal CT perfusion parameter for assessing infarct core. Stroke 2011;42: 3435–40.

35. Bivard A, McElduff P, Spratt N, et al. Defining the extent of irreversible brain ischemia using perfusion computed tomography. Cerebrovasc Dis 2011;31: 238–45.

36. Lev MH. CT perfusion. AJNR News Digest 2016. Available at: http://ajnrdigest.org/ct-perfusion/.

37. Copen WA, Morais LT, Wu O, et al. In acute stroke, can CT perfusion-derived cerebral blood volume maps substitute for diffusion-weighted imaging in identifying the ischemic core? PLoS One 2015;10: e0133566.

38. Schaefer PW, Souza L, Kamalian S, et al. Limited reliability of computed tomographic perfusion acute infarct volume measurements compared with diffusion-weighted imaging in anterior circulation stroke. Stroke 2015;46:419–24.

39. Copen WA, Deipolyi AR, Schaefer PW, et al. Exposing hidden truncation-related errors in acute stroke perfusion imaging. AJNR Am J Neuroradiol 2015;36:638–45.

40. Copen WA, Rezai Gharai L, Barak ER, et al. Existence of the diffusion-perfusion mismatch within 24 hours after onset of acute stroke: dependence on proximal arterial occlusion. Radiology 2009;250: 878–86.

41. Wintermark M, Sanelli PC, Albers GW, et al. Imaging recommendations for acute stroke and transient ischemic attack patients: a joint statement by the american society of neuroradiology, the American college of radiology, and the society of neurointerventional surgery. AJNR Am J Neuroradiol 2013; 34:E117–27.

42. Lev MH, Segal AZ, Farkas J, et al. Utility of perfusion-weighted CT imaging in acute middle cerebral artery stroke treated with intra-arterial thrombolysis: prediction of final infarct volume and clinical outcome. Stroke 2001;32:2021–8.

43. Leslie-Mazwi TM, Hirsch JA, Falcone GJ, et al. Endovascular stroke treatment outcomes after patient selection based on magnetic resonance imaging and clinical criteria. JAMA Neurol 2016;73:43–9.

44. Nederkoorn PJ, van der Graaf Y, Hunink MG. Duplex ultrasound and magnetic resonance angiography compared with digital subtraction angiography in carotid artery stenosis: a systematic review. Stroke 2003;34:1324–32.

45. Gonzalez RG, Copen WA, Schaefer PW, et al. The massachusetts general hospital acute stroke imaging algorithm: an experience and evidence based approach. J Neurointerv Surg 2013; 5(Suppl 1):i7–12.

46. Souza LC, Yoo AJ, Chaudhry ZA, et al. Malignant cta collateral profile is highly specific for large admission dwi infarct core and poor outcome in acute stroke. AJNR Am J Neuroradiol 2012;33:1331–6.

47. Bouslama M, Bowen MT, Haussen DC, et al. Selection paradigms for large vessel occlusion acute ischemic stroke endovascular therapy. Cerebrovasc Dis 2017;44:277–84.

48. Kamalian SK, Boulter DJ, Lev MH, et al. Stroke differential diagnosis and mimics: Part 1. Appl Radiol 2015;44:26–39.

49. Jauch EC, Saver JL, Adams HP Jr, et al. Guidelines for the early management of patients with acute ischemic stroke: a guideline for healthcare professionals from the american heart association/american stroke association. Stroke 2013;44:870–947.

50. Powers WJ, Derdeyn CP, Biller J, et al. 2015 American heart association/American stroke association focused update of the 2013 guidelines for the early management of patients with acute ischemic stroke regarding endovascular treatment: a guideline for healthcare professionals from the American heart association/american stroke association. Stroke 2015;46:3020–35.

51. National Institute of Neurological Disorders and Stroke rt-PA Stroke Study Group. Tissue plasminogen activator for acute ischemic stroke. N Engl J Med 1995;333:1581–7.

52. Hacke W, Kaste M, Bluhmki E, et al. Thrombolysis with alteplase 3 to 4.5 hours after acute ischemic stroke. N Engl J Med 2008;359:1317–29.

53. Riedel CH, Zimmermann P, Jensen-Kondering U, et al. The importance of size: Successful recanalization by intravenous thrombolysis in acute anterior stroke depends on thrombus length. Stroke 2011; 42:1775–7.

54. Berkhemer OA, Fransen PS, Beumer D, et al. A randomized trial of intraarterial treatment for acute ischemic stroke. N Engl J Med 2015;372:11–20.

55. Jovin TG, Chamorro A, Cobo E, et al. Thrombectomy within 8 hours after symptom onset in ischemic stroke. N Engl J Med 2015;372:2296–306.

56. Saver JL, Goyal M, Bonafe A, et al. Stent-retriever thrombectomy after intravenous t-pa vs. T-pa alone in stroke. N Engl J Med 2015;372:2285–95.

57. Campbell BC, Mitchell PJ, Kleinig TJ, et al. Endovascular therapy for ischemic stroke with perfusion-imaging selection. N Engl J Med 2015;372:1009–18.

58. Broderick JP, Palesch YY, Demchuk AM, et al. Endovascular therapy after intravenous t-pa versus t-pa alone for stroke. N Engl J Med 2013;368:893–903.

59. Ciccone A, Valvassori L, Nichelatti M, et al. Endovascular treatment for acute ischemic stroke. N Engl J Med 2013;368:904–13.

The Patient with Thunderclap Headache

Ajay Malhotra, MD, MMM[a],*, Xiao Wu, BS[b], Dheeraj Gandhi, MD[c], Pina Sanelli, MD, MPH[d]

KEYWORDS

• Thunderclap headache • Subarachnoid hemorrhage • Lumbar puncture • Intracranial aneurysm

KEY POINTS

• Thunderclap headache (sudden onset of severe headache reaching maximal intensity within seconds to a minute) can have multiple causes, but aneurysmal rupture causing subarachnoid hemorrhage is the primary concern.
• Noncontrast CT performed within 6 hours of onset is very sensitive for subarachnoid hemorrhage, but the sensitivity decreases with time.
• Further work-up for subarachnoid hemorrhage should be guided by the pattern of blood on noncontrast CT head.

Headache is an extremely common symptom and annually more than 70% of the United States population may have a headache.[1] Headache accounts for approximately 2% of all emergency department (ED) visits.[2] Most episodes of headache are benign and do not require emergent imaging.[3] Clinical decision rules have been proposed to identify patients with acute nontraumatic headache who need further investigation.[4] Despite high sensitivity for subarachnoid hemorrhage (SAH), they suffer from poor specificity and are applicable to only a minority of ED patients with headache.[5] In a 2006 study, 14% of patients presenting with headache underwent neuroimaging, and only 5.5% of the imaged patients received a pathologic diagnosis.[2]

Thunderclap headache (TCH) is defined as sudden-onset unruptured intracranial aneurysm (UIA) of severe headache reaching maximal intensity within seconds to a minute.[6] The term TCH was initially used in reference to pain associated with a UIA, but multiple causes have since been described (**Boxes 1 and 2, Table 1**).[6,7] Aneurysmal rupture resulting in SAH is the primary concern, given the high morbidity and mortality associated with this condition.[8] It accounts, however, for only 4% to 12% of acute, severe headaches.[9–12] Primary TCH is a diagnosis of exclusion when all other underlying causes have been eliminated. Primary TCH can recur intermittently but is generally associated with a benign outcome.[6] This review discusses the differential diagnosis of TCH and details the

Disclosure Statement: The authors have nothing to disclose.
[a] Department of Radiology and Biomedical Imaging, Yale School of Medicine, The Imaging Clinical Effectiveness and Outcomes Research, Northwell Health, 55 York Street, New Haven, CT 06511, USA; [b] Department of Radiology and Biomedical Imaging, Yale School of Medicine, 55 York Street, New Haven, CT 06511, USA; [c] Interventional Neuroradiology, University of Maryland School of Medicine, 22 South Greene Street, Room N2e23, Baltimore, MD 21201, USA; [d] Department of Radiology, The Imaging Clinical Effectiveness and Outcomes Research, Northwell Health, NSUH, 300 Community Drive, Manhasset, NY 11030, USA
* Corresponding author.
E-mail address: ajay.malhotra@yale.edu

Neuroimag Clin N Am 28 (2018) 335–351
https://doi.org/10.1016/j.nic.2018.03.002

Box 1
Etiology of spontaneous convexity/sulcal subarachnoid hemorrhage

- Cerebral amyloid angiopathy
- RCVS
- AVMs, dural fistulae
- Cavernomas
- CVT
- Moyamoya disease
- Arterial dissection/stenosis
- Nonvascular causes—such as brain tumors and abscesses
- Coagulation disorders

Table 1
Causes of thunderclap headache

Findings on CT and Cerebrospinal Fluid	Causes of Thunderclap Headache
Usually detected by noncontrast CT	• SAH (most cases detected by noncontrast CT done within 24 h of symptom onset) • Intracerebral hematoma • Intraventricular hemorrhage • Acute subdural hematoma • Cerebral infarcts (after 3 h) • Tumors (eg, third-ventricle colloid cyst)
Usually detected by analysis of CSF after normal CT	• SAH • Meningitis
Possibly presenting with normal CT results and normal or near-normal results of analysis of CSF	• Intracranial venous thrombosis • Dissection of cervical arteries (extracranial or intracranial—carotid or vertebral) • Pituitary apoplexy • RCVS with or without posterior reversible encephalopathy syndrome • Symptomatic aneurysm without evidence of subarachnoid haemorrhage (painful third nerve paralysis) • Intracranial hypotension • Cardiac cephalalgia due to myocardial ischaemia (very rare)

Data from Kumar S, Goddeau RP Jr, Selim MH, et al. Atraumatic convexal subarachnoid hemorrhage: clinical presentation, imaging patterns, and etiologies. Neurology 2010;74(11):893–9.

diagnostic assessment of patients presenting with TCH.

DETECTION OF SUBARACHNOID HEMORRHAGE

SAH results most commonly from rupture of an intracranial aneurysm.[13] Headache associated with SAH typically lasts a few days; it is atypical for the headache to resolve in less than 2 hours.[14] Loss of consciousness can occur in a third of patients with SAH.[10] Other symptoms may include nausea, vomiting, dizziness, photophobia, neck stiffness, delirium, and seizures.[15] Prompt

Box 2
Other names for reversible cerebral vasoconstriction syndrome

- Isolated benign cerebral vasculitis
- Acute benign cerebral angiopathy
- Reversible cerebral segmental vasoconstriction
- Call or Call-Fleming syndrome
- CNS pseudovasculitis
- Benign angiopathy of the CNS
- Postpartum angiopathy
- Migraine angiitis
- Migrainous vasospasm
- Primary TCH
- Drug-induced vasospasm
- Cerebral vasculopathy
- Vasospasm in fatal migrainous infarction

diagnosis of acute SAH is critical because initial misdiagnosis and subsequent rebleeding correspond with a poor prognosis and up to 70% mortality.[16] SAH may go undiagnosed in 5% of patients during ED visits, with lower acuity patients at higher risk.[17]

Physical examination is of limited utility for assessment of patients with suspected SAH.[11] Noncontrast CT is the initial diagnostic test for suspected SAH. The sensitivity of CT for detecting acute SAH is 90% to 100% when performed within 24 hours but decreases with time as blood is progressively diluted by normal cerebrospinal fluid (CSF) flow.[12,18,19] In patients presenting with TCH and normal neurologic examination, a normal brain CT within 6 hours of headache onset is extremely specific in ruling out aneurysmal SAH.[20] Beyond 6 hours, the reported sensitivity of CT is 89%.[21] Patients with atypical features (syncope and seizures), focal neurologic deficits, or CT performed beyond 6 hours of onset do need further work-up after a negative noncontrast CT Head.

Negative CT in patients with SAH is often attributed to delayed clinical presentation, very small volumes of initial hemorrhage, or a low hematocrit.[22] Certain locations, such as the interpeduncular cistern, and small, focal convexity bleeds are more likely overlooked.[23] Posterior temporal horn dilatation has been reported as a prevalent finding in 66% to 84% of SAH cases, even in the absence of visible hemorrhage.[24] Mark and colleagues[25] reported that in 9 of 18 previously reported CT-negative SAH cases confirmed on lumbar puncture (LP) and read by non-neuroradiologists, SAH could be identified in subsequent review.

Because early-generation CTs did not detect SAH in up to 5% patients, traditional teaching has emphasized the need to perform LP to exclude SAH.[21] The diagnosis in these cases is made by LP and the presence of red blood cells (RBCs) and/or bilirubin (as established by visual or spectrophotometric analysis).[25] LP is associated, however, with patient anxiety and discomfort and can be complicated by postprocedure headache in 15% to 20% of patients.[26] In addition, LP may be contraindicated if a patient has a bleeding disorder or increased intracranial pressure. Traumatic taps, which occur in 10% to 15% of patients, may lead to unnecessary vascular imaging and other downstream consequences.[27] Identifying xanthochromia from breakdown of hemoglobin in CSF is considered pathognomonic for SAH but requires up to 12 hours to develop and may be false positive due to ex vivo hemolysis or hyperbilirubinemia.[8] Visible xanthochromia has reported sensitivity of 85% for SAH and specificity of 97%.[21] Perry and colleagues[28] reported a sensitivity of 93% and a specificity of 91% for threshold RBCs less than 2000×10^6/L in the final tube of CSF collected to distinguish traumatic LP from aneurysmal SAH. Even when applying the recommended cut-offs of RBCs greater than 2000×10^6/L CSF and absence of xanthochromia for further investigation of SAH, there is still a false-positive rate of approximately 10%.[25,28,29] Despite the recommendations, multicenter observational studies report that fewer than half of acute headache patients undergo LP after a negative CT, and, of these, less than 1 in 100 LPs are deemed "true positive."[4] Change in practice has been proposed wherein an LP can be withheld in a patient with a negative CT performed less than 6 hours after symptom onset.[30]

CT angiography (CTA) has been proposed to replace LP after a negative noncontrast CT in patients with acute-onset headache, due to wide availability, noninvasive testing, and improved sensitivity for detection of intracranial aneurysms.[31] A recent meta-analysis reported the pooled sensitivity and specificity for CTA to detect aneurysms of 98% and 100%, respectively[32]; 75% of patients in a recent survey favored undergoing a CTA instead of LP after a nondiagnostic noncontrast CT.[33] The utility and cost-effectiveness of CTA to replace LP in this situation, however, have been questioned.[34–36] CTA is associated with radiation risks and requires administration of iodine-based contrast, which can be nephrotoxic. There is an approximately 3.2% prevalence of unruptured aneurysms in the general, non–high-risk population.[37] More recent studies with liberal use of magnetic resonance angiography (MRA) report a prevalence as high as 7% in large, population-based studies.[38] A significant proportion (up to 87.6%) of incidental UIAs have been reported to be small, measuring less than 3 mm to 4 mm.[39] Small aneurysms (<7 mm) uncommonly cause symptoms and are most frequently incidentally detected.[40,41] No studies have sufficiently correlated presentation with headache with change in risk of spontaneous hemorrhage in unruptured aneurysms, and most headaches in UIAs are not directly related to the aneurysm.[42] Treatment or imaging surveillance of these incidentally detected UIAs is not without significant costs and complications.[43] Although CTA is frequently performed in clinical practice, current guidelines still recommend LP as the next diagnostic test after initial negative head CT.

MR imaging can be sensitive for the detection of SAH; T2 fluid-attenuated inversion recovery (FLAIR) is sensitive in the acute phase, and subarachnoid blood products display sulcal hyperintensity.[44] It may fail, however, to demonstrate blood in tight cisterns, and there are multiple causes of sulcal hyperintensity on FLAIR other than hemorrhage.[45,46] T2* sequence has been demonstrated as having a sensitivity of 94% within 4 days of ictus, but a 100% sensitivity between 4 days and 14 days, with a high specificity.[47] MR imaging is not recognized, however, as sufficiently sensitive to discard LP.[48]

FURTHER WORK-UP OF SUBARACHNOID HEMORRHAGE

Multidetector CTA is an accurate and sufficient tool for detecting and characterizing aneurysms in the setting of acute SAH.[49,50] CTA has largely replaced digital subtraction angiography (DSA) for detection of intracranial aneurysms in most patients.[51] The reported sensitivity, specificity, and accuracy of aneurysm detection with modern-generation scanners have improved dramatically.[52] When CTA is negative, DSA is still performed at many institutions due to concern that an intradural aneurysms may be missed.

The pattern and distribution of blood on noncontrast CT, however, determine the etiology and possible role for repeat angiography after a negative CTA.[53]

ANEURYSMAL SUBARACHNOID HEMORRHAGE

Ruptured aneurysms account for 85% of SAH cases; 10% to 43% of patients with aneurysmal SAH have a history of a sentinel headache or warning leak days to weeks before detection of aneurysm rupture.[54] The most common locations for aneurysm are anterior communicating artery, middle cerebral artery bifurcation, posterior communicating artery, and the terminal basilar artery.[55] High volume of hemorrhage localized to the basilar cisterns is indicative of aneurysmal SAH, and patterns of hemorrhage help predict site of aneurysm[56] (**Fig. 1**). Although SAH usually occurs at the same location as cerebral aneurysm, location of SAH is not always a reliable indicator of site of aneurysm rupture, with the exception of

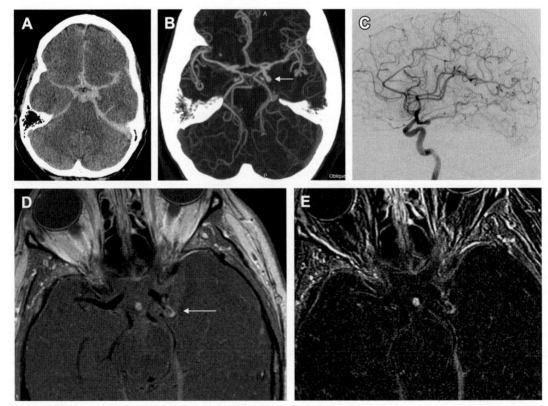

Fig. 1. Diffuse SAH in the basal cisterns, sylvian fissures and interhemispheric fissure on axial noncontrast CT (*A*). Axial CTA maximum intensity projection (*B*) shows a lobulated posterior communicating artery aneurysm directed posteriorly (*arrow*) and confirmed on DSA (*C*). Vessel wall MR imaging (*D, E*) shows wall enhancement at the tip of the aneurysm (*arrow*), indicating likely site of rupture.

anterior cerebral or anterior communicating artery aneurysms.[57] A significant percentage (15%–20%) of SAH patients have no aneurysm detected on initial vascular imaging.[53] An aneurysm may not be depicted on the initial angiographic study for several reasons: very small size, presence of intraluminal thrombus, adjacent hematoma, aneurysms on arterial dissections, suboptimal image quality due to technical reasons or in uncooperative patients, or missed diagnosis due to error.[58] Aneurysms that may potentially be missed on initial CTA include those at the skull base, small bifurcation aneurysms, those on a curve of a vessel, perforator aneurysms, and small, infectious, or myxomatous aneurysms.[51] The sensitivity of CTA for detection of aneurysms depends on the arterial attenuation of vessels.[59] Repeat DSA is recommended in patients with diffuse, nonperimesencephalic pattern of SAH, although the timing of repeat angiography is subject to debate.[60] Even in patients with negative initial 3-D rotational angiography for aneurysmal-type SAH, repeat 3-D rotational angiography may show a ruptured aneurysm in 1 in 4 patients.[58]

Cranial MR imaging performed within 72 hours, or on a delayed basis, for an angiogram-negative SAH has a low diagnostic yield and is not routinely recommended.[61,62] High-resolution vessel wall–MR imaging has so far not been shown to alter management in angiogram-negative SAH patients, although it is increasingly used to identify the ruptured lesion when a CTA reveals multiple aneurysms.[63]

PERIMESENCEPHALIC HEMORRHAGE

Two-thirds of the nonaneurysmal SAH patients may have perimesencephalic hemorrhage with blood confined to the perimesencephalic cisterns.[53] Perimesencephalic hemorrhage is blood confined to the interpeduncular, prepontine, ambient, quadrigeminal, or premedullary cisterns, with possible extension to the proximal stems of the sylvian fissure but no deep extension into the anterior interhemispheric fissure or lateral aspect of sylvian fissures (**Fig. 2**). Perimesencephalic hemorrhage patients usually have a good clinical grade at presentation, no neurologic deficits, and generally a good prognosis.[64] Because approximately 10% of posterior circulation aneurysms can present with a perimesencephalic bleeding pattern, initial angiographic imaging is essential.[65] In patients meeting the strict imaging criteria of perimesencephalic hemorrhage, however, initial negative CTA has been shown reliable and cost-

effective in excluding aneurysms, without need for further angiographic work-up.[66,67] Recurrence is extremely rare and does not reveal aneurysms on further imaging, and patients have a good prognosis compared with aneurysmal SAH.[68] American Heart Association/American Stroke Association guidelines suggest that DSA may not be necessary if a classic perimesencephalic pattern of hemorrhage is present and CTA may suffice.[69]

PERIPHERAL, CONVEXITY SUBARACHNOID HEMORRHAGE

Subarachnoid blood restricted to 1 or more cerebral sulci without extension to the basal cisterns, ventricles, or sylvian and interhemispheric fissures represents a distinct group of patients with nontraumatic SAH.[51] Reversible cerebral vasoconstriction syndrome (RCVS) is increasingly recognized as the most common cause of convexity SAH in patients 60 years or younger, with amyloid angiopathy the leading cause in older patients.[70] Amyloid angiopathy patients typically do not present with recurrent headaches.[71] Cerebral venous thrombosis (CVT) and arterial dissection can also present with TCH and small, convexity bleeds and do not show up on CT or CSF analysis. MR imaging and craniocervical angiography may be needed in these cases. Mycotic and oncotic aneurysms in the distal vasculature can also present as convexity, sulcal SAH. Cross-sectional imaging has a poor sensitivity in detection of abnormalities in distal vasculature, including aneurysms, dissections, and dural arteriovenous fistulae, and conventional angiography is frequently needed.[72]

REVERSIBLE CEREBRAL VASOCONSTRICTION SYNDROME

RCVS is characterized by severe headaches, with or without acute neurologic symptoms, and diffuse segmental constriction of cerebral arteries that resolves spontaneously within 3 months.[73] More than half of cases occur postpartum or after exposure to adrenergic or serotonergic drugs.[71] Many patients have a history of migraine, and acute migraine treatments (triptans and ergots) can precipitate RCVS or aggravate the vasoconstriction when the TCH is mistaken for a migraine attack.[71,74] Severe headaches typically are short lived (usually lasting 1–3 hours) and recur for 1 week to 2 weeks, with a self-limiting course, and no new symptoms typically occur after 1 month.[75] Triggering event for the headache maybe

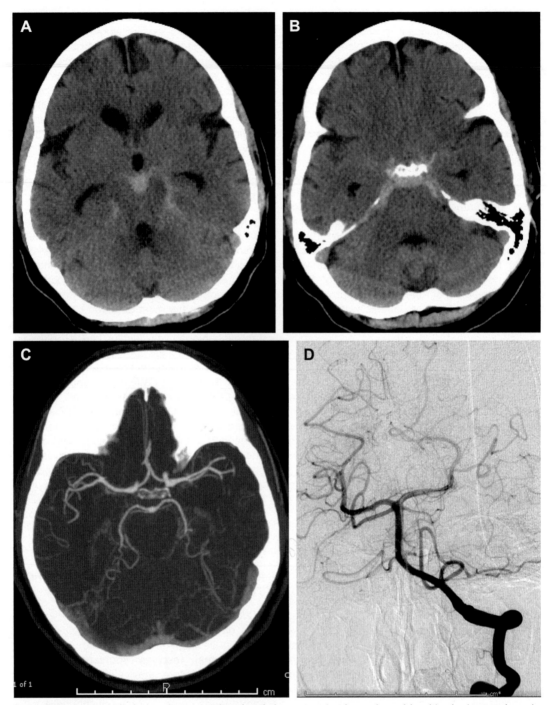

Fig. 2. Perimesencephalic hemorrhage. Axial CT (*A*, *B*) demonstrating hyperdense blood in the interpeduncular, ambient, and prepontine cisterns. CTA (*C*) and DSA (*D*) did not reveal any vascular etiology for the perimesencephalic blood.

sexual activity, straining during defecation, stressful or emotional situations, coughing, sneezing, showering, and sudden bending down.[71] The course is uniphasic, but the manifestations can vary from pure cephalgia to rare catastrophic forms complicated by ischemic and hemorrhagic strokes.[76] The clinicoradiologic features tend to be dynamic with cerebral vasoconstriction at its peak on angiograms obtained 2 weeks to 3 weeks after clinical onset.[71]

Brain scans of many patients with RCVS do not show focal abnormalities despite presence of diffuse vasoconstriction on angiography, especially on initial imaging.[77] The spectrum of imaging findings described are reversible edema, convexity SAH, intracerebral hemorrhage, and cerebral infarction.[71] Parenchymal hemorrhages are more frequently single than multiple and lobar than deep. They occur early in the course of RCVS and are associated with focal deficits.[78] Cerebral infarctions typically occur in arterial watershed regions and occur later than hemorrhagic strokes in the course of RCVS.[75] Edema is an early manifestation of RCVS, with distribution similar to that of posterior reversible encephalopathy syndrome and usually totally reverses within 1 month of onset, earlier than does vasoconstriction.[71] Reversible brain edema occurs in 8% to 38% of all cases of RCVS, whereas multifocal cerebral vasoconstriction has been noted in more than 85% of patients with posterior reversible encephalopathy syndrome.[79]

The arteriopathy is typically bilateral and diffuse and frequently disproportionate and distant to the small, focal amount of subarachnoid blood.[80] The imaging findings of SAH along with cerebral vasoconstriction can be easily confused with other entities, such as vasospasm after aneurysmal SAH and vasculitis. The clinical features, CSF characteristics, and distinctive pattern of imaging on DSA, however, can generally easily help with characterization. Arterial changes in RCVS are typically widespread, involving smaller/distal vessels, and disproportionately excessive compared with small amount of SAH seen on the CT or MR imaging. In contrast, vasospasm is typically observed in patients with higher Fisher scale grade SAH patients, predominates in the large vessels of circle of Willis, and generally peaks between days 4 and 12 after SAH. In RCVS patients, initial angiographic study maybe normal if performed early, even in presence of brain edema or hemorrhage. Maximum vasoconstriction has been reported in branches of middle cerebral arteries after 2 weeks of clinical onset[81] (Fig. 3). The arterial narrowing is not fixed, with new constrictions seen on subsequent angiography often affecting more proximal vessels.[71] High-resolution MR imaging vessel wall imaging may help distinguish RCVS (uniform wall thickening with negligible to mild enhancement) from central nervous system (CNS) vasculitis (concentric or eccentric wall enhancement).[82]

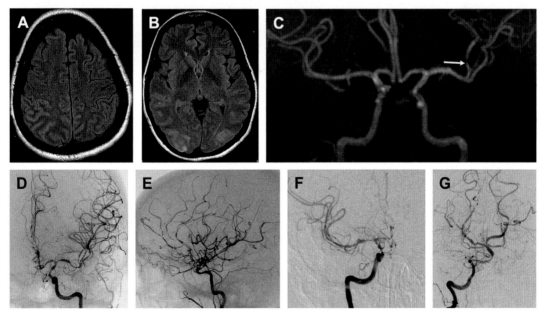

Fig. 3. RCVS. MR imaging FLAIR images (A, B) demonstrating sulcal hyperintensity due to SAH and cortical-subcortical edema in posterior distribution. Time-of-flight MRA (C) showing areas of irregularity and narrowing most prominent in left M2 (arrow). DSA performed at 3 weeks (D–G) showing beading with more prominent areas of stenosis and beading involving more proximal circle of Willis.

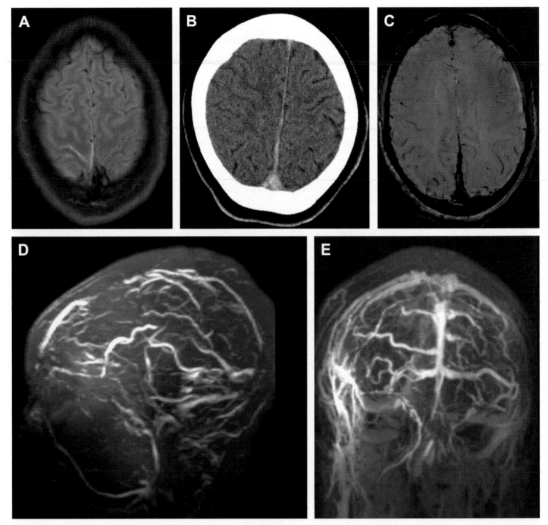

Fig. 4. Cerebral venous sinus thrombosis. A 32-year-old, recent postpartum woman with acute, severe headache. SAH seen on FLAIR (*A*). Thrombus in the superior sagittal sinus seen as hyperdensity on CT (*B*) and hypointense signal on susceptibility-weighted imaging (*C*). Noncontrast (*D*) and postcontrast MR venogram (*E*) demonstrate extensive venous sinus thrombosis.

PRIMARY ANGIITIS OF THE CENTRAL NERVOUS SYSTEM

Primary CNS angiitis usually has an insidious onset in contrast to RCVS. Headaches are not typically thunderclap and are followed by stepwise deterioration with focal deficits, infarcts, or cognitive decline.[71] TCH rarely is seen with a ruptured aneurysm associated with vasculitis. Abnormal results of CSF analysis are seen in 80% of patients with primary angiitis, whereas they are normal or near normal in patients with RCVS.[6] MR imaging is abnormal in most cases and shows several small deep or superficial infarcts of different ages, with or without white matter abnormalities and/or parenchymal enhancing lesion.[83] High-resolution black-blood MRA may depict concentric or eccentric areas of vessel wall enhancement. Arterial irregularities typically involve the third-order or fourth-order branches of the circle of Willis. These irregular areas of narrowing are not as dynamic and do not change or improve as rapidly as in RCVS.[77]

CEREBRAL VENOUS THROMBOSIS

Although headaches are a common presentation in patients with CVT, only 2% to 10% have TCH as predominant symptom.[84] Headaches are frequently persistent and exacerbated by

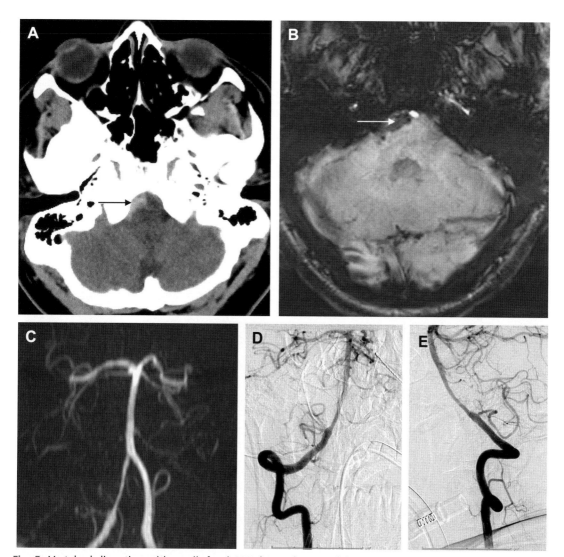

Fig. 5. Vertebral dissection with small, focal SAH (*arrows*) on CT (*A*) and susceptibility-weighted imaging (*B*). Time-offlight maximum intensity projection MRA (*C*) shows abrupt change in caliber of right vertebral artery distal to posterior inferior cerebellar artery origin, which was confirmed on DSA right vertebral injection frontal (*D*) and lateral (*E*) views.

increased intracranial pressure (caused by coughing, sneezing, or Valsalva maneuver) or in recumbent position; 10% of patients with CVT can present with SAH, usually focal and localized to few convexity sulci.[85] It is uncommon, however, to see SAH as a sole imaging finding in CVT. CT abnormalities can be seen in 90% of patients with focal neurologic deficits and include venous infarcts, edema, or hyperdensity within the occluded sinus (**Fig. 4**). Hemorrhage in venous thrombosis is typically cortical with subcortical extension. MR imaging with venography is commonly needed for diagnosis of CVT and should be considered when clinically concerned for venous thrombosis.[6] CT venography is a reasonable alternative. DSA is generally not necessary for diagnosis but is generally used in treatment of refractory patients that are considered for endovenous thrombolysis.

CERVICAL ARTERY DISSECTION

Headache is reported in 60% to 95% of patients with arterial dissections and up to 20% present with TCHs.[86] Neck pain is frequently associated. Associated findings include amaurosis fugax, Horner syndrome, pulsatile tinnitus, dysgeusia, diplopia, and other stroke manifestations.[6] Dissections resulting in SAH are more common in the posterior circulation and in children.[87] Brain CT and LP are usually normal and ultrasound, CTA, or MRA should be considered when clinically concerned for dissection. Angiographic features include luminal narrowing, vessel irregularity, wall thickening/mural hematoma, intimal flap, and pseudoaneurysm formation (Fig. 5). Up to 7% of patients with arterial dissections can present with self-limiting, convexity SAH.[88]

SPONTANEOUS INTRACRANIAL HYPOTENSION

Spontaneous intracranial hypotension usually presents as orthostatic headaches, which

worsen when upright and improves after lying down. However, 15% of spontaneous intracranial hypotension patients can present with TCH.[71] Brain MR imaging reveals diffuse pachymeningeal thickening and enhancement, in addition to brain sagging and cerebellar tonsillar descent (Fig. 6). Crowding of the posterior fossa, reduction in prepontine space, descent of optic chiasm, and subdural collections may also be present.[89]

ARTERIOVENOUS MALFORMATION

Less than 5% of ruptured arteriovenous malformations (AVMs) can present as SAH without intracerebral hematoma.[13] SAH as a presentation is more likely when aneurysms occur in

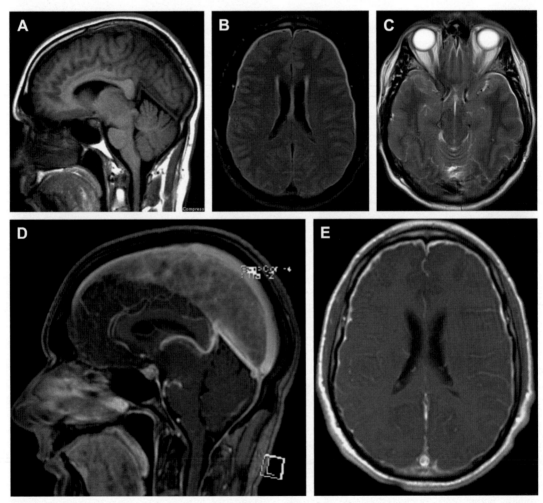

Fig. 6. Sagittal T1WI (*A*) shows brain sagging with effacement of suprasellar and prepontine cisterns, cerebellar tonsillar ectopia, and sharp angulation at the junction of internal cerebral veins with straight sinus. Bilateral subdural collections seen on FLAIR (*B*) and axial T2 (*C*) with effacement of basal cisterns and deformation of brainstem. Sagittal postcontrast image (*D*) shows pituitary engorgrment and prominent venous sinuses. Diffuse pachymeningeal enhancement on axial postcontrast image (*E*).

association with AVM. These aneurysms can be characterized as (1) proximal or distal, flow related, (2) intranidal, or (3) unrelated.[90] Flow-related aneurysms occur more frequently, but intranidal aneurysms present with bleeding more often. Serpiginous hyperdense structures representing dilated vasculature in the periphery of brain parenchyma, with or without associated calcifications, on unenhanced CT should raise concern for an AVM. This can be easily confirmed with CTA or MR imaging of the brain that reveals typical cluster of vessels/nidus (**Fig. 7**). AVMs often require assessment with DSA for better characterization and identification of associated aneurysms, and, to understand the flow-dynamics. DSA is also performed as an adjunct to embolization.

DURAL ARTERIOVENOUS FISTULA

Tentorial dural arteriovenous fistulas can cause a pattern of basilar hemorrhage that is indistinguishable from aneurysmal SAH.[13] SAH and/or associated parenchymal bleed, however, can occur in other types of tentorial dural arteriovenous fistulas, especially those considered high-grade lesions (Borden II and III). These lesions are associated with cortical venous reflux/drainage.[91] CTA/MRA may demonstrate venous sinus thrombosis and dilated, abnormal vessels. Conventional angiography is often needed, however, to diagnose and characterize the fistula and as an adjunct to plan endovascular therapy. A vast majority of these lesions lend themselves to endovascular embolization techniques.

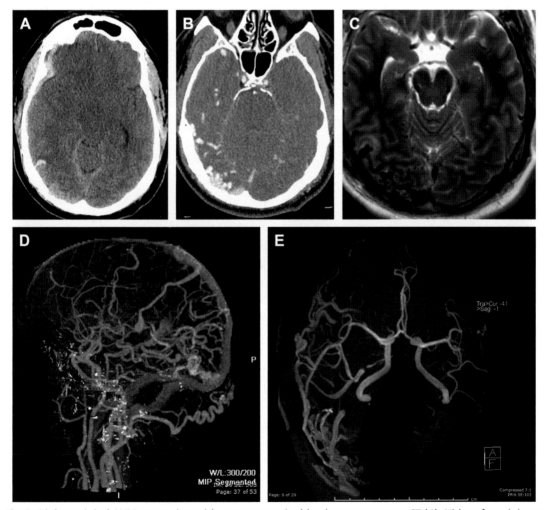

Fig. 7. Right occipital AVM presenting with acute convexity bleed on noncontrast CT (*A*). Nidus of serpiginous vessels on CTA (*B*) and axial T2-weighted image (*C*). CTA maximum intensity projections (*D*) and time-of-flight MRA (*E*) show predominant arterial supply of the AVM from right occipital and middle meningeal artery.

ISCHEMIC STROKE

Headaches occur in approximately 25% of patients with stroke and are more common with large ischemic stroke, in the territory of posterior circulation, in patients with migraine, and in younger patients.[92] TCH presentation, however, is rare with stroke.[93]

PITUITARY APOPLEXY

Hemorrhage or infarction of the pituitary gland rarely presents as TCH.[94] This may occur with or without a known history of pituitary tumor. Pregnancy, general anesthesia, bromocriptine therapy, and pituitary irradiation are other known risk factors.[6] These can easily be overlooked on CT and often detected and characterized on MR imaging (**Fig. 8**).

THIRD-VENTRICLE COLLOID CYST

Colloid cysts at the anterosuperior third ventricle can present with abrupt-onset headache that frequently is relieved by recumbency.[95] Most are oval or rounded and situated at the foramen of Munro (**Fig. 9**). A majority are hyperdense on CT and hypointense on T2-weighted images, and 50% are hyperintense on T1-weighted images.

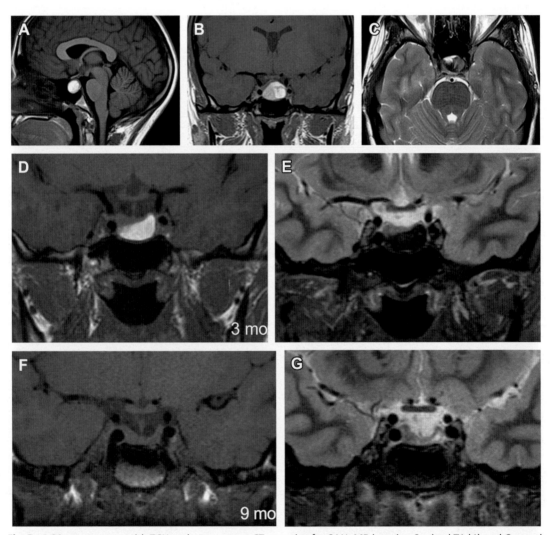

Fig. 8. A 30-year woman with TCH and noncontrast CT negative for SAH. MR imaging Sagittal T1 (*A*) and Coronal; T1-weighted (*B*) images show sellar heterogeneous, T1 hyperintense lesion with pituitary enlargement. Axial T2-weighted image (*C*) shows corresponding patchy low T2 signal. Follow-up Cor T1 (*D*) and T2-weighted (*E*) images done at 3 months and at 9 months (*F, G*) show progressive decrease in size and resolution of pituitary hemorrhage.

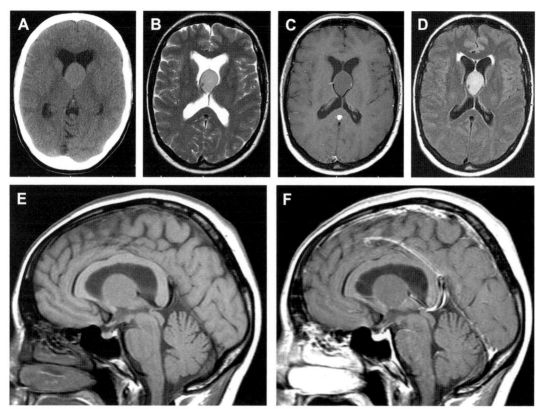

Fig. 9. Colloid cyst. Circumscribed, oval lesion in the midline at level of foramen of Monro—hyperdense on CT (*A*), hypointense on T2 (*B*), and no contrast enhancement on axial contrast image (*C*). Obstructive dilatation of the lateral ventricles and mild subependymal CSF flow on FLAIR (*D*). Sagittal T1 (*E*) and postcontrast (*F*) images show the lesion in the anterosuperior third ventricle. Remaining ventricular system is normal in size.

SUMMARY

TCH can have potentially catastrophic consequences and should be managed as a medical emergency. Initial assessment must be focused on excluding SAH. Imaging work-up depends on the time since onset of symptoms. Noncontrast CT is highly sensitive and specific in the first 6 hours to 12 hours. CSF evaluation by LP has high sensitivity when LP is done 12 hours to 2 weeks after SAH in patients with negative CT.[96] LP is an invasive procedure, and some studies have proposed a CT/CTA algorithm to replace CT/LP.[97] Utility of CTA, however, in this context is not established, especially given the incidental detection of intracranial aneurysms.[34] This possibility should be discussed with patients before offering CTA, given the implication for subsequent aneurysmal treatment and/or imaging surveillance. MR imaging should be considered in patients with TCH who have negative CT and CSF analysis. CTA is sensitive for detection of intracranial aneurysm in patients with known SAH. In CTA-negative patients, further work-up should be decided based on the pattern of distribution of blood on CT. Repeat angiography should be considered in patients with aneurysmal SAH but may be of limited utility in perimesencephalic SAH.

REFERENCES

1. Medina LS, D'Souza B, Vasconcellos E. Adults and children with headache: evidence-based diagnostic evaluation. Neuroimaging Clin N Am 2003;13(2): 225–35.
2. Goldstein JN, Camargo CA Jr, Pelletier AJ, et al. Headache in United States emergency departments: demographics, work-up and frequency of pathological diagnoses. Cephalalgia 2006;26(6): 684–90.
3. Jordan JE. Headache. AJNR Am J Neuroradiol 2007;28(9):1824–6.
4. Perry JJ, Stiell IG, Sivilotti ML, et al. Clinical decision rules to rule out subarachnoid hemorrhage for acute headache. JAMA 2013;310(12):1248–55.
5. Bellolio MF, Hess EP, Gilani WI, et al. External validation of the Ottawa subarachnoid hemorrhage clinical

decision rule in patients with acute headache. Am J Emerg Med 2015;33(2):244–9.

6. Schwedt TJ, Matharu MS, Dodick DW. Thunderclap headache. Lancet Neurol 2006;5(7):621–31.

7. Day JW, Raskin NH. Thunderclap headache: symptom of unruptured cerebral aneurysm. Lancet 1986; 2(8518):1247–8.

8. Edlow JA, Caplan LR. Avoiding pitfalls in the diagnosis of subarachnoid hemorrhage. N Engl J Med 2000;342(1):29–36.

9. Landtblom AM, Fridriksson S, Boivie J, et al. Sudden onset headache: a prospective study of features, incidence and causes. Cephalalgia 2002;22(5): 354–60.

10. Linn FH, Wijdicks EF, van der Graaf Y, et al. Prospective study of sentinel headache in aneurysmal subarachnoid haemorrhage. Lancet 1994;344(8922): 590–3.

11. Ramirez-Lassepas M, Espinosa CE, Cicero JJ, et al. Predictors of intracranial pathologic findings in patients who seek emergency care because of headache. Arch Neurol 1997;54(12):1506–9.

12. Morgenstern LB, Luna-Gonzales H, Huber JC Jr, et al. Worst headache and subarachnoid hemorrhage: prospective, modern computed tomography and spinal fluid analysis. Ann Emerg Med 1998; 32(3 Pt 1):297–304.

13. van Gijn J, Rinkel GJ. Subarachnoid haemorrhage: diagnosis, causes and management. Brain 2001; 124(Pt 2):249–78.

14. Linn FH, Rinkel GJ, Algra A, et al. Headache characteristics in subarachnoid haemorrhage and benign thunderclap headache. J Neurol Neurosurg Psychiatry 1998;65(5):791–3.

15. Hasan D, Schonck RS, Avezaat CJ, et al. Epileptic seizures after subarachnoid hemorrhage. Ann Neurol 1993;33(3):286–91.

16. Verweij RD, Wijdicks EF, van Gijn J. Warning headache in aneurysmal subarachnoid hemorrhage. A case-control study. Arch Neurol 1988; 45(9):1019–20.

17. Vermeulen MJ, Schull MJ. Missed diagnosis of subarachnoid hemorrhage in the emergency department. Stroke 2007;38(4):1216–21.

18. Perry JJ, Stiell IG, Sivilotti ML, et al. Sensitivity of computed tomography performed within six hours of onset of headache for diagnosis of subarachnoid haemorrhage: prospective cohort study. BMJ 2011; 343:d4277.

19. Backes D, Rinkel GJ, Kemperman H, et al. Time-dependent test characteristics of head computed tomography in patients suspected of nontraumatic subarachnoid hemorrhage. Stroke 2012;43(8): 2115–9.

20. Dubosh NM, Bellolio MF, Rabinstein AA, et al. Sensitivity of early brain computed tomography to exclude aneurysmal subarachnoid hemorrhage: a systematic review and meta-analysis. Stroke 2016; 47(3):750–5.

21. Carpenter CR, Hussain AM, Ward MJ, et al. Spontaneous subarachnoid hemorrhage: a systematic review and meta-analysis describing the diagnostic accuracy of history, physical examination, imaging, and lumbar puncture with an exploration of test thresholds. Acad Emerg Med 2016;23(9):963–1003.

22. Edlow JA, Malek AM, Ogilvy CS. Aneurysmal subarachnoid hemorrhage: update for emergency physicians. J Emerg Med 2008;34(3):237–51.

23. Strub WM, Leach JL, Tomsick T, et al. Overnight preliminary head CT interpretations provided by residents: locations of misidentified intracranial hemorrhage. AJNR Am J Neuroradiol 2007;28(9): 1679–82.

24. Hosoya T, Yamaguchi K, Adachi M, et al. Dilatation of the temporal horn in subarachnoid haemorrhage. Neuroradiology 1992;34(3):207–9.

25. Mark DG, Sonne DC, Jun P, et al. False-negative interpretations of cranial computed tomography in aneurysmal subarachnoid hemorrhage. Acad Emerg Med 2016;23(5):591–8.

26. Evans RW. Complications of lumbar puncture. Neurol Clin 1998;16(1):83–105.

27. Shah KH, Richard KM, Nicholas S, et al. Incidence of traumatic lumbar puncture. Acad Emerg Med 2003;10(2):151–4.

28. Perry JJ, Alyahya B, Sivilotti ML, et al. Differentiation between traumatic tap and aneurysmal subarachnoid hemorrhage: prospective cohort study. BMJ 2015;350:h568.

29. Mark DG, Kene MV, Offerman SR, et al. Validation of cerebrospinal fluid findings in aneurysmal subarachnoid hemorrhage. Am J Emerg Med 2015; 33(9):1249–52.

30. Blok KM, Rinkel GJ, Majoie CB, et al. CT within 6 hours of headache onset to rule out subarachnoid hemorrhage in nonacademic hospitals. Neurology 2015;84(19):1927–32.

31. McCormack RF, Hutson A. Can computed tomography angiography of the brain replace lumbar puncture in the evaluation of acute-onset headache after a negative noncontrast cranial computed tomography scan? Acad Emerg Med 2010;17(4):444–51.

32. Westerlaan HE, van Dijk JM, Jansen-van der Weide MC, et al. Intracranial aneurysms in patients with subarachnoid hemorrhage: CT angiography as a primary examination tool for diagnosis–systematic review and meta-analysis. Radiology 2011;258(1):134–45.

33. Hess EP, Grudzen CR, Thomson R, et al. Shared decision-making in the emergency department: respecting patient autonomy when seconds count. Acad Emerg Med 2015;22(7):856–64.

34. Malhotra A, Wu X, Kalra VB, et al. Cost-effectiveness analysis of follow-up strategies for thunderclap

headache patients with negative noncontrast CT. Acad Emerg Med 2016;23(3):243–50.

35. Wu X, Kalra VB, Durand D, et al. Utility analysis of management strategies for suspected subarachnoid haemorrhage in patients with thunderclap headache with negative CT result. Emerg Med J 2016;33(1):30–6.

36. Wu X, Kalra VB, Forman HP, et al. Cost-effectiveness analysis of CTA and LP for evaluation of suspected SAH after negative non-contrast CT. Clin Neurol Neurosurg 2016;142:104–11.

37. Vlak MH, Algra A, Brandenburg R, et al. Prevalence of unruptured intracranial aneurysms, with emphasis on sex, age, comorbidity, country, and time period: a systematic review and meta-analysis. Lancet Neurol 2011;10(7):626–36.

38. Li MH, Chen SW, Li YD, et al. Prevalence of unruptured cerebral aneurysms in Chinese adults aged 35 to 75 years: a cross-sectional study. Ann Intern Med 2013;159(8):514–21.

39. Murayama Y, Takao H, Ishibashi T, et al. Risk analysis of unruptured intracranial aneurysms: prospective 10-year cohort study. Stroke 2016;47(2):365–71.

40. Wardlaw JM, White PM. The detection and management of unruptured intracranial aneurysms. Brain 2000;123(Pt 2):205–21.

41. Malhotra A, Wu X, Forman HP, et al. Growth and rupture risk of small unruptured intracranial aneurysms: a systematic review. Ann Intern Med 2017; 167(1):26–33.

42. Thompson BG, Brown RD Jr, Amin-Hanjani S, et al. Guidelines for the management of patients with unruptured intracranial aneurysms: a guideline for healthcare professionals from the American Heart Association/American Stroke Association. Stroke 2015;46(8):2368–400.

43. Malhotra A, Wu X, Forman HP, et al. Management of tiny unruptured intracranial aneurysms: a comparative effectiveness analysis. JAMA Neurol 2018; 75(1):27–34.

44. Noguchi K, Ogawa T, Inugami A, et al. Acute subarachnoid hemorrhage: MR imaging with fluid-attenuated inversion recovery pulse sequences. Radiology 1995;196(3):773–7.

45. Shimoda M, Hoshikawa K, Shiramizu H, et al. Problems with diagnosis by fluid-attenuated inversion recovery magnetic resonance imaging in patients with acute aneurysmal subarachnoid hemorrhage. Neurol Med Chir (Tokyo) 2010; 50(7):530–7.

46. Stuckey SL, Goh TD, Heffernan T, et al. Hyperintensity in the subarachnoid space on FLAIR MRI. AJR Am J Roentgenol 2007;189(4):913–21.

47. Mitchell P, Wilkinson ID, Hoggard N, et al. Detection of subarachnoid haemorrhage with magnetic resonance imaging. J Neurol Neurosurg Psychiatry 2001;70(2):205–11.

48. Mohamed M, Heasly DC, Yagmurlu B, et al. Fluid-attenuated inversion recovery MR imaging and subarachnoid hemorrhage: not a panacea. AJNR Am J Neuroradiol 2004;25(4):545–50.

49. Agid R, Lee SK, Willinsky RA, et al. Acute subarachnoid hemorrhage: using 64-slice multidetector CT angiography to "triage" patients' treatment. Neuroradiology 2006;48(11):787–94.

50. Westerlaan HE, Gravendeel J, Fiore D, et al. Multi-slice CT angiography in the selection of patients with ruptured intracranial aneurysms suitable for clipping or coiling. Neuroradiology 2007;49(12): 997–1007.

51. Agid R, Andersson T, Almqvist H, et al. Negative CT angiography findings in patients with spontaneous subarachnoid hemorrhage: when is digital subtraction angiography still needed? AJNR Am J Neuroradiol 2010;31(4):696–705.

52. Yang ZL, Ni QQ, Schoepf UJ, et al. Small intracranial aneurysms: diagnostic accuracy of CT angiography. Radiology 2017;285(3):941–52.

53. Rinkel GJ, van Gijn J, Wijdicks EF. Subarachnoid hemorrhage without detectable aneurysm. A review of the causes. Stroke 1993;24(9):1403–9.

54. Polmear A. Sentinel headaches in aneurysmal subarachnoid haemorrhage: what is the true incidence? A systematic review. Cephalalgia 2003;23(10): 935–41.

55. van Gijn J, Kerr RS, Rinkel GJ. Subarachnoid haemorrhage. Lancet 2007;369(9558):306–18.

56. Karttunen AI, Jartti PH, Ukkola VA, et al. Value of the quantity and distribution of subarachnoid haemorrhage on CT in the localization of a ruptured cerebral aneurysm. Acta Neurochir (Wien) 2003;145(8):655–61 [discussion: 661].

57. van der Jagt M, Hasan D, Bijvoet HW, et al. Validity of prediction of the site of ruptured intracranial aneurysms with CT. Neurology 1999;52(1):34–9.

58. Bechan RS, van Rooij WJ, Peluso JP, et al. Yield of repeat 3D angiography in patients with aneurysmal-type subarachnoid hemorrhage. AJNR Am J Neuroradiol 2016;37(12):2299–303.

59. Ramgren B, Siemund R, Nilsson OG, et al. CT angiography in non-traumatic subarachnoid hemorrhage: the importance of arterial attenuation for the detection of intracranial aneurysms. Acta Radiol 2015;56(10):1248–55.

60. Bakker NA, Groen RJ, Foumani M, et al. Repeat digital subtraction angiography after a negative baseline assessment in nonperimesencephalic subarachnoid hemorrhage: a pooled data meta-analysis. J Neurosurg 2014;120(1):99–103.

61. Woodfield J, Rane N, Cudlip S, et al. Value of delayed MRI in angiogram-negative subarachnoid haemorrhage. Clin Radiol 2014;69(4):350–6.

62. Maslehaty H, Petridis AK, Barth H, et al. Diagnostic value of magnetic resonance imaging in

perimesencephalic and nonperimesencephalic subarachnoid hemorrhage of unknown origin. J Neurosurg 2011;114(4):1003–7.

63. Coutinho JM, Sacho RH, Schaafsma JD, et al. High-resolution vessel wall magnetic resonance imaging in angiogram-negative non-perimesencephalic subarachnoid hemorrhage. Clin Neuroradiol 2017;27(2): 175–83.

64. Brilstra EH, Hop JW, Rinkel GJ. Quality of life after perimesencephalic haemorrhage. J Neurol Neurosurg Psychiatry 1997;63(3):382–4.

65. Alen JF, Lagares A, Lobato RD, et al. Comparison between perimesencephalic nonaneurysmal subarachnoid hemorrhage and subarachnoid hemorrhage caused by posterior circulation aneurysms. J Neurosurg 2003;98(3):529–35.

66. Kalra VB, Wu X, Matouk CC, et al. Use of follow-up imaging in isolated perimesencephalic subarachnoid hemorrhage: a meta-analysis. Stroke 2015; 46(2):401–6.

67. Kalra VB, Wu X, Forman HP, et al. Cost-effectiveness of angiographic imaging in isolated perimesencephalic subarachnoid hemorrhage. Stroke 2014; 45(12):3576–82.

68. Malhotra A, Wu X, Borse R, et al. Should patients be counseled about possible recurrence of perimesencephalic subarachnoid hemorrhage? World Neurosurg 2016;94:580.e17-22.

69. Connolly ES Jr, Rabinstein AA, Carhuapoma JR, et al. Guidelines for the management of aneurysmal subarachnoid hemorrhage: a guideline for healthcare professionals from the American Heart Association/American Stroke Association. Stroke 2012; 43(6):1711–37.

70. Kumar S, Goddeau RP Jr, Selim MH, et al. Atraumatic convexal subarachnoid hemorrhage: clinical presentation, imaging patterns, and etiologies. Neurology 2010;74(11):893–9.

71. Ducros A. Reversible cerebral vasoconstriction syndrome. Lancet Neurol 2012;11(10):906–17.

72. Walkoff L, Brinjikji W, Rouchaud A, et al. Comparing magnetic resonance angiography (MRA) and computed tomography angiography (CTA) with conventional angiography in the detection of distal territory cerebral mycotic and oncotic aneurysms. Interv Neuroradiol 2016;22(5):524–8.

73. Calabrese LH, Dodick DW, Schwedt TJ, et al. Narrative review: reversible cerebral vasoconstriction syndromes. Ann Intern Med 2007;146(1): 34–44.

74. Singhal AB, Caviness VS, Begleiter AF, et al. Cerebral vasoconstriction and stroke after use of serotonergic drugs. Neurology 2002;58(1):130–3.

75. Ducros A, Boukobza M, Porcher R, et al. The clinical and radiological spectrum of reversible cerebral vasoconstriction syndrome. A prospective series of 67 patients. Brain 2007;130(Pt 12):3091–101.

76. Chen SP, Fuh JL, Lirng JF, et al. Recurrent primary thunderclap headache and benign CNS angiopathy: spectra of the same disorder? Neurology 2006; 67(12):2164–9.

77. Singhal AB, Hajj-Ali RA, Topcuoglu MA, et al. Reversible cerebral vasoconstriction syndromes: analysis of 139 cases. Arch Neurol 2011;68(8): 1005–12.

78. Ducros A, Fiedler U, Porcher R, et al. Hemorrhagic manifestations of reversible cerebral vasoconstriction syndrome: frequency, features, and risk factors. Stroke 2010;41(11):2505–11.

79. Bartynski WS, Boardman JF. Catheter angiography, MR angiography, and MR perfusion in posterior reversible encephalopathy syndrome. AJNR Am J Neuroradiol 2008;29(3):447–55.

80. Ansari SA, Rath TJ, Gandhi D. Reversible cerebral vasoconstriction syndromes presenting with subarachnoid hemorrhage: a case series. J Neurointerv Surg 2011;3(3):272–8.

81. Chen SP, Fuh JL, Wang SJ, et al. Magnetic resonance angiography in reversible cerebral vasoconstriction syndromes. Ann Neurol 2010;67(5):648–56.

82. Obusez EC, Hui F, Hajj-Ali RA, et al. High-resolution MRI vessel wall imaging: spatial and temporal patterns of reversible cerebral vasoconstriction syndrome and central nervous system vasculitis. AJNR Am J Neuroradiol 2014;35(8):1527–32.

83. Hajj-Ali RA, Singhal AB, Benseler S, et al. Primary angiitis of the CNS. Lancet Neurol 2011;10(6): 561–72.

84. Cumurciuc R, Crassard I, Sarov M, et al. Headache as the only neurological sign of cerebral venous thrombosis: a series of 17 cases. J Neurol Neurosurg Psychiatry 2005;76(8):1084–7.

85. Boukobza M, Crassard I, Bousser MG, et al. Radiological findings in cerebral venous thrombosis presenting as subarachnoid hemorrhage: a series of 22 cases. Neuroradiology 2016;58(1):11–6.

86. Mitsias P, Ramadan NM. Headache in ischemic cerebrovascular disease. Part I: clinical features. Cephalalgia 1992;12(5):269–74.

87. Krings T, Choi IS. The many faces of intracranial arterial dissections. Interv Neuroradiol 2010;16(2): 151–60.

88. Fukuma K, Ihara M, Tanaka T, et al. Intracranial cerebral artery dissection of anterior circulation as a cause of convexity subarachnoid hemorrhage. Cerebrovasc Dis 2015;40(1–2):45–51.

89. Rahman M, Bidari SS, Quisling RG, et al. Spontaneous intracranial hypotension: dilemmas in diagnosis. Neurosurgery 2011;69(1):4–14 [discussion: 14].

90. Redekop G, TerBrugge K, Montanera W, et al. Arterial aneurysms associated with cerebral arteriovenous malformations: classification, incidence, and risk of hemorrhage. J Neurosurg 1998;89(4):539–46.

91. Gandhi D, Chen J, Pearl M, et al. Intracranial dural arteriovenous fistulas: classification, imaging findings, and treatment. AJNR Am J Neuroradiol 2012; 33(6):1007–13.

92. Tentschert S, Wimmer R, Greisenegger S, et al. Headache at stroke onset in 2196 patients with ischemic stroke or transient ischemic attack. Stroke 2005;36(2):e1–3.

93. Schwedt TJ, Dodick DW. Thunderclap stroke: embolic cerebellar infarcts presenting as thunderclap headache. Headache 2006;46(3):520–2.

94. Randeva HS, Schoebel J, Byrne J, et al. Classical pituitary apoplexy: clinical features, management and outcome. Clin Endocrinol (Oxf) 1999;51(2):181–8.

95. Armao D, Castillo M, Chen H, et al. Colloid cyst of the third ventricle: imaging-pathologic correlation. AJNR Am J Neuroradiol 2000;21(8): 1470–7.

96. Vermeulen M, Hasan D, Blijenberg BG, et al. Xanthochromia after subarachnoid haemorrhage needs no revisitation. J Neurol Neurosurg Psychiatry 1989; 52(7):826–8.

97. Thomas LE, Czuczman AD, Boulanger AB, et al. Low risk for subsequent subarachnoid hemorrhage for emergency department patients with headache, bloody cerebrospinal fluid, and negative findings on cerebrovascular imaging. J Neurosurg 2014; 121(1):24–31.

Approach to Imaging in Patients with Spontaneous Intracranial Hemorrhage

Peter G. Kranz, MD*, Michael D. Malinzak, MD, PhD,
Timothy J. Amrhein, MD

KEYWORDS

- Intracranial hemorrhage • Spontaneous • Hematoma • Imaging • Brain • Hypertension
- Amyloid angiopathy

KEY POINTS

- The approach to spontaneous intracranial hemorrhage (ICH) must both address emergent considerations that may prompt or guide immediate action and identify etiology of the hemorrhage.
- Understanding anatomic differences in the deep portions of the brain and the lobar brain helps predict the etiology of the hemorrhage and guide imaging selection.
- Various imaging modalities have different strengths in identifying individual etiologies of ICH. Knowledge of these strengths helps guide appropriate imaging selection.

INTRODUCTION

Spontaneous (ie, nontraumatic) intracerebral hemorrhage (ICH) is a potentially devastating neurologic event that requires emergent diagnosis and management. It is estimated that 10% to 15% of all new clinical strokes are due to ICH, with an incidence of 40,000 to 67,000 cases per year in the United States.[1,2] Mortality from ICH is high; 30-day mortality rates are 35% to 52%, with half of those deaths occurring within the first 2 days.[1] Rapid diagnosis and aggressive management are critical to reducing morbidity and mortality. Imaging plays a pivotal role in establishing the diagnosis of ICH, identifying the cause of hemorrhage, and identifying complications of acute ICH that guide management.

When a patient presents with spontaneous ICH, the role of imaging is 2-fold: first, imaging must rapidly provide information that immediately establishes the diagnosis and guides interventions intended to stabilize the patient, and, second,

imaging helps determine the etiology of the hemorrhage, which can be important in both acute management and preventing rebleeding. It is, therefore, useful to have a conceptual approach to imaging that addresses both of these goals. The authors advocate the use of a primary survey intended to define factors that are expected to immediately guide the emergent stabilization and management of the patient and a secondary survey aimed at determining the etiology of the hemorrhage.[3]

This review describes anatomy, imaging techniques, and the diagnostic approach relevant to spontaneous ICH within the brain parenchyma. Additionally, it reviews the information that needs to be communicated emergently as part of the primary survey. Finally, it summarizes imaging features of the most common causes of spontaneous ICH and discusses how these features combine with clinical information to produce a patient-centered approach to the selection of imaging, as part of the secondary survey.

Disclosures: None.
Department of Radiology, Duke University Medical Center, Box 3808, Durham, NC 27710, USA
* Corresponding author.
E-mail address: peter.kranz@duke.edu

neuroimaging.theclinics.com

NORMAL ANATOMY AND IMAGING TECHNIQUE
Anatomy

Hemorrhage tends to occur in specific and sometimes predictable locations in the brain, depending on the etiology of the hemorrhage. Understanding how various anatomic factors contribute to the risk of hemorrhage, therefore, is instructive in assigning the etiology of spontaneous ICH. The most fundamental distinction to understand in terms of cerebral anatomy when it comes to ICH is the difference between deep brain and lobar hemorrhage.

The deep brain structures are composed of the basal ganglia (including the caudate nucleus, putamen, and globus pallidus), the thalamus, pons, and dentate nuclei of the cerebellum. Hypertension, the most common cause of spontaneous brain hemorrhage, has a predilection for the deep brain structures. It is believed that this predilection is related to the particular anatomy of the blood vessels that perfuse these regions. Specifically, the deep structures are supplied by small penetrating arteries that arise directly off of medium-caliber vessels.[4] As a result of this rapid transition in caliber of the vessels, the perfusion pressure in the small perforators is higher than the pressure in the vessels that irrigate the lobar portions of the brain, which originate more distally in the arterial supply. This difference in perfusion pressure becomes even more exaggerated in the setting of hypertension.[5]

In the penetrating vessels of the deep brain structures, chronic exposure to high intra-arterial pressure results in destruction of the smooth muscle cells in the vascular wall and results in the formation of microaneurysms, termed Charcot-Bouchard aneurysms.[4,6] Together, these changes make the vessel fragile and more prone to rupture. The lenticulostriate perforating vessels that supply the basal ganglia are 1 example of such vessels and are 1 of the most frequent sites of hypertensive hemorrhage.

Although the basal ganglia are commonly involved in cases of hypertensive hemorrhage, it is important to realize that infratentorial locations are vulnerable to hypertensive hemorrhage as well. In particular, the pons and the dentate nuclei of the cerebellum are frequent sites of bleeding. The pons is perfused by very small penetrating arteries that arise directly off of the relatively larger basilar artery and thus are vulnerable to the same perfusional stresses exerted on the lenticulostriate perforating vessels.

The dentate nucleus is a deep gray nucleus located in the medial cerebellum notable for its convoluted, serrated margin (**Fig. 1**). As a metabolically active gray matter structure, it too has an abundant blood supply supplied by small perforating vessels, which predispose it to hypertensive hemorrhage. Because of its proximity to the fourth ventricle, hypertensive hemorrhages centered in the dentate nucleus often extend into the ventricle and can be mistaken for a primary subarachnoid or intraventricular hemorrhage (IVH) if the parenchymal component is not appreciated.

In contrast, the supratentorial white matter in the more peripheral or lobar portions of the brain is irrigated by penetrating long medullary arteries. These long medullary arteries arise further from the circle of Willis compared with the perforating vessels in the deep brain structures and, therefore, experience lower perfusion pressures.[7] They course from their origins in the pial vasculature into the deep white matter of the centrum semiovale and periventricular white matter, where they are provide end-arterial supply.[8] Exposure to chronic hypertension is associated with increasing vascular tortuosity, which increases the overall vessel length, in turn further decreasing perfusion pressures distally.[5,7,9] These factors combine to make hypertensive hemorrhage less likely in the lobar portions of the brain. Rather, hemorrhages here are more likely to be due to other entities, including amyloid angiopathy, arteriovenous malformations (AVM), tumors, and other etiologies. Generally speaking, then, imaging is more likely to reveal underlying lesions in lobar hemorrhages and less likely to identify lesions in the deep portions of the brain, where hypertensive hemorrhages predominate.

Imaging Technique

As first-line imaging, noncontrast computed tomography (NCT) is by far the most common modality used to diagnose ICH and is highly sensitive for the detection of acute blood products.[10] NCT provides very rapid imaging and is widely available. The American College of Radiology Practice Parameters recommend that brain computed tomography (CT) obtained for new focal neurologic deficit or suspected parenchymal hemorrhage include at minimum contiguous or overlapping axial slices of no greater than 5-mm thickness.[11]

MR imaging has also been shown sensitive for the detection of acute hemorrhage and has the benefit of being more sensitive for acute ischemia and chronic hemorrhage than NCT.[12,13] Nevertheless, its use as an initial, first-line imaging test is limited to a few centers because of issues of scanner availability, scan time, patient contraindications to MR imaging, and challenges associated

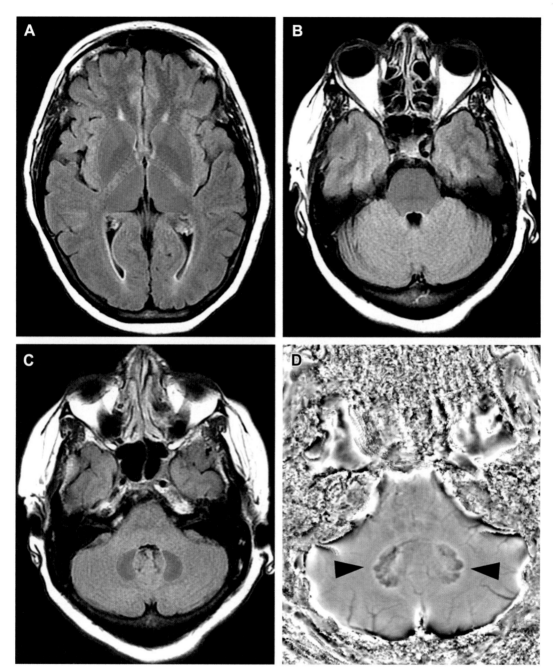

Fig. 1. Sites of hypertensive hemorrhage. Axial FLAIR MR images with superimposed shaded areas indicating the most common sites of ICH in hypertensive patients, including (*A*) the basal ganglia and thalami, (*B*) the pons, and (*C*) the dentate nuclei of the cerebellum. Axial image from phase map of SWI (*D*) more clearly depicts the dentate nuclei (*arrowheads*) as low signal structures in the medial cerebellum with a serrated margin.

with managing a critically ill patient in the environment of the MR imaging suite.

Once a diagnosis of ICH has been made, CT angiography (CTA) and MR imaging are valuable tools in defining the etiology of the hemorrhage and informing prognosis, as part of the secondary survey.

CTA excels in defining arterial vascular lesions and can help detect active bleeding that may result in hematoma expansion. It has been found 96% sensitive for the detection of vascular malformations in the setting of ICH.[14] Helical scan technique on modern multidetector scanners using a slice thickness of no greater than 1.5 mm is required. Intravenous contrast material is administered using a power injector at a rate of 4 mL or 5 mL per second through an antecubital intravenous line that is 20-gauge or larger. Image acquisition is timed to maximize opacification of the intracranial arterial vasculature; optimal timing of the scan after contrast injection is established via an initial test bolus (10–15 mL) or by using automated or semiautomated scan triggering.

Although digital subtraction angiography (DSA) is the gold standard for the assessment of the cerebral arterial vasculature due to its superior imaging resolution and ability to detect arteriovenous shunting, it is invasive and has a higher risk profile than CTA. Therefore, DSA is now most commonly reserved for the setting of a high clinical suspicion and a negative CTA or to further evaluate and treat a known lesion.

MR imaging is superior at detecting nonarterial causes, such as central nervous system (CNS) neoplasms, metastases, cavernomas, ischemia, and cerebral amyloid angiopathy (CAA). Although NCT has excellent sensitivity for acute hemorrhage, MR imaging is more sensitive for the detection of microhemorrhages and chronic hemorrhage[12] and can often provide a better estimate of the age of blood products than NCT.[15] The optimal protocol for evaluating ICH involves several key sequences. Anatomic imaging with fast spin-echo T2 and FLAIR imaging is useful for defining the hematoma extent, any adjacent lesions, and regional vascular flow-voids that may suggest an arterial lesion. Postcontrast T1-weighted imaging is important to detect enhancing lesions, such as tumors. Precontrast T1-weighted precontrast images are required both to evaluate for blood products and to determine whether hyperintense signal seen on postcontrast images is related to blood products or actual enhancement. Diffusion-weighted images help determine if there is ischemia surrounding the hematoma that might point to hemorrhagic transformation of an ischemic infarct.

Finally, a sequence sensitive to magnetic susceptibility artifacts (either a T2*-weighted gradient-echo [GRE] sequence or a susceptibility-weighted imaging [SWI] sequence) is critical to looking for evidence of microhemorrhages (ie, hemorrhages <10 mm in size) separate from the main hematoma.[16] These sequences lack the 180° refocusing pulse found with spin-echo sequences, resulting in increased dephasing compared with spin-echo sequences when magnetic field inhomogeneities are present. As a result, these sequences are exquisitely sensitive for the detection of hemosiderin, which is highly paramagnetic and leads to magnetic field inhomogeneity. SWI sequences make use of phase information in addition to T2*-weighting and are more sensitive for the detection of microhemorrhage than GRE sequences (**Fig. 2**).[17]

IMAGING FINDINGS
Primary Survey

The purpose of the primary survey in a patient with ICH is to rapidly identify factors that inform or have an impact on the acute stabilization and management of the patient. These factors can be remembered using the mnemonic, BLEED, as depicted in **Box 1**.[3]

B: how big is the hemorrhage
Hematoma volume is 1 of the most powerful and widely used predictors of mortality in patients

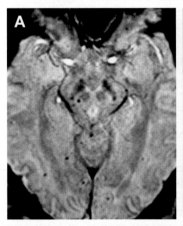 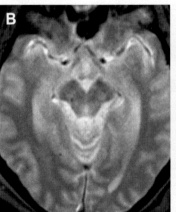 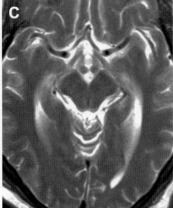

Fig. 2. Comparison of SWI and GRE images for the detection of microhemorrhages. Axial SWI (*A*) and GRE image (*B*) in a patient with amyloid angiopathy show multiple small punctate hypointense foci representing microhemorrhages. These are not seen on fast spin-echo T2-weighted image (*C*). Note that more microhemorrhages are visible on the SWI than on the GRE image.

Box 1
What the referring physician needs to know: elements of the primary survey

B	How *Big* is the hemorrhage
L	*Location* of the hemorrhage
E	*Edema* and associated mass effect
E	*Extension* of hemorrhage into the ventricles and hydrocephalus
D	*Displacement* of critical brain structures and herniation

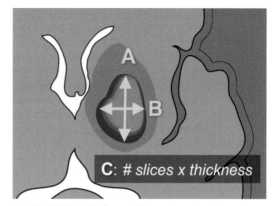

Fig. 3. ABC/2 rule for quickly estimating the volume of a hematoma. "A" represents the greatest axial diameter of the hematoma, "B" is a perpendicular diameter on the same axial slice, and "C" is the cranio-caudal diameter (estimated by multiplying the number of axial slices containing hematoma by the slice thickness). Multiplying these values together and dividing by 2 approximates the volume of an ellipsoid.

with ICH; 30-day mortality rates for patients with smaller hemorrhages of less than 30 cm³ are less than 20%, whereas hemorrhages with volumes greater than 60 cm³ are associated with 30-day mortality rates of greater than 90%.[18] Additionally, patients with hematoma volumes of greater than 30 cm³ are unlikely to be functionally independent at 30 days.[18] Providing a volume of hemorrhage is, therefore, informative in predicting prognosis. Hematoma volume can be rapidly and easily calculated without the need for cumbersome volumetric analysis by using the ABC/2 method.[19,20] In this method, the greatest axial dimension of the hematoma is measured (A), a perpendicular diameter on the same slice is measured (B), and the craniocaudal dimension (C) can be measured off of reformatted images (if available) or estimated by counting the number of slices where the hematoma is present and multiplying that number by the slice thickness (eg, C equals 3 cm for a hematoma present on 6 slices with a slice thickness of 5 mm) **(Fig. 3)**. The hematoma volume is estimated by multiplying these 3 dimensions together and diving by 2, which estimates the simplified volume of an ellipse. This method is well-validated, quickly accomplished, and sufficiently accurate for use in routine clinical practice.[19,20]

L: location of the hemorrhage
Hematoma location, in addition to predicting etiology, is important for informing prognosis and guiding immediate management. Morbidity and mortality are worse among patients with hemorrhages in the deep structures of the supratentorial brain compared with the lobar brain, and greater still when the hemorrhage is located in the cerebellum or brainstem.[1] Because of its anatomically confined volume, hemorrhage in the posterior fossa may prompt emergent surgical craniotomy and decompression.[21] American Heart Association/American Stroke Association guidelines support urgent surgical decompression of posterior fossa hematoma where brainstem compression

or fourth ventricular compression resulting in hydrocephalus is present (class 1; level of evidence B).[22]

E: edema
Perihematomal edema (PHE) is an often-overlooked component of ICH on CT but can be very important. A large volume of baseline PHE is predictive of poor functional outcomes in patients with ICH.[23] PHE grows most rapidly in the first 2 days after hemorrhage, increasing in volume by 75% within the first 24 hours.[24,25] In some patients, the edema associated with ICH results in greater mass effect than the hematoma itself and can result in early neurologic deterioration.[26] Clinically, symptomatic increases in PHE may trigger interventions designed to lower intracranial pressure, including head elevation, sedation, osmotic diuretics, and/or cerebrospinal fluid drainage.[26] Consequently, the degree of mass effect from PHE should be part of the routine assessment, with particular attention given to increases from scan to scan.

E: extension of hemorrhage into the ventricles and hydrocephalus
When ICH is located close to the ventricular system, expansion of the hematoma may breach the ventricular wall, resulting in IVH. This occurs in approximately 45% of cases of ICH.[22] IVH is a strong independent risk factor for mortality and poor functional outcome.[27] Blood within the ventricular system can cause hydrocephalus due to localized clot obstructing CSF flow within the ventricles or by traveling distally in the CSF and

decreasing CSF resorption at the level of the arachnoid granulations. Hydrocephalus can contribute to rapid increases in intracranial pressures and, therefore, is critical to identify early on. Scrutiny of the temporal horns of the lateral ventricles may help identify early hydrocephalus, because variability in the caliber of this portion of the ventricles is less than in the body of the lateral ventricles, which are more frequently enlarged an ex vacuo basis. When hydrocephalus is present, it should be rapidly communicated to the clinical team, because it may prompt emergent placement of a ventriculostomy catheter.[28] Intraventricular fibrinolytic therapy or endoscopic clot removal are interventions for IVH that are the subject of recent clinical trials and may be used at some centers.[22]

D: displacement of critical brain structures and herniation

Mass effect from the hematoma and the surrounding edema results in asymmetric forces on the brain. Although these may be localized to the region around the hematoma, particularly with small lobar hematomas, larger or deep hematomas may result in midline shift or herniation. The herniation pattern depends on the location of the hematoma: anterior temporal lobe hematomas may result in uncal herniation (**Fig. 4**); those near the midline or in the frontal lobes may cause subfalcine herniation, whereas those in the posterior fossa may cause ascending transtentorial herniation or downward cerebellar tonsillar herniation. Mass effect on the ventricular system may cause localized compression of the ventricular lumen, resulting in a trapped ventricle or generalized obstructive hydrocephalus, depending on the location of compression. If mass effect is pronounced, decompressive craniectomy, possibly with hematoma evacuation, may be pursued.[29]

CT Angiography Spot Sign

CTA is used to evaluate for arterial causes of ICH and, therefore, is principally important as part of the secondary survey. It has been recognized, however, that arterial extravasation can be identified during some CTA studies that can predict imminent expansion of the hematoma and can, therefore, in some cases be considered part of the primary survey. This arterial extravasation manifests as a focus of contrast enhancement within or at the periphery of the hematoma (**Fig. 5**) and has been termed the *CTA spot sign*. The presence of 1 or more spot signs predicts hematoma expansion and poor clinical outcome.[30] To be classified as a spot sign, a focus of contrast must be greater than or equal to 120 Hounsfield units and discontinuous from adjacent vascular structures.[31] This sign is seen in 40% to 70% of patients in the first 3 hours after hemorrhage onset but decreases substantially thereafter.[30,31] When present, this finding should be communicated to the care team because of its association with clinical deterioration.

Secondary Survey

The purpose of the secondary survey is to consider the potential etiology of an ICH, which can have prognostic as well as treatment implications, and is essential to preventing rebleeding. Patient characteristics, such as age, gender, and medical history (eg, known primary malignancy or hypertension), in conjunction with the appearance of the ICH on the initial NCT may suggest certain underlying causes of ICH. This may help guide the decision making with regard to further imaging or may lead to a decision not to obtain any further imaging if hypertensive hemorrhage is suspected. Familiarity with the most common demographic presentations and imaging findings associated with the major etiologies of ICH is, therefore, essential when conducting the secondary survey (**Box 2**).

Etiologies of Spontaneous Intracranial Hemorrhage

Primary intracranial hemorrhage: hypertensive hemorrhage and cerebral amyloid angiopathy
Hypertensive hemorrhage Uncontrolled hypertension is the most common cause of spontaneous

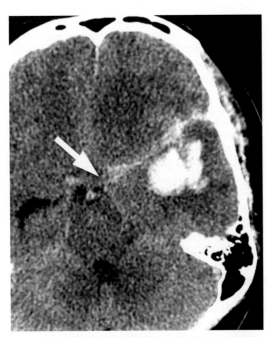

Fig. 4. Herniation due to ICH. Axial NCT image shows an anterior temporal lobe hematoma causing uncal herniation (*arrow*). Herniation is a complication that is important to identify during the primary survey.

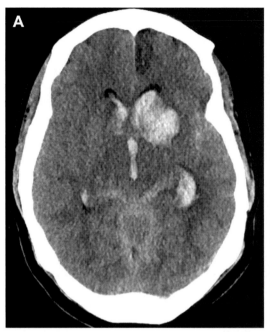 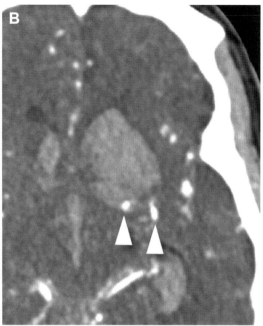

Fig. 5. CTA spot sign. (*A*) Axial NCT image shows a hypertensive hemorrhage centered in the left caudate, with extension into the ventricles. (*B*) Axial image from CTA shows 2 round foci of contrast enhancement (*arrowheads*) that are not connected to nearby vessels, consistent with CTA spot signs.

ICH, accounting for approximately 65% of ICH cases.[32,33] A history of poorly controlled hypertension in a patient presenting with ICH certainly prompts consideration of this diagnosis, but a

---

Box 2
Differential diagnosis of spontaneous intracranial hemorrhage

Primary ICH

  Hypertension

  CAA

Secondary ICH—vascular pathology

  AVM

  Cavernoma

  Adherent aneurysm

  Vasculitis

  Moyamoya disease

Secondary ICH—vascular occlusion

  Hemorrhagic transformation of infarction

  Dural venous sinus thrombosis

Secondary ICH—nonvascular pathology

  Tumor, primary or metastatic

  Drugs (cocaine, amphetamines)

  Coagulopathy

---

complete medical history may be unavailable at the time of presentation, and many patients may have clinically silent hypertension prior to presentation with ICH.[34–36] Demographic and imaging clues may, therefore, be important in establishing this diagnosis.

The 2 most important factors that predict a hypertensive etiology of ICH are hematoma location and patient age. Hypertensive hemorrhage typically affects the deep structures of the brain, including the basal ganglia (35%–40%), thalamus (10%–20%), cerebellar dentate nucleus (5%–10%), and pons (5%–10%).[3,4,14,33,37]

Although hypertension is the single most common cause of spontaneous ICH, it becomes substantially less common in patients under 45 years old, because this patient population is less likely to suffer from chronic hypertension.[38,39] Younger patients, therefore, should be worked up for the presence of an underlying lesion even when presenting with hemorrhage in a typical location for hypertension. Lobar hemorrhages, on the other hand, are uncommon locations for hypertensive ICH, accounting for less than 20% of hypertensive hemorrhages and should, therefore, be viewed as suspicious for the presence of an alternative diagnosis, such as amyloid angiopathy (in older patients) or other secondary cause of hemorrhage.[3,32]

Generally speaking, hypertension produces bland-appearing hematomas that are homogeneous, ovoid, and associated with a thin halo of edema that parallels the contours of the hematoma and progressively enlarges over several days after the hemorrhage (**Fig. 6**).[3,38] Certain chronic brain changes may also help to suggest a history of uncontrolled hypertension. Hypertensive microangiopathy, known as leukoaraiosis, affects the periventricular white matter and pons, producing patchy areas of hypoattenuation on CT and T2 hyperinensity on MR imaging.[40] Lacunar infarcts may also suggest long-standing hypertension.

Microhemorrhages seen on T2*-weighted sequences, such as GRE and SWI, are particularly useful suggesting chronic hypertensive microangiopathy. These microhemorrhages also have a strong predilection for the brainstem and deep gray structures, just like the larger parenchymal hematomas associated with hypertensive ICH (**Fig. 7**).[40–42]

Cerebral amyloid angiopathy CAA occurs almost exclusively in patients older than 60, with the prevalence of the condition increasing in the later decades of life.[43] It has been estimated to be present in 10% to 40% of elderly brains,[44] leading some investigators to question whether it should be considered an expected part of aging rather than a disease per se.[45] In CAA, the β-amyloid peptide deposits in the media of small arteries

and capillaries of the cortex and leptomeninges.[46,47] This deposition results in luminal narrowing and occlusion, weakening of the vascular walls, and microaneurysm formation.[43,44] Chronic ischemia and inflammation contribute to white matter atrophy and cortical damage.[43,44] These pathologic changes make vessels prone to rupture, either into the brain parenchyma (when the affected vessels are located deeper in the brain) or into the subarachnoid space (when the vessels are more superficially located). CAA has been found one of the most common causes of atraumatic convexal subarachnoid hemorrhage (SAH) in the elderly.[48]

The radiologic hallmark of CAA is a lobar distribution of microhemorrhages, seen best on T2*-weighted imaging, in an elderly patient.[41,46] In particular, the periphery of the occipital and temporal lobes seem to be common sites of CAA involvement (**Fig. 8**).[43,44,49,50] CAA less commonly produces cerebellar hemorrhage, and hemorrhage within the deep gray structures or brainstem is atypical.[37]

In addition to age and hemorrhage location, 2 other imaging findings may suggest CAA. White matter atrophy and regions of T2-weighted signal hyperintensity are often present in CAA and likely reflect vaso-occlusive events,[43] although this pattern may overlap with the leukoaraiosis seen

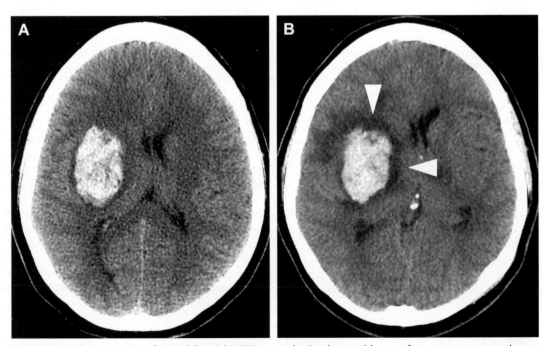

Fig. 6. Expected progression of PHE. (*A*) Axial NCT image obtained several hours after symptom onset shows a hypertensive hemorrhage centered in the right putamen. There is a very thin halo of PHE that parallels the contours of the hematoma, the expected pattern with an acute hypertensive hematoma. (*B*) Axial NCT obtained 2 days later shows concentric expansion of the edema (*arrowheads*).

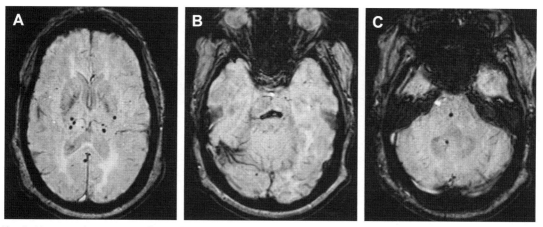

Fig. 7. Hypertensive pattern of microhemorrhages. Axial susceptibility-weighted MR images at the level of the basal ganglia (*A*), pons (*B*), and dentate nuclei (*C*) show low signal foci of chronic microhemorrhage. These microhemorrhages are in the same locations where larger hematomas are seen in hypertensive ICH.

with chronic hypertension. Involvement of the leptomeningeal vessels with subsequent SAH, which may be clinically silent or unrecognized, may produce cortical hemosiderin deposits, which appear as thin gyriform hypointensities coating the cortical surface on T2*-weighted imaging.[3,32]

Apart from defining the etiology in a patient with ICH, the identification of CAA may be important because some clinicians may choose to withhold anticoagulation in these patients, particularly with the newer direct factor Xa inhibitors, for which

there are no specific reversal agents currently widely available.[51]

Secondary intracranial hemorrhage due to vascular pathology: arteriovenous malformation, cavernomas, adherent aneurysm, vasculitis, and moyamoya disease

Arteriovenous malformation AVMs are direct connections between arteries and veins within the brain parenchyma or pia. There is no normal intervening capillary network. These high-flow

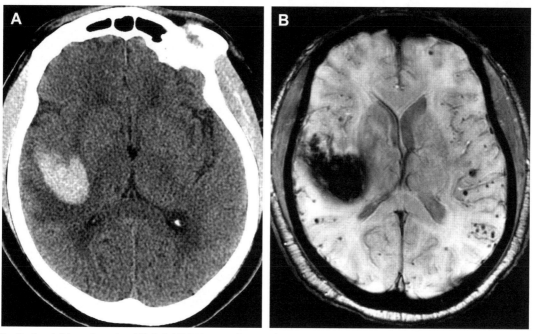

Fig. 8. Amyloid angiopathy. (*A*) Axial NCT image shows a hematoma in the right temporal lobe. This lobar location is not typical of hypertensive hemorrhage. (*B*) Axial SWI shows multiple microhemorrhages in the periphery of the brain, sparing the deep brain structures. This pattern is typical of amyloid angiopathy.

vascular lesions consequently develop elevated intravascular pressures on the venous side of the lesion, with resultant vascular dilatation and proliferation. In patients with previously unruptured AVMs, the annual risk of ICH is 1% to 4%.[52,53] After the first episode of bleeding, the recurrent hemorrhage rate is 7% to 18% in the first year and 2% to 4% in every following year.[54–56] Treatment can reduce hemorrhage risk and may entail catheter embolization, resection, radiation, and medical management. Recognition of these lesions on imaging is, therefore, important.

Studies have found that 47% to 63% of patients with spontaneous ICH under 45 years of age are eventually discovered to have a vascular lesion, and approximately half of these are AVMs.[57,58] In 1 study, 100% of pediatric patients 10 years old and younger presenting with spontaneous ICH were found to have an underlying vascular lesion.[57] Thus, in younger patients presenting with spontaneous ICH, an AVM should be suspected as the most likely etiology, regardless of where the hematoma is located, and imaging should be tailored to maximizing detection of vascular lesions first (Fig. 9).

On cross-sectional imaging, AVMs are characterized by the presence of a tangle of blood vessels with enlarged feeding arteries and draining veins. These vessels may even be appreciated on NCT if the lesion is very large. On MR imaging, flow voids are seen within the nidus of the AVM and are often well depicted on T2-weighted images as very low signal, serpentine structures. No solid parenchymal mass should be present, although there may be gliotic brain tissue adjacent to the AVM that demonstrates T2 hyperintensity and volume loss.

Vascular imaging (including CTA, magnetic resonance angiography, or conventional catheter angiography) is particularly well suited to depicting the vascular nidus and feeding and draining vessels. Abnormally enlarged vessels may be seen even if the nidus itself is partially obscured by hematoma.[14] It is important to search for aneurysms within the nidus, on feeding vessels more proximally, or for venous stenoses in the draining veins, because these may increase the risk of rebleeding. The Spetzler-Martin grading system (Table 1) is a widely used scale that helps predict the morbidity of potential surgical treatment.[59]

Cavernoma Cavernomas, also called cavernous angiomas, are composed of thin-walled vascular spaces. In contrast to high-flow AVMs, cavernomas are low-flow vascular lesion and are, therefore, not associated with arterial feeding vessels or arteriovenous shunting.

Cavernomas can occur anywhere in the brain and are usually smaller than 1 cm, although giant cavernomas can be seen.[60] They are prone to recurrent hemorrhage, with an annual hemorrhage risk of 0.6% to 7.0%.[32,61] They may be solitary lesions, or in cases of familiar syndromes, may be multiple. Although most commonly sporadic, they may also be acquired after radiation therapy to the brain. Cavernomas can be diagnosed at any age but are a particularly common cause of ICH in patients under 45 years.[39]

On NCT, cavernomas appear as mildly hyperattenuating lesions, with a density greater than that of normal brain but less than that of an acute hematoma. There may be internal foci of calcification. On MR imaging, the presence of internal hemorrhage of different ages produces a characteristic

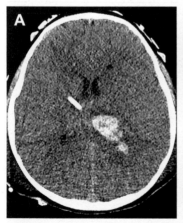
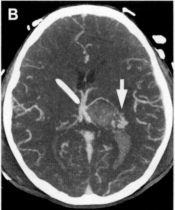
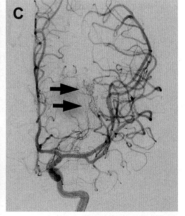

Fig. 9. AVM. (*A*) Axial NCT image in a 5-year-old boy shows a hematoma in the left corona radiata with intraventricular extension. (*B*) Axial maximum intensity projection image of a CTA shows a tangle of blood vessels along the lateral margin of the hematoma (*arrow*), with deep venous drainage. (*C*) Frontal projection of a dignital subtraction angiogram shows the nidus of the AVM arising from branches of the left middle cerebral artery.

Table 1
Spetzler-Martin grading scale for arteriovenous malformations

Feature	Points[a]
Size of nidus	
Small (<3 cm)	1
Medium (3–6 cm)	2
Large (>6 cm)	3
Eloquence of brain[b]	
Noneloquent	0
Eloquent	1
Deep venous drainage	
Superficial	0
Deep	1

[a] Points are totaled from each feature, resulting in a total score of 1 to 5. Higher scores predict higher morbidity with surgical resection.
[b] Eloquent areas: sensorimotor, language, and visual centers, hypothalamus, thalamus, internal capsule, brainstem, cerebellar peduncles, cerebellar nuclei.

multiloculated, mulberry-like appearance. A hypointense hemosiderin ring completely encircling the lesion is seen on T2-weighted images and shows blooming on T2*-weighted images.[40] T2*-weighted images may also can reveal additional subclinical lesions in patients with multiple cavernomas.[37] Internally, the locules are often T1 hyperintense but may vary depending on the age of the internal blood products (**Fig. 10**). As low-flow lesions, they typically show little or no arterial phase enhancement and thus are typically occult on angiographic studies.[3,38] Some delayed internal enhancement may be seen on postcontrast MR imaging. In some cases, contrast-enhanced imaging may reveal the presence of an associated developmental venous anomaly (DVA), which appears as an anomalous draining vein with a characteristic medusa head of radiating smaller veins. The discovery of a DVA next to a hematoma should suggest a cavernoma as the etiology of the hemorrhage,[62] but the DVA should not be mistaken for an arterial feeding vessel from an AVM.

Adherent aneurysm Although most ruptured aneurysms produce purely SAH, aneurysms of the major intracranial arteries may produce ICH when the jet of blood is directed toward the brain parenchyma or when the aneurysm is adherent to the pia (**Fig. 11**).[63] This cause of ICH should be considered in the setting where there is a large volume of SAH associated with a peripheral parenchymal hematoma.[3,32] In such cases, the hematoma tends to be near common aneurysm sites, such as the anterior communicating artery, middle cerebral artery bifurcation, or posterior inferior cerebellar artery, and, therefore, are found in close proximity to the suprasellar cistern or sylvian fissure.[64] Although rare, in the setting of infective endocarditis or meningitis, mycotic aneurysms of small intraparenchymal arteries can produce ICH, sometimes without prominent SAH. Hematomas due to other causes that are located near the surface of the brain can extend into the subarachnoid space and, therefore, not all cases of SAH associated with ICH are aneurysm related, particularly when the volume of SAH is small compared with the volume of the hematoma.

Vasculitis Cerebral vasculitis is an uncommon cause of ICH and can be primary or secondary. Primary angiitis of the CNS is a disease restricted to the CNS and characterized histologically by the infiltration of inflammatory cells into the walls of small and medium-sized vessels.[65] Secondary vasculitis denotes a vasculitis that occurs as the result of a systemic condition or an infectious process. Hemorrhage can complicate up to 10% of cases of cerebral vasculitis.[66,67]

Brain parenchymal findings suggestive of vasculitis include patchy white matter lesions, often affecting the subcortical U-fibers, or cortical infarctions; the precise distribution of lesions depends on the size of the vessels involved. Diffusion restriction is variable. Brain parenchymal or leptomeningeal enhancement is also variably present. The classic angiographic appearance of CNS vasculitis is alternating segments of concentric stenosis and dilation, producing a beaded appearance.[65–67] The sensitivity of vascular imaging for detecting CNS vasculitis, however, may be as low as 40%, especially when the condition is confined to small vessels, where lesions predominate in the white matter but spare the cortex.[65] Vasculitis should be a consideration when hemorrhage occurs in young or middle aged patients with systemic symptoms or suggestive neuroimaging features, particularly if multifocal microhemorrhages are present in patients less than 60 years of age.

Moyamoya disease Moyamoya disease most commonly affects children and young adults and can occur sporadically or in association with several congenital and hematologic disorders. It is characterized by steno-occlusive lesions of the largest intracranial arteries, in particular the distal portions of the internal cerebral arteries, the carotid termini, and the proximal anterior cerebral and middle cerebral arteries, with formation of collateral vessels in the basal

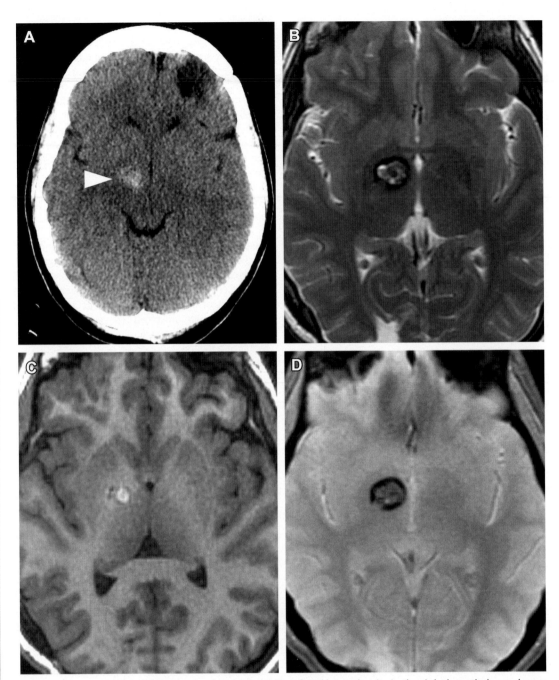

Fig. 10. Cavernoma. (*A*) Axial NCT image shows a focal ill-defined hyperdensity in the right hypothalamus (*arrowhead*). The attenuation is not as high as is seen with acute hematoma, and there is no surrounding edema. This density is typical of cavernomas. Encephalomalacia in the left frontal lobe is present form a previous hemorrhage in this patient with multiple familial cavernomas. (*B*) Axial T2-weighted MR image shows the characteristic hypointense hemosiderin ring related to prior hemorrhage. (*C*) Axial T1-weighted MR image shows internal loculations containing T1 hyperintense blood breakdown products. (*D*) Axial GRE MR image shows blooming of the hypointense rim due to susceptibility effects of hemosiderin.

brain parenchyma.[68] Infarctions in the watershed territories may be present. The collateral vessels are prone to aneurysm formation and rupture, with hemorrhage occurring in approximately 20% of cases.[69,70] Angiographic imaging demonstrate the characteristic enhancing blush of numerous small collaterals surrounding the affected large arteries (**Fig. 12**).

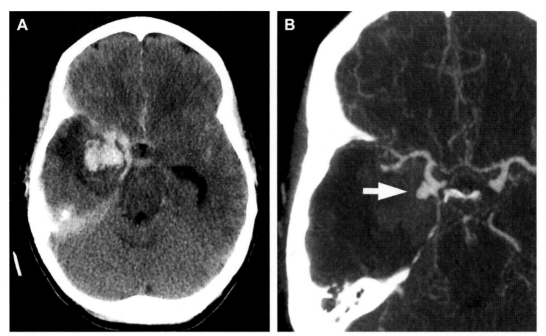

Fig. 11. Hemorrhage due to adherent aneurysm. (*A*) Axial NCT image shows a hematoma in the medial right temporal lobe with a large component of adjacent SAH. (*B*) Axial maximum intensity projection image of a CTA shows an aneurysm (*arrow*) arising from the carotid terminus, projecting into the parenchymal hematoma.

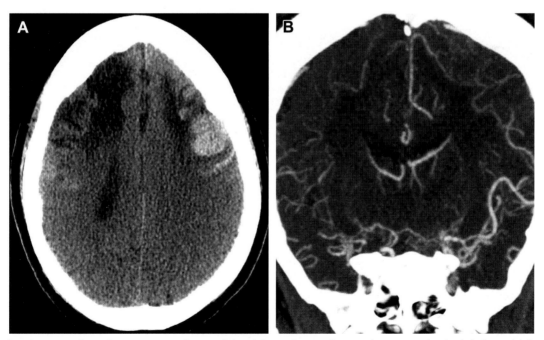

Fig. 12. Hemorrhage in moyamoya disease. (*A*) Axial NCT image shows a hematoma in the left frontal lobe with a small volume of associated SAH. An old infarct is seen in the right superficial anterior cerebral artery–middle cerebral artery watershed territory. (*B*) Coronal maximum intensity projection image of a CTA shows occlusion of the bilateral supraclinoid internal carotid arteries, with extensive small collateral vessels.

Secondary intracranial hemorrhage due to acute vascular occlusion: hemorrhagic transformation of arterial infarcts and venous ischemia

Hemorrhagic transformation of arterial infarctions On NCT, a hematoma associated with cytotoxic edema and loss of gray-white differentiation suggests hemorrhagic transformation of an acute arterial infarct (**Fig. 13**). MR imaging can be used to evaluate for restricted diffusion in a vascular distribution around the hematoma. Increased risk of hemorrhage is associated with cardioembolic infarctions, larger infarctions, leukoariosis, and a hyperdense middle cerebral artery sign; clinical risk factors for hemorrhagic transformation include advanced age, uncontrolled hypertension, and use of anticoagulants or thrombolytics.[71–74]

Dural venous sinus thrombosis Venous sinus thrombosis or cortical vein thrombosis impairs venous drainage from the brain parenchyma, leading to venous congestion and edema. If the venous congestion is sufficient to impair arterial inflow into the affected tissue, infarction may result.[75] Increased intravascular pressures can cause rupture of small vessels and hemorrhage.[76] Characteristic hematoma locations include subcortical portions of the parasagittal frontal and parietal lobes (drained by the superior sagittal sinus), the posterior temporal lobes (drained by the vein of Labbé and transverse sinus) and the thalami (drained by the deep venous system) (**Fig. 14**). The venous sinuses should be scrutinized on NCT in patients with spontaneous ICH for the hyperdense dural sinus sign, with the caveat that this sign is not highly sensitive for dural venous sinus thrombosis.[77] Dedicated venous sinus imaging using CT venography or magnetic resonance venography can be performed in patients with hypercoagulable states or suggestive imaging findings.

Secondary intracranial hemorrhage due to nonvascular pathology: tumors, drugs, coagulopathy

Hemorrhagic tumors Metastatic disease is the most common source of tumor-related brain hemorrhage.[78] Metastatic cancers especially prone to hemorrhaging include renal cell carcinoma, thyroid carcinoma, choriocarcinoma, and melanoma.[79] Due to very high prevalence, however, lung and breast carcinomas produce the majority of metastasis-associated hemorrhages. The most common primary brain tumor to produce hemorrhage is glioblastoma multiforme.[80]

Hematomas with internal heterogeneity, irregular margins, or unusually thick or asymmetric rinds of edema can suggest the possibility of underlying malignancy.[81,82] MR imaging is the

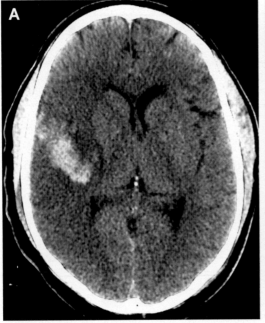
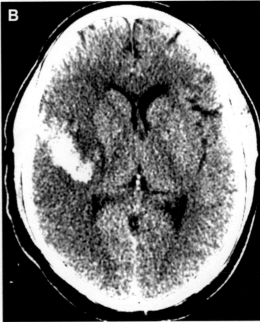

Fig. 13. Hemorrhagic transformation of infarction. (*A*) Axial NCT image obtained at the time of presentation to an emergency department shows a hematoma in the right temporal lobe and posterior insula. (*B*) Axial NCT image at the same anatomic level but displayed with a narrow window width (ie, stroke window settings) more clearly shows the cytotoxic edema in right middle cerebral artery territory.

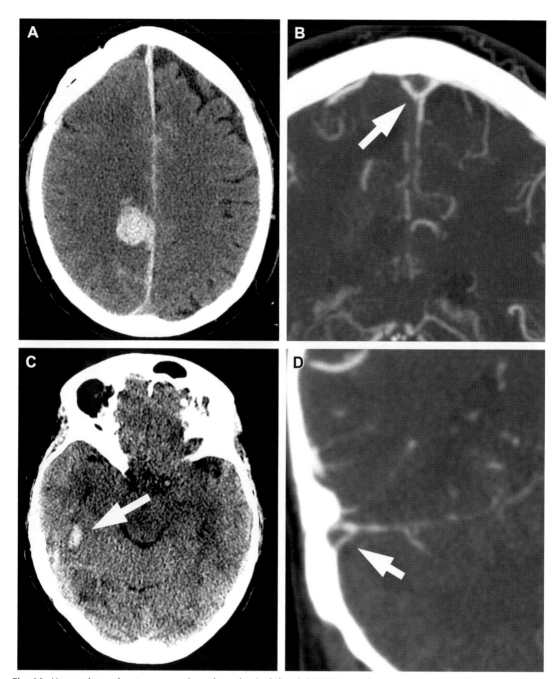

Fig. 14. Hemorrhage due to venous sinus thrombosis. (*A*) Axial NCT image shows a parenchymal hematoma in the right medial frontal lobe, with small amounts of associated subarachnoid and subdural hemorrhage. (*B*) Coronal CT venogram image in the same patient shows thrombosis of the superior sagittal sinus (*arrow*). (*C*) Axial NCT image from a second patient shows a hemorrhage in the right posterior temporal lobe (*arrow*). (*D*) Coronal CT venogram image from the second patient shows thrombosis of the right transverse sinus (*arrow*).

preferred modality for evaluating for suspected brain tumors. CTA may miss tumors because of the arterial timing of the contrast and should not be used to exclude the possibility of a tumor. On MR imaging, large hematomas can partially obscure smaller tumors, and, therefore, the margin of a hematoma should be carefully scrutinized for nodular or masslike enhancement. A caveat is that enhancement may be present around any hematoma, even non-neoplastic hemorrhages, due

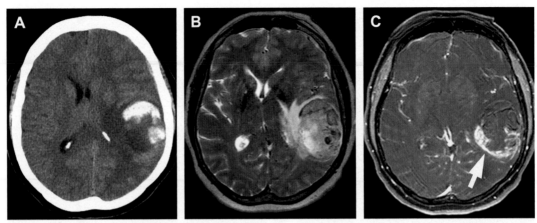

Fig. 15. Hemorrhage due to primary brain tumor. (*A*) Axial NCT image shows a hematoma in the left temporal lobe. The hematoma is heterogeneous, and there is extensive adjacent vasogenic edema, suggesting the presence of an underlying lesion. (*B*) Axial T2-weighted MR image shows a large mass associated with the hematoma. (*C*) Axial postcontrast T1-weighted image shows solid nodular enhancement along the posterior aspect of the mass (*arrow*). This enhancing area was biopsied, revealing a diagnosis of glioblastoma multiforme.

to breakdown of the blood-brain barrier, but in these cases the enhancement should correspond to areas where a hemosiderin rim is seen. If there is nodular enhancement that is not associated with a hemosiderin rim, or if the hemosiderin rim is incomplete around the margin the hematoma, a tumor may be suspected (**Fig. 15**).[82] If an underlying malignancy is suspected but not clearly demonstrated on contrast-enhanced MR imaging, a repeat contrast-enhanced MR imaging can be performed after several weeks to allow for hematoma involution.

Cocaine and amphetamines Illicit use of cocaine and amphetamines is an important cause of ICH and is more prevalent in younger patients. These drugs are sympathomimetic, can generate extreme hypertension, and often produce hemorrhages in the deep gray nuclei and pons that are indistinguishable from primary hypertensive ICH (**Fig. 16**).[83,84] Cocaine has additional procoagulant effects and chronic cocaine use is also associated with lobar hemorrhages, leukoariosis, arterial infarctions, aneurysm formation, and CNS vasculitis.[84–86]

Coagulopathy Coagulopathic patients are at increased risk for ICH and, when hemorrhage occurs, are at higher risk of poor outcomes.[33,87–89] Imaging findings suggestive of coagulopathy can aid timely recognition and reversal of the coagulopathic state. Fluid-fluid levels, also called hematocrit levels, within hematomas should raise suspicion for coagulopathy (**Fig. 17**).[90] Irregularly shaped and multiple simultaneous hematomas have also been associated with coagulopathic ICH.[32]

Patient-centered Imaging Selection

When spontaneous ICH is discovered on an initial imaging test, such as NCT, consideration of a few key clues derived from patient demographics and imaging features of the hematoma can help narrow the differential diagnosis and guide the selection of

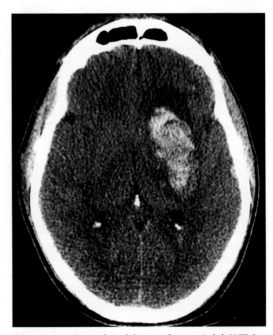

Fig. 16. Cocaine-related hemorrhage. Axial NCT image in a 33-year-old man shows a large hematoma in the left basal ganglia. Although this is a common site for hemorrhage due to chronic hypertension, this would be an unusual etiology in a patient of this age. Drug screen revealed recent cocaine use.

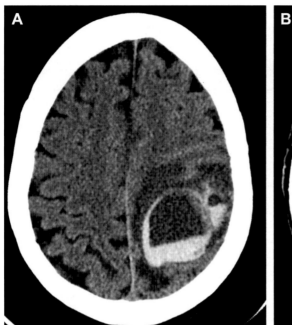
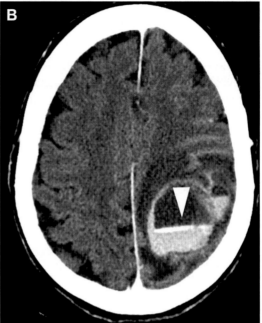

Fig. 17. Hematocrit level in a coagulopathic patient. (A) Axial NCT image from a patient on heparin shows a large left frontal lobe hematoma with a fluid-fluid, or hematocrit, level due dependent settling to unclotted blood. (B) Axial image obtained after contrast administration shows contrast layering within the hematoma (arrowhead), also due to failure of the blood to form a solid clot.

the next appropriate imaging test. General suggestions for the approach to imaging after ICH is identified are provided in **Box 3**.

Note that these are broad suggestions and may be altered to fit an individual patient or practice; current guidelines allow for clinical judgment in determining what additional imaging, if any, is appropriate once ICH has been identified.[22]

The most informative considerations are

1. Patient age
2. Hematoma location
3. Presence of specific imaging features on the presenting NCT that are atypical for hypertensive hemorrhage: heterogeneity of the hematoma, widespread PHE, a hematocrit level, and extensive SAH

Similarly, a clinical decision rule for obtaining brain MR imaging in patients with ICH using only 3 factors—age, presence of hypertension, and hematoma location—correctly predicted 100% of patients who had a subsequent etiology identified on their scans.[91]

As discussed previously, multiple studies have demonstrated that younger patients (in particular those under the age of 55) are much more likely to have a vascular lesion as the etiology for spontaneous ICH.[39,57,92,93] These patients are the most likely to benefit from CTA.[93] One study found that

the diagnostic yield of CTA in the setting of spontaneous ICH was 47% in patients aged 18 years to 45 years but dropped to 15% in patients aged 46 years to 70 years and revealed a vascular lesion in only 4% in patients aged 71 years to 94 years.[94]

Because of the predilection of the deep brain structures for hypertensive hemorrhage, location is another strong consideration in selection of imaging. In an older patient with known hypertension and hemorrhage in a deep brain structure, it may be the case that no additional imaging modality is required apart from NCT. Lobar location clearly increases the diagnostic yield of additional imaging, however. Lobar location was associated with a 20% diagnostic yield of CTA compared with a 2% yield for deep gray matter hemorrhage.[94]

Atypical imaging findings present on the initial NCT may prompt further evaluation with CTA or MR imaging. Because hypertensive hemorrhages are typically smoothly marginated and uniform, hemorrhages that have markedly irregular contours, ill-defined margins, or internal heterogeneous density should be regarded as suspicious for an underlying lesion (**Fig. 18**).[82] Hypertensive hemorrhage usually shows a halo of PHE that parallels the contours of the hematoma and concentrically expands over several days after the ictus. Patients who demonstrate large or asymmetric areas of edema that do not parallel the contours

Box 3
Patient-centered imaging selection after intracranial hemorrhage is identified on noncontrast CT

	Most Common Etiologies of Intracranial Hemorrhage	Highest-Yield Next Step After Initial Noncontrast CT[a]
Common scenarios		
Older patient, hypertensive, deep location, no atypical imaging features	Hypertension	NCT alone may be sufficient; additional imaging at discretion of the care team
Elderly patient, lobar location, no atypical imaging features	Amyloid angiopathy, tumor	MR imaging brain
Young patient, any location	AVM, cavernoma	CTA first; MR imaging brain if negative
Special considerations for atypical NCT features		
Extensive or asymmetric vasogenic edema at presentation	Tumor	MR imaging brain
Hematocrit level	Coagulopathy	Laboratory assessment of coagulopathy
Large amount of SAH + inferior frontal, temporal, cerebellar hematoma location	Adherent aneurysm	CTA
Heterogeneous hematoma	AVM or tumor	CTA first in younger patient, MR imaging in older patient

[a] These suggestions are based on the most common ICH etiologies. Subsequent imaging may be necessary if no etiology for ICH is identified.

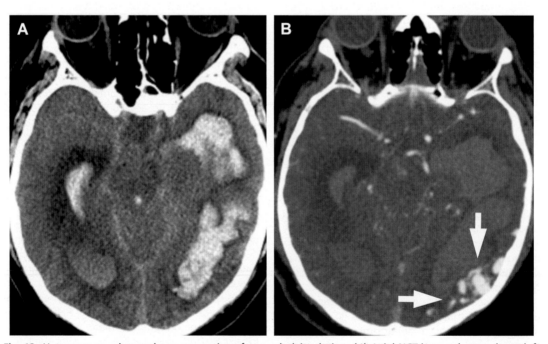

Fig. 18. Heterogeneous hemorrhage suggestive of an underlying lesion. (*A*) Axial NCT image shows a large left temporal lobe hematoma with heterogeneous margins and intraventricular extension. (*B*) Axial image from CTA in the same patient reveals an AVM along the posterior aspect of the hematoma (*arrows*).

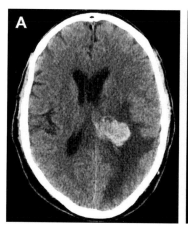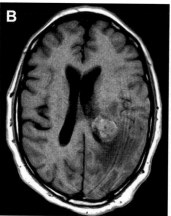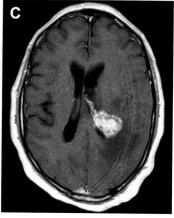

Fig. 19. Vasogenic edema pattern suggests an underlying lesion. (*A*) Axial NCT image obtained at the time of initial presentation shows a hematoma in the left corona radiata. There is extensive surrounding edema which does not parallel the contours of the hematoma, suggestive of an underlying lesion. Axial T1-weighted precontrast (*B*) and postcontrast (*C*) images show an enhancing mass at this location. Biopsy revealed metastatic lung cancer.

of the hematoma on initial presentation should undergo further imaging with MR imaging, because this may be a marker of vasogenic edema surrounding a preexisting tumor (**Fig. 19**).[3,22] The presence of a hematocrit level within a hematoma is highly suggestive of an underlying coagulopathy, often iatrogenic, particularly in patients taking coumadin.[90] Hemorrhage into a necrotic tumor can rarely also produce this finding[81] but is much less common than coagulopathy, in the authors' experience. Finally, the presence of a large volume of SAH in the setting of spontaneous brain parenchymal ICH may indicate the presence of a ruptured adherent aneurysm and would be an indication for vascular imaging.

SUMMARY

Spontaneous ICH is a commonly encountered neurologic emergency. Imaging plays important roles in both guiding the emergent stabilization of patients with ICH and in elucidating the etiology of the hemorrhage to prevent rebleeding. A thorough understanding of the factors that have an impact on immediate management, the causes of hemorrhage, and the strengths of various imaging techniques in addressing these 2 concerns is vital to crafting a patient-centered approach to this condition.

REFERENCES

1. Broderick J, Connolly S, Feldmann E, et al, American Heart Association, American Stroke Association Stroke Council, High Blood Pressure Research Council, Quality of Care and Outcomes in Research Interdisciplinary Working Group. Guidelines for the management of spontaneous intracerebral hemorrhage in adults: 2007 update: a guideline from the American Heart Association/American Stroke Association Stroke Council, High Blood Pressure Research Council, and the Quality of Care and Outcomes in Research Interdisciplinary Working Group. Stroke 2007;38:2001–23.

2. Caceres JA, Goldstein JN. Intracranial hemorrhage. Emerg Med Clin North Am 2012;30(3):771–94.

3. Kranz PG, Amrhein TJ, Provenzale JM. Spontaneous brain parenchymal hemorrhage: an approach to imaging for the emergency room radiologist. Emerg Radiol 2015;22(1):53–63.

4. Sutherland GR, Auer RN. Primary intracerebral hemorrhage. J Clin Neurosci 2006;13(5):511–7.

5. Blanco PJ, Müller LO, Spence JD. Blood pressure gradients in cerebral arteries: a clue to pathogenesis of cerebral small vessel disease. Stroke Vasc Neurol 2017;50(24):1524–35.

6. Wakai S, Nagai M. Histological verification of microaneurysms as a cause of cerebral haemorrhage in surgical specimens. J Neurol Neurosurg Psychiatry 1989;52(5):595–9.

7. Moody DM, Bell MA, Challa VR. Features of the cerebral vascular pattern that predict vulnerability to perfusion or oxygenation deficiency: an anatomic study. AJNR Am J Neuroradiol 1990;11(3):431–9.

8. Akashi T, Takahashi S, Mugikura S, et al. Ischemic white matter lesions associated with medullary arteries: classification of MRI findings based on the anatomic arterial distributions. AJR Am J Roentgenol 2017;209(3):W160–8.

9. Hiroki M, Miyashita K, Oda M. Tortuosity of the white matter medullary arterioles is related to the severity of hypertension. Cerebrovasc Dis 2002;13(4):242–50.

10. Expert Panel on Neurologic Imaging, Salmela MB, Mortazavi S, Jagadeesan BD, et al. ACR appropriateness criteria(R) cerebrovascular disease. J Am Coll Radiol 2017;14(5S):S34–61.

11. American College of Radiology. ACR–ASNR–SPR practice parameter for the performance of computed tomography (CT) of the brain. 2015. Available at: https://www.acr.org/Quality-Safety/Standards-Guidelines/Practice-Guidelines-by-Modality/CT. Accessed September 17, 2017.

12. Kidwell CS, Chalela JA, Saver JL, et al. Comparison of MRI and CT for detection of acute intracerebral hemorrhage. JAMA 2004;292(15):1823–30.

13. Chalela JA, Kidwell CS, Nentwich LM, et al. Magnetic resonance imaging and computed tomography in emergency assessment of patients with suspected acute stroke: a prospective comparison. Lancet 2007;369(9558):293–8.

14. Khosravani H, Mayer SA, Demchuk A, et al. Emergency noninvasive angiography for acute intracerebral hemorrhage. AJNR Am J Neuroradiol 2013; 34(8):1481–7.

15. Bradley WG Jr. MR appearance of hemorrhage in the brain. Radiology 1993;189(1):15–26.

16. Chavhan GB, Babyn PS, Thomas B, et al. Principles, techniques, and applications of T2*-based MR imaging and its special applications. Radiographics 2009;29(5):1433–49.

17. Tong KA, Ashwal S, Holshouser BA, et al. Hemorrhagic shearing lesions in children and adolescents with posttraumatic diffuse axonal injury: improved detection and initial results. Radiology 2003;227(2):332–9.

18. Broderick JP, Brott TG, Duldner JE, et al. Volume of intracerebral hemorrhage. A powerful and easy-to-use predictor of 30-day mortality. Stroke 1993; 24(7):987–93.

19. Huttner HB. Comparison of ABC/2 estimation technique to computer-assisted planimetric analysis in warfarin-related intracerebral parenchymal hemorrhage. Stroke 2006;37(2):404–8.

20. Kothari RU, Brott T, Broderick JP, et al. The ABCs of measuring intracerebral hemorrhage volumes. Stroke 1996;27(8):1304–5.

21. Amar AP. Controversies in the neurosurgical management of cerebellar hemorrhage and infarction. Neurosurg Focus 2012;32(4):E1.

22. Hemphill JC, Greenberg SM, Anderson CS, et al. Guidelines for the management of spontaneous intracerebral hemorrhage: a guideline for healthcare professionals from the American Heart Association/American Stroke Association. Stroke 2015;46(7): 2032–60.

23. Gebel JM Jr, Jauch EC, Brott TG, et al. Relative edema volume is a predictor of outcome in patients with hyperacute spontaneous intracerebral hemorrhage. Stroke 2002;33(11):2636–41.

24. Venkatasubramanian C, Mlynash M, Finley-Caulfield A, et al. Natural history of perihematomal edema after intracerebral hemorrhage measured by serial magnetic resonance imaging. Stroke 2011;42(1):73–80.

25. Inaji M, Tomita H, Tone O, et al. Chronological changes of perihematomal edema of human intracerebral hematoma. Acta Neurochir Suppl 2003;86: 445–8.

26. Balami JS, Buchan AM. Complications of intracerebral haemorrhage. Lancet Neurol 2012;11(1):101–18.

27. Hanley DF. Intraventricular hemorrhage: severity factor and treatment target in spontaneous intracerebral hemorrhage. Stroke 2009;40(4):1533–8.

28. Fewel ME, Thompson BG, Hoff JT. Spontaneous intracerebral hemorrhage: a review. Neurosurg Focus 2003;15(4):E1.

29. Gupta A, Sattur MG, Aoun RJN, et al. Hemicraniectomy for ischemic and hemorrhagic stroke: facts and controversies. Neurosurg Clin N Am 2017; 28(3):349–60.

30. Brouwers HB, Falcone GJ, McNamara KA, et al. CTA spot sign predicts hematoma expansion in patients with delayed presentation after intracerebral hemorrhage. Neurocrit Care 2012;17(3):421–8.

31. Delgado Almandoz JE, Yoo AJ, Stone MJ, et al. The spot sign score in primary intracerebral hemorrhage identifies patients at highest risk of in-hospital mortality and poor outcome among survivors. Stroke 2010;41(1):54–60.

32. Wang QT, Tuhrim S. Etiologies of intracerebral hematomas. Curr Atheroscler Rep 2012;14(4):314–21.

33. Keep RF, Hua Y, Xi G. Intracerebral haemorrhage: mechanisms of injury and therapeutic targets. Lancet Neurol 2012;11(8):720–31.

34. Woo D, Sauerbeck LR, Kissela BM, et al. Genetic and environmental risk factors for intracerebral hemorrhage, preliminary results of a population-based study. Stroke 2002;33:1190–6.

35. Woo D, Haverbusch M, Sekar P, et al. Effect of untreated hypertension on hemorrhagic stroke. Stroke 2004;35:1703–8.

36. Qureshi AI, Suri MF, Mohammad Y, et al. Isolated and borderline isolated systolic hypertension relative to long-term risk and type of stroke: a 20-year follow-up of the national health and nutrition survey. Stroke 2002;33(12):2781–8.

37. Greenberg SM, Vernooij MW, Cordonnier C, et al. Cerebral microbleeds: a guide to detection and interpretation. Lancet 2009;8:165–74.

38. Fischbein NJ, Wijman CA. Nontraumatic intracranial hemorrhage. Neuroimaging Clin N Am 2010;20(4): 469–92.

39. Ruiz-Sandoval JL, Cantu C, Barinagarrementeria F. Intracerebral hemorrhage in young people: analysis

of risk factors, location, causes, and prognosis. Stroke 1999;30(3):537–41.

40. Koennecke HC. Cerebral microbleeds on MRI: prevalence, associations, and potential clinical implications. Neurology 2006;66(2):165–71.

41. Vernooij MW, van der Lugt A, Ikram MA, et al. Prevalence and risk factors of cerebral microbleeds: the Rotterdam scan study. Neurology 2008;70(14):1208–14.

42. Kinoshita T, Okudera T, Tamura H, et al. Assessment of lacunar hemorrhage associated with hypertensive stroke by echo-planar gradient-echo T2*-weighted MRI. Stroke 2000;31(7):1646–50.

43. Viswanathan A, Greenberg SM. Cerebral amyloid angiopathy in the elderly. Ann Neurol 2011;70(6):871–80.

44. Zhang-Nunes SX, Maat-Schieman ML, van Duinen SG, et al. The cerebral beta-amyloid angiopathies: hereditary and sporadic. Brain Pathol 2006;16(1):30–9.

45. Soffer D. Cerebral amyloid angiopathy–a disease or age-related condition. Isr Med Assoc J 2006;8(11):803–6.

46. Pezzini A, Padovani A. Cerebral amyloid angiopathy-related hemorrhages. Neurol Sci 2008;29(Suppl 2):S260–3.

47. Knudsen KA, Rosand J, Karluk D, et al. Clinical diagnosis of cerebral amyloid angiopathy: validation of the Boston criteria. Neurology 2001;56(4):537–9.

48. Kumar S, Goddeau RP, Selim MH, et al. Atraumatic convexal subarachnoid hemorrhage. Neurology 2010;74(11):893–9.

49. Ropper AH, Davis KR. Lobar cerebral hemorrhages: acute clinical syndromes in 26 cases. Ann Neurol 1980;8:141–7.

50. Rosand J, Muzikansky A, Kumar A, et al. Spatial clustering of hemorrhages in probable cerebral amyloid angiopathy. Ann Neurol 2005;58:459–62.

51. Makris M, Van Veen JJ, Tait CR, et al, British Committee for Standards in Haematology. Guideline on the management of bleeding in patients on antithrombotic agents. Br J Haematol 2013;160(1):35–46.

52. Ondra SL, Troupp H, George ED, et al. The natural history of symptomatic arteriovenous malformations of the brain: a 24-year follow-up assessment. J Neurosurg 1990;73(3):387–91.

53. Laakso A, Dashti R, Juvela S, et al. Risk of hemorrhage in patients with untreated Spetzler-Martin grade IV and V arteriovenous malformations: a long-term follow-up study in 63 patients. Neurosurgery 2011;68(2):372–7.

54. Al-Shahi R, Warlow C. A systematic review of the frequency and prognosis of arteriovenous malformations of the brain in adults. Brain 2001;124:1900–26.

55. Hernesniemi J, Dashti R, Juvela S, et al. Natural history of brain arteriovenous malformations: a long-term follow-up study of risk of hemorrhage in 238 patients. Neurosurgery 2008;63(5):823–9.

56. Mattle HP, Schroth G, Seiler RW. Dilemmas in the management of patients with arteriovenous malformations. J Neurol 2000;247:917–28.

57. Zhu XL, Chan MS, Poon WS. Spontaneous intracranial hemorrhage: which patients need diagnostic cerebral angiography? A prospective study of 206 cases and review of the literature. Stroke 1997;28(7):1406–9.

58. Kirkman MA, Tyrrell PJ, King AT, et al. Imaging in young adults with intracerebral hemorrhage. Clin Neurol Neurosurg 2012;114(10):1297–303.

59. Spetzler RF, Martin NA. A proposed grading system for arteriovenous malformations. J Neurosurg 1986;65(4):476–83.

60. Al-Shahi Salman R, Berg MJ, Morrison L, et al. Hemorrhage from cavernous malformations of the brain: definition and reporting standards. Stroke 2008;39(12):3222–30.

61. Washington CW, McCoy KE, Zipfel GJ. Update on the natural history of cavernous malformations and factors predicting aggressive clinical presentation. Neurosurg Focus 2010;29(3):E7.

62. Töppera R, Jürgensa E, Reulb J, et al. Clinical significance of intracranial developmental venous anomalie. J Neurol Neurosurg Psychiatry 1999;67:234–8.

63. Masson RL, Day AL. Aneurysmal intracerebral hemorrhage. Neurosurg Clin N Am 1992;3(3):539–50.

64. Tokuda Y, Inagawa T, Katoh Y, et al. Intracerebral hematoma in patients with ruptured cerebral aneurysms. Surg Neurol 1995;43(3):272–7.

65. Hajj-Ali RA, Singhal AB, Benseler S, et al. Primary angiitis of the CNS. Lancet Neurol 2011;10(6):561–72.

66. Salvarani C, Brown RD, Calamia KT, et al. Primary central nervous system vasculitis: analysis of 101 patients. Ann Neurol 2007;65(5):442–51.

67. Suri V, Kakkar A, Sharma MC, et al. Primary angiitis of the central nervous system: a study of histopathological patterns and review of the literature. Folia Neuropathol 2014;52(2):187–96.

68. Scott RM, Smith ER. Moyamoya disease and moyamoya syndrome. N Engl J Med 2009;360:1226–37.

69. Saeki N, Nakazaki S, Kubota M, et al. Hemorrhagic type moyamoya disease. Clin Neurol Neurosurg 1997;99(Suppl 2):S196–201.

70. Burke GM, Burke AM, Sherma AK, et al. Moyamoya disease: a summary. Neurosurg Focus 2009;26(4):E11.

71. Lansberg MG, Thijs VN, Bammer R, et al. Risk factors of symptomatic intracerebral hemorrhage after tPA therapy for acute stroke. Stroke 2007;38(8):2275–8.

72. Khatri P, Wechsler LR, Broderick JP. Intracranial hemorrhage associated with revascularization therapies. Stroke 2007;38(2):431–40.

73. Singer OC, Humprich MC, Fiehler J, et al. Risk for symptomatic intracerebral hemorrhage after thrombolysis assessed by diffusion-weighted magnetic resonance imaging. Ann Neurol 2008;63(1):52–60.

74. Smith EE, Rosand J, Knudsen KA, et al. Leukoariosis is associated with warfarin-related hemorrhage following ischemic stroke. Neurology 2002;59:193–7.

75. Makkat S, Stadnik T, Peeters E, et al. Pathogenesis of venous stroke: evaluation with diffusion- and perfusion-weighted MRI. J Stroke Cerebrovasc Dis 2003;12(3):132–6.

76. English JD, Fields JD, Le S, et al. Clinical presentation and long-term outcome of cerebral venous thrombosis. Neurocrit Care 2009;11(3):330–7.

77. Provenzale JM, Kranz PG. Dural sinus thrombosis: sources of error in image interpretation. Am J Roentgenol 2011;196(1):23–31.

78. Cestari DM, Weine DM, Panageas KS, et al. Stroke in patients with cancer: incidence and etiology. Neurology 2004;62(11):2025–30.

79. Katz JM, Segal AZ. Incidence and etiology of cerebrovascular disease in patients with malignancy. Curr Atheroscler Rep 2005;7(4):280–8.

80. Licata B, Turazzi S. Bleeding cerebral neoplasms with symptomatic hematoma. J Neurosurg Sci 2003;47(4):201–10.

81. Morris BS, Nagar AM, Morani AC, et al. Blood-fluid levels in the brain. Br J Radiol 2007;80(954):488–98.

82. Atlas SW, Grossman RI, Gomori JM, et al. Hemorrhagic intracranial malignant neoplasms: spin-echo MR imaging. Radiology 1987;164(1):71–7.

83. Toossi S, Hess CP, Hills NK, et al. Neurovascular complications of cocaine use at a tertiary stroke center. J Stroke Cerebrovasc Dis 2010;19(4):273–8.

84. Restrepo CS, Rojas CA, Martinez S, et al. Cardiovascular complications of cocaine: imaging findings. Emerg Radiol 2009;16(1):11–9.

85. Pozzi M, Roccatagliata D, Sterzi R. Drug abuse and intracranial hemorrhage. Neurol Sci 2008;29(Suppl 2):S269–70.

86. Martin-Schild S, Albright KC, Hallevi H, et al. Intracerebral hemorrhage in cocaine users. Stroke 2010; 41(4):680–4.

87. Fang MC, Go AS, Chang Y, et al. Death and disability from warfarin-associated intracranial and extracranial hemorrhages. Am J Med 2007;120(8): 700–5.

88. Cucchiara B, Messe S, Sansing L, et al. Hematoma growth in oral anticoagulant related intracerebral hemorrhage. Stroke 2008;39(11):2993–6.

89. Quinones-Hinojosa A, Gulati M, Singh V, et al. Spontaneous intracerebral hemorrhage due to coagulation disorders. Neurosurg Focus 2003;15(4):E3.

90. Livoni JP, McGahan JP. Intracranial fluid-blood levels in the anticoagulated patient. Neuroradiology 1983;25(5):335–7.

91. Kamel H, Navi BB, Hemphill JC. A rule to identify patients who require magnetic resonance imaging after intracerebral hemorrhage. Neurocrit Care 2011; 18(1):59–63.

92. Griffiths PD, Beveridge CJ, Gholkar A. Angiography in non-traumatic brain haematoma. Acta Radiol 2016;38(5):797–802.

93. Bekelis K, Desai A, Zhao W, et al. Computed tomography angiography: improving diagnostic yield and cost effectiveness in the initial evaluation of spontaneous nonsubarachnoid intracerebral hemorrhage. J Neurosurg 2012;117(4):761–6.

94. Delgado Almandoz JE, Schaefer PW, Forero NP, et al. Diagnostic accuracy and yield of multidetector CT angiography in the evaluation of spontaneous intraparenchymal cerebral hemorrhage. AJNR Am J Neuroradiol 2009;30(6):1213–21.

Acute Neurologic Syndromes Beyond Stroke
The Role of Emergent MR Imaging

Edward K. Sung, MD, Chad Farris, MD,
Mohamad Abdalkader, MD, Asim Mian, MD*

KEYWORDS

• Diffusion • Nonischemic • Infection • Trauma • Toxic • Metabolic

KEY POINTS

- MR imaging is an important diagnostic tool in the assessment of injured or acutely ill patients in the emergency setting.
- MR imaging with diffusion-weighted imaging is important for the evaluation of nonischemic disorders.
- Various infectious, traumatic, toxic/metabolic, and other processes can show diffusion abnormalities, and should not be confused for acute ischemia.

INTRODUCTION

The use of MR imaging in the emergency setting for injured or acutely ill patients is crucial for the diagnosis, treatment, and follow-up for a variety of different disorders. Specifically, diffusion-weighted imaging (DWI) has played a critical role in patients who are suspected to have an acute stroke. DWI, however, can also be used to diagnose other nonischemic disorders that may be life threatening and may otherwise go undetected. These disorders can include infectious processes (cerebral abscesses, subdural/epidural empyemas, viral encephalitis), trauma (diffuse axonal injury [DAI]), and toxic/metabolic abnormalities (carbon monoxide [CO] poisoning, medication-induced toxicity, opioid toxicity), among other entities. These disorders may be erroneously attributed to changes related to ischemia or infarct, but a proper clinical history and findings on other MR sequences becomes essential for accurate diagnosis and treatment of patients in the emergency setting. This article describes some selected cases with diffusion abnormality that can be encountered in the emergency setting (**Table 1**).

INFECTIOUS PROCESSES
Cerebral Abscess

A cerebral abscess can be fatal if not diagnosed and treated in a timely fashion. The most common associated clinical symptoms are headaches (90%) and fevers (50%). These abscesses are typically secondary to sinusitis, mastoiditis, or otitis media or can be acquired by immunocompromised patients. Although the location is variable, these lesions are typically found in the frontal and temporal lobes at the gray-white junction, and may be associated with the presence of tortuous subcortical vessels that can serve as a nidus for this infection.[1,2] The 4 stages of cerebral abscess are early and late cerebritis followed by early and late capsule.

MR imaging typically shows a centrally T2/fluid-attenuated inversion recovery (FLAIR) hyperintense or heterogeneous-appearing lesion with surrounding edema and well-defined peripheral enhancement with the enhancing capsule being thin along the medial or white matter aspect of the lesion because of decreased vascularity in this location. They can also show peripheral T1

Department of Radiology, Boston University Medical Center, 820 Harrison Avenue, FGH Building, 3rd Floor, Boston, MA 02118, USA
* Corresponding author.
E-mail address: Asim.Mian@bmc.org

Neuroimag Clin N Am 28 (2018) 375–395
https://doi.org/10.1016/j.nic.2018.03.012
1052-5149/18/© 2018 Elsevier Inc. All rights reserved.

Table 1
Selected cases with diffusion abnormality

Disorder	Clinical Context	Imaging Findings	Take-Home Points
Cerebral abscess	• Patients with sinusitis, mastoiditis, or immunocompromised • Headaches, fevers	• Peripherally enhancing, centrally necrotic cystic lesion • Central restricted diffusion	• Cystic lesion with peripheral enhancement and central restricted diffusion in the proper clinical context is typically abscess
Empyema	• Patients with sinusitis, mastoiditis, or thrombophlebitis	• Peripherally enhancing collection in the epidural or subdural space • Central restricted diffusion	• Empyema typically develops as an extension of an extracranial infection • Underlying meningitis or cerebritis is more typically seen with subdural empyema rather than epidural empyema
Herpes encephalitis	• HSV-1 in adults • HSV-2 in neonates • Headaches, fever, altered mentation, seizures	• Early: asymmetric cortical restricted diffusion in temporal lobes, insula, inferior frontal lobes, or cingulate gyri • Subacute: T2 hyperintensity, gyral swelling, enhancement, hemorrhage	• MR imaging abnormalities in the temporal lobes should raise concern for HSV encephalitis • Rapid empiric treatment with acyclovir is needed to minimize the high mortality of HSV encephalitis
DAI	• High-speed trauma with acceleration and sudden deceleration	• Multiple foci of restricted diffusion in the white matter • Multiple T2/FLAIR hyperintense lesions • Scattered hemorrhagic lesions on GRE or SWI	• Most (~80%) DAI lesions are nonhemorrhagic • Multiple DWI hyperintense lesions in high-speed trauma is DAI, and usually not infarct
CO poisoning	• Accidental or intentional exposure to CO	• Isolated restricted diffusion in the globus pallidus is the earliest imaging finding and is seen in the ultra-acute phase • Restricted diffusion can be seen in the cerebral white matter in all phases • Globus pallidus atrophy is seen in the chronic phase	• Imaging findings vary based on the time of imaging relative to the time of exposure to CO • Restricted diffusion in the globus pallidus is the first finding in the ultra-acute phase • Atrophy of gray matter structures in the chronic phase is commonly seen in patients with persistent neurologic symptoms

Opioid toxicity	• Confusion and delirium with other neurologic symptoms in the setting of exogenous opioid use	• Abnormal signal intensity and restriction diffusion of the globus pallidus and less frequently the medial temporal lobes or cerebellum • Lack of mass effect and enhancement	• Bilateral, symmetric restriction diffusion of the globus pallidus, medial temporal lobes, or cerebellum warrants consideration of opioid toxicity, and should elicit appropriate screening
Methotrexate toxicity	• Children with acute lymphoblastic leukemia on methotrexate	• T2 and FLAIR hyperintensities and restriction diffusion within the deep periventricular white matter	• Abnormal signal intensity and restricted diffusion of the deep periventricular white matter in patients receiving methotrexate
Metronidazole toxicity	• Any patient taking metronidazole	• DWI and T2/FLAIR hyperintensity in the dentate nucleus is the most common finding with no postcontrast enhancement • Restricted diffusion on DWI imaging in the splenium	• Dose and duration of metronidazole are not correlated with neurotoxicity • Usually reversible, but not always • Dentate nucleus is almost always involved • Splenium is usually involved with corpus callosum involvement
Central pontine myelinolysis	• Rapid correction of hyponatremia in alcoholic, malnourished, transplant, and severely burned patients	• Abnormal signal intensity and restriction diffusion of the central pons • Lack of mass effect and enhancement	• Restricted diffusion involving the central part of the pons in the setting of rapid correction of hyponatremia
Tumefactive demyelinating lesion	• Patient with multiple neurologic symptoms commonly including motor, sensory, and/or cognitive symptoms • Known history of multiple sclerosis	• T2/FLAIR hyperintense lesion >2 cm in the white matter • Different enhancement patterns, but incomplete ring is most suggestive • Peripheral rim of restricted diffusion can be seen	• Peripheral rim of restricted diffusion can be seen • Discontinuous peripheral enhancement is the most suggestive feature • History of multiple sclerosis or multiple additional white matter lesions suggests diagnosis • Brain biopsy may still be necessary to rule out malignancy, especially in the cases of a single initial lesion
Epidermoid cyst	• Often incidental findings • Nonspecific symptoms such as headache • Potential symptoms caused by mass effect	• Cystic structure that can appear similar to CSF • Central restricted diffusion • Mass effect on surrounding brain	• Extra-axial cystic lesion similar to arachnoid cyst, but with central restricted diffusion • Most commonly in cerebellopontine angle, followed by fourth ventricle and sellar region

(continued on next page)

Table 1
(continued)

Disorder	Clinical Context	Imaging Findings	Take-Home Points
Seizure-related changes	• Patients with recent seizure, either iso-lated event or in the setting of epilepsy	• T2/FLAIR hyperintensity is most common and it occurs in the area of the seizure activity • Restricted diffusion in the site of T2/FLAIR hyperintensity is common • Mild gadolinium enhancement can be seen	• MR imaging findings are usually reversible • Imaging finding can occur anywhere based on where the seizure occurred, but the hippocampus is most commonly involved
Dural venous sinus thrombosis	• Most common risk factors are immediate postpartum period, oral hormonal contraception, and coagulation disorders (factor V Leiden most commonly)	• Filling defects on MRV and contrast-enhanced T1 sequences are most sensitive • DWI, T2, and FLAIR hyperintensity • GRE hypointensity or blooming	• Imaging study of choice is MRV or CTV • 3D T1 contrast-enhanced sequences can have excellent sensitivity • Presence of signal abnormality in 1 con-ventional sequence or DWI in a given scan is sensitive, but not specific

Abbreviations: CSF, cerebrospinal fluid; CTV, computed tomography venogram; FLAIR, fluid-attenuated inversion recovery; GRE, gradient recalled echo; HSV, herpes simplex virus; MRV, MR venogram; SWI, susceptibility-weighted imaging.

and T2 shortening caused by hemorrhage, proteinaceous material, and free radicals.[3] DWI is particularly useful because cerebral abscesses show restricted diffusion caused by increased viscosity and cellularity of pus compared with necrotic tumors, which do not typically have restricted diffusion[4] (**Fig. 1**).

Empyema

Empyema is a purulent collection that can develop in the subdural or epidural space, usually seen as an extension of infection from sinusitis, mastoiditis, or thrombophlebitis.[1,5] Symptoms of fever, headache, meningismus, and neurologic deficits can vary depending on the location of the empyema, with more severe symptoms typically seen with subdural empyemas given the increased propensity for the adjacent brain parenchyma to become affected (caused by lack of the dura mater to provide an additional layer of separation from the brain).[1] Treatment can vary depending on the size and location of the empyema as well as the severity of symptoms, ranging from conservative management with antibiotic therapy to surgical evacuation.

MR imaging is the imaging modality of choice to diagnose an empyema, showing an extra-axial collection with T2 hyperintensity, peripheral enhancement, and central restricted diffusion[1,5] (**Fig. 2**), similar in pathophysiology to cerebral abscesses. Empyemas also typically appear mildly hyperintense on FLAIR images because of the internal complexity. Particularly with subdural empyemas, there may be inflammation of the adjacent meninges and brain parenchyma, manifesting as leptomeningeal enhancement and cortical swelling with T2/FLAIR hyperintensity, respectively.

Herpes Encephalitis

Herpes simplex virus (HSV) infection can result in encephalitis, either caused by primary infection or viral reactivation. HSV encephalitis is usually caused by HSV-2 in neonates and HSV-1 in adults.[1,5,6] Typical patient presentation can include fever, headaches, altered mentation, various neurologic deficits, and seizures. Early diagnosis and treatment with acyclovir is essential, because mortalities of untreated HSV encephalitis can exceed 70%.[1,7] Diagnosis relies on imaging and HSV polymerase chain reaction testing of the cerebrospinal fluid (CSF).[5,8]

MR imaging is most sensitive for detecting abnormalities in HSV encephalitis. Early imaging findings can include asymmetric cortical restricted diffusion involving the temporal lobes, insula, inferior frontal lobes, and cingulate gyri (**Fig. 3**), caused by cytotoxic edema. Subacute imaging findings can include T2 hyperintensity, gyral swelling, and enhancement, as well as presence of susceptibility artifact indicating hemorrhage.[5] Presence of these imaging findings in acutely ill patients should raise concern for HSV encephalitis, with rapid empiric treatment with acyclovir to minimize mortality.

TRAUMATIC INJURY
Diffuse Axonal Injury

DAI is found in patients with traumatic brain injury in the setting of trauma with angular or rotational

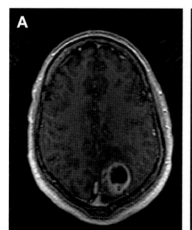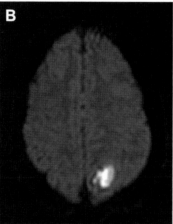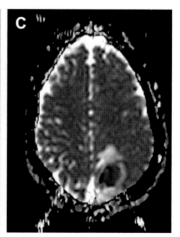

Fig. 1. A 42-year-old man on steroids for sarcoid presenting with fever and headaches. Brain MR imaging with postcontrast T1-weighted axial image (*A*) shows a peripherally enhancing, centrally cystic lesion in the left parieto-occipital lobe. DWI (*B*) and apparent diffusion coefficient (ADC) (*C*) axial images show restricted diffusion of the lesion. Findings are consistent with brain abscess, confirmed with surgical drainage.

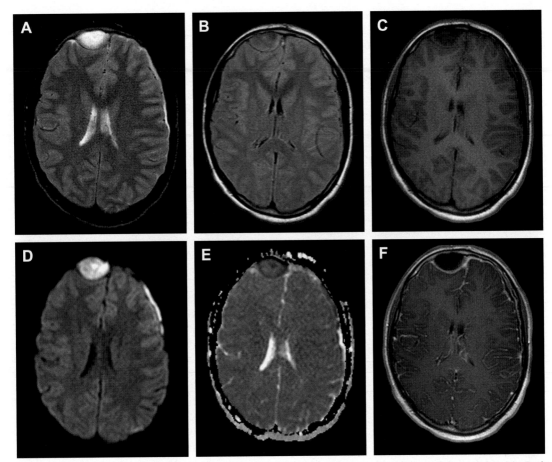

Fig. 2. A 14-year-old boy presenting with fever and altered mental status in the setting of frontal sinusitis. Brain MR imaging with T2-weighted (*A*), FLAIR (*B*), and T1-weighted (*C*) axial images shows a T2 hyperintense, FLAIR isointense, and T1 hypointense epidural collection in the right anterior frontal convexity, which shows restricted diffusion on DWI (*D*) and ADC (*E*) images, and peripheral enhancement on T1 postcontrast (*F*) images. Findings are consistent with an epidural empyema. There is also a thin subdural empyema along the left frontal convexity showing similar imaging characteristics.

acceleration and sudden deceleration causing shearing injury to the myelin sheath of axons, which are typically located at the gray-white matter junction. Tearing of the axons is uncommon and usually seen in severe cases. A clinical hallmark of DAI is the sudden loss of consciousness at the time of the trauma, with the patient being in a persistent and prolonged coma depending on the degree of DAI and other concomitant injuries.[1]

Initial imaging findings of DAI on noncontrast head computed tomography (CT) may be nonspecific and even normal despite the patient's poor neurologic presentation. However, follow-up imaging in 24 to 48 hours, specifically with MR imaging, can show multiple, focal FLAIR and T2 hyperintense lesions, some of which may show susceptibility artifact on gradient or susceptibility-weighted imaging consistent with

hemorrhagic lesions[9] (**Fig. 4**). Only 20% of lesions associated with DAI are hemorrhagic. The distribution of these lesions is typically at the gray-white matter interface, dorsolateral brainstem, pons, and corpus callosum.[10]

Some lesions associated with DAI also show restricted diffusion. Although the mechanism of this is unclear, it is postulated that the restricted diffusion may be from glutamate excitotoxicity of glial cells. In addition, a study has also shown a direct correlation between the number of diffusion-weighted signal abnormalities and the neurologic disability of the patient.[11]

TOXIC AND METABOLIC ABNORMALITIES
Carbon Monoxide Poisoning

CO poisoning is a common problem in the United States, with an estimated 50,000 related

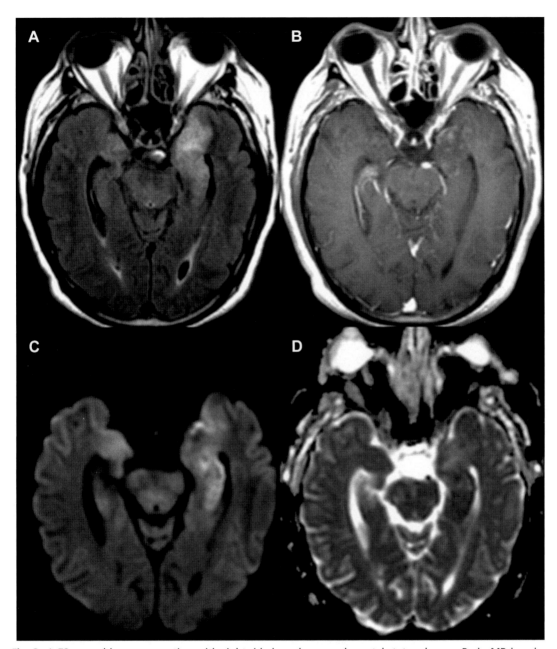

Fig. 3. A 73-year-old man presenting with right-sided weakness and mental status change. Brain MR imaging with FLAIR axial image (*A*) shows abnormal hyperintensity in the medial left temporal lobe, and also minimally in the medial right temporal lobe. Postcontrast T1-weighted axial image (*B*) shows minimal heterogeneous enhancement in the medial left temporal lobe. DWI (*C*) and ADC (*D*) axial images show restricted diffusion in these regions. Findings are consistent with HSV encephalitis confirmed with CSF analysis.

emergency department visits yearly and causing 1319 deaths in 2014.[12] CO poisoning can be accidental or intentional, with approximately 15,000 intentional CO poisonings yearly, which account for about two-thirds of the deaths.[12] CO gas is colorless, odorless, and most commonly produced by incomplete combustion of carbon compounds, with faulty furnaces, fires, and engine exhaust being common sources.[12] Many of the detrimental effects of CO are related to its ability to reduce oxygen delivery to tissues, impair oxidative phosphorylation in cells, and contribute to free radical formation.[12] Damage to the central nervous system in CO poisoning occurs by a combination

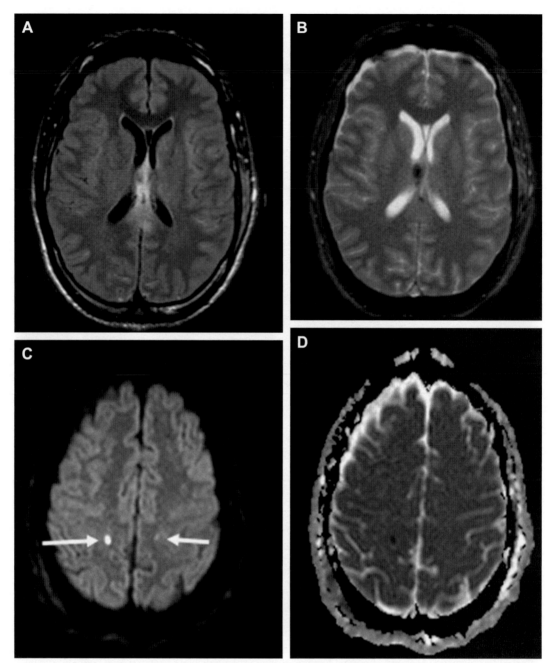

Fig. 4. A 22-year-old man presenting after trauma from high-speed motor vehicle accident. Brain MR imaging with FLAIR (*A*) and gradient recalled echo (GRE) (*B*) images show abnormal hyperintensity of the corpus callosum with susceptibility artifact consistent with hemorrhage. DWI (*C*) and ADC (*D*) images show foci of restricted diffusion (*arrows*) in the bilateral parietal white matter without corresponding susceptibility artifact. Findings are consistent with hemorrhagic and nonhemorrhagic lesions in DAI.

of hypoxic injury and triggered inflammation that leads to oxidative stress, necrosis, apoptosis, and central nervous system demyelination that may be reversible.[13] Central nervous system damage or malfunction from CO poisoning can contribute to observable impaired cognitive function with carboxyhemoglobin (COHb) levels as low as 5%, and long-term sequelae of CO poisoning occur in up to 50% of patients with a COHb of 10%, with a delayed symptom onset of 3 weeks on average.[13] Hyperbaric oxygen therapy is the best currently available therapy for treatment of CO poisoning, with 100% normobaric oxygen therapy being the best option if hyperbaric therapy is not available or during transit to a hyperbaric-capable facility.[12]

MR imaging findings associated with CO poisoning have been known to evolve over time after the initial exposure, with one earlier study describing the typical findings on conventional MR imaging in the acute phase with imaging occurring within the first week of presentation after exposure.[14] This study showed that the globus pallidus was the most common site of abnormal signal, typically with increased T2 signal unless there was increased T1 signal suggesting hemorrhage, and bilateral involvement occurring in nearly 50% of cases involving the globus pallidus[14] (Fig. 5). Areas of increased T2 signal were also seen less commonly in the following areas in

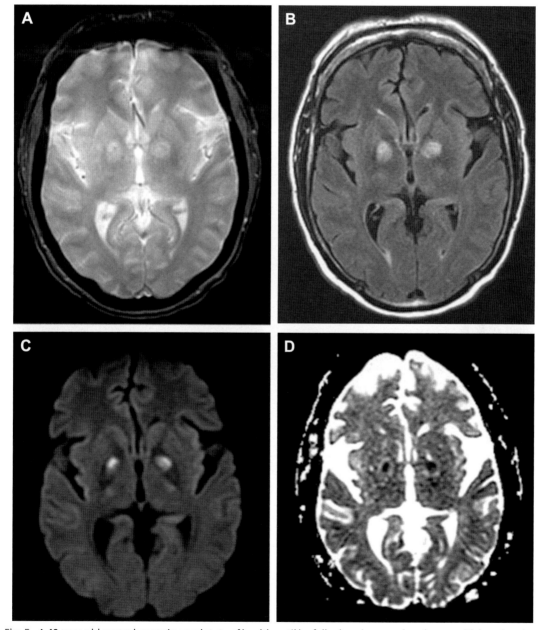

Fig. 5. A 49-year-old man who was in usual state of health until he fell asleep in an enclosed room with burning charcoal for warmth. Patient was found to have altered mental status the following morning. Brain MR imaging with T2-weighted (A) and FLAIR (B) axial images show abnormal hyperintensity in the bilateral globus pallidi, with evidence of restricted diffusion on DWI (C) and ADC (D) axial images. Findings are consistent with acute CO poisoning.

order of decreasing frequency: hemispheric white matter, cerebral cortex not involving the medial temporal lobe in the region of the hippocampus, the medial temporal lobe in the region of the hippocampus, and the cerebellum.[14]

A subsequent review divided imaging findings into ultra-acute (within 24 hours of CO inhalation), acute (24 hours to 7 days after CO inhalation), subacute (7–21 days after CO inhalation), and chronic (≥22 days after CO inhalation), and also described advanced imaging techniques, including DWI.[15] The first finding seen in the globus pallidus in the ultra-acute phase seems to be increased signal on DWI and a reduced apparent diffusion coefficient (ADC), which can be seen before an increase in T2 signal intensity, which may not occur until the acute phase, and notably the DWI signal decreases by the subacute phase, likely caused by necrosis.[15] The globus pallidus can appear small in the chronic phase because of necrosis.[15] The central hemispheric white matter can show increased DWI signal and reduced ADC in the ultra-acute phase, which can persist even into the chronic phase with associated increase in T2 signal that may suggest progressive demyelination.[15] In the chronic phase, atrophy is the main imaging finding to suggest prior gray matter damage from CO poisoning, and atrophy of the cerebral cortex and hippocampus have been commonly reported in patients with persistent neurologic symptoms after CO poisoning.[15]

Opioid Toxicity

The misuse of opioids (fentanyl, methadone, and heroin) is a serious public health problem.[16] Opioid-induced encephalopathy is an acute condition characterized by confusion and delirium with concomitant other neurologic symptoms in the setting of exogenous opioid use, and in the absence of primary structural brain disease.[17,18]

The physiologic and pathophysiologic effects of opioids are attributed to the activation of mu, delta, and kappa opioid receptors throughout the nervous systems.[19] The mechanism of opioid-associated brain injury is not completely understood, but it may be caused by neurotoxicity secondary to hypoxic/ischemic events affecting areas of high energy demand in the brain,[20] such as cardiac arrest or respiratory depression causing hypoxia, ischemia, and pulmonary edema. There is resulting leukoencephalopathy with spongiform changes. However, history of cardiorespiratory arrest is not present in all of the reported cases.[21]

Imaging findings in opioid-induced encephalopathy are characterized by bilateral and symmetric involvement of the globus pallidus and less frequently the medial temporal lobes or cerebellum.[22] For instance, involvement of the globus pallidus has been consistently described in heroin or methadone users, whereas cerebellar involvement has been described in the setting of methadone toxicity and heroin overdose.[23]

These changes are characterized by increased signal intensity on T2 and FLAIR images and decreased signal intensity on T1 images on MR imaging. On DWI, these changes show restricted diffusion caused by cytotoxic edema secondary to ischemic/hypoxic incident affecting these areas of high energy demand (**Fig. 6**). There is usually no mass effect or enhancement of the involved areas. The bilateral and symmetric distribution in addition to the lack of mass effect and the absence of enhancement are usually helpful to rule out other potential causes of restricted diffusion.[1,22,24]

Methotrexate Toxicity

Methotrexate is a main component of many chemotherapeutic regimens for acute lymphoblastic leukemia (ALL) of childhood.[25] Although effective, it can cause significant neurotoxicity characterized clinically by acute or subacute neurologic symptoms, such as seizure, stroke, and behavioral changes, usually occurring within 2 weeks of receiving methotrexate (administered either intravenously or intrathecally).[26]

The exact histologic and pathophysiologic neurotoxicity of methotrexate is unclear. Metabolic encephalopathy including focal demyelination or microinfarctions secondary to direct toxic effects of adenosine accumulation, increased homocysteine levels, or alterations of biopterin metabolism have been described as potential mechanisms leading to cytotoxic edema predominantly in the cerebral white matter.[26–28]

Imaging findings of methotrexate neurotoxicity include white matter T2 and FLAIR hyperintensities within the deep periventricular white matter on MR imaging (**Fig. 7**). These lesions are characterized by increased signal intensity on DWI with decreased signal intensity on the ADC map sequences, indicating cytotoxic edema, as described earlier.[29–31] Methotrexate-induced leukoencephalopathy is not necessarily irreversible; the diffusion abnormalities in acute methotrexate neurotoxicity reflect cerebral dysfunction but not necessarily structural injury.[32,33]

Metronidazole Toxicity

Metronidazole is a commonly used antibiotic for treatment of anaerobic and protozoal

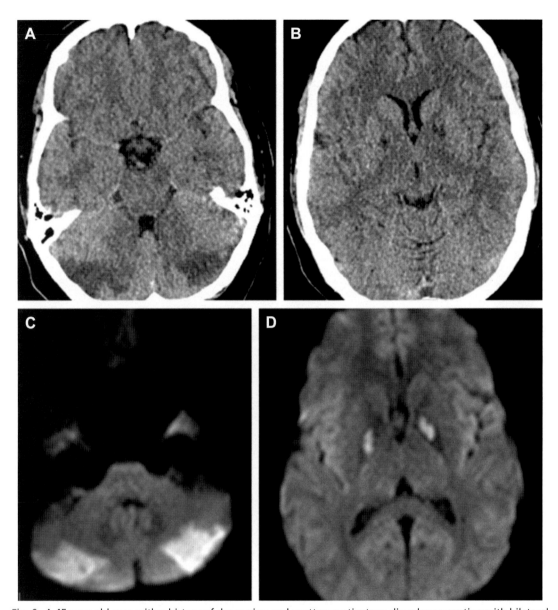

Fig. 6. A 45-year-old man with a history of depression and posttraumatic stress disorder presenting with bilateral lower extremity numbness, unsteady gait, bowel and bladder incontinence, and seizurelike activity. Urine toxicology was positive for cocaine, fentanyl, and opioids. Axial head CT images through the posterior fossa (*A*) and basal ganglia (*B*) show abnormal hypodensity in the bilateral cerebellar hemispheres as well as the bilateral globus pallidi. Brain MR imaging with DWI (*C, D*) images through these same regions show restricted diffusion. Findings are consistent with opioid toxicity.

infections.[34] Metronidazole is known to rarely induce central nervous system toxicity that can manifest as cerebellar dysfunction, altered mental status, and seizure.[35] A review of case reports found no clear association between the duration or dose of metronidazole that resulted in central nervous system toxicity.[35] Treatment of metronidazole-induced central nervous system toxicity is discontinuation of the medication and

supportive care. Almost all patients with metronidazole-induced central nervous system toxicity improve or completely recover after stopping the medication, but it is not always reversible.[35,36]

Alterations of the appearance of the brain on MR imaging in a patient with metronidazole-induced central nervous system toxicity was first described in 1995 and showed symmetric

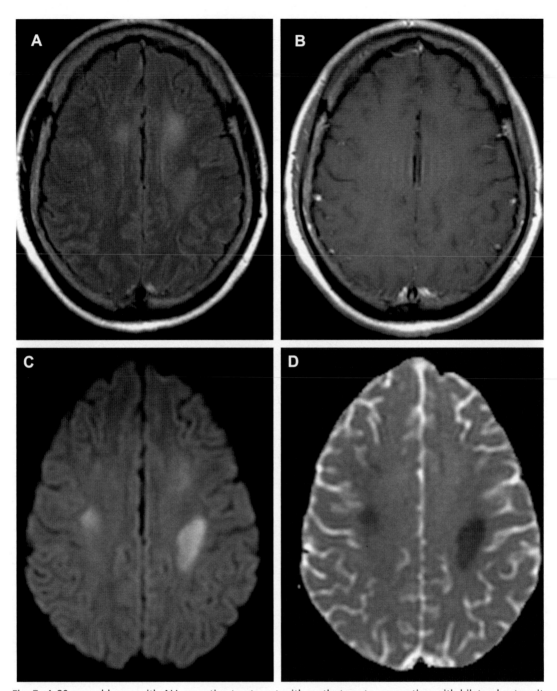

Fig. 7. A 20-year-old man with ALL on active treatment with methotrexate, presenting with bilateral extremity weakness. Brain MR imaging with FLAIR (*A*) and postcontrast T1-weighted (*B*) axial images show abnormal hyperintensity in the bilateral frontoparietal white matter without any enhancement. DWI (*C*) and ADC (*D*) axial images show restricted diffusion. Findings are consistent with methotrexate toxicity.

increased T2 signal within the supratentorial white matter, including the corpus callosum, and within the cerebellum, including the cerebellar deep gray nuclei[34] (**Fig. 8**). Multiple subsequent reports have further delineated the signal abnormalities seen in patients with

metronidazole-induced central nervous system toxicity.[35,37,38] An initial report on DWI signal changes showed increased DWI signal within the dentate nuclei with a corresponding increase in the ADC, which was consistent with T2 shinethrough. A later study of more patients showed

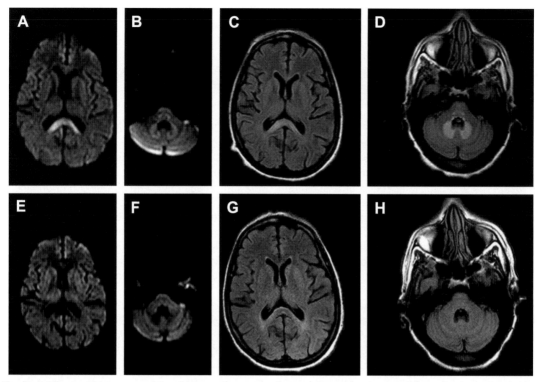

Fig. 8. A 58-year-old woman with a history of recently diagnosed rectal cancer and liver abscesses, presenting with ataxia, nystagmus, dysmetria, dysarthria, and generalized weakness. Brain MR imaging shows DWI hyperintensity in the splenium of the corpus callosum (*A*) and dentate nuclei (*B*), with FLAIR hyperintensity also seen in the splenium of the corpus callosum (*C*) and dentate nuclei (*D*) on initial presentation. After cessation of taking the metronidazole, all symptoms resolved, and follow-up MR imaging showed normalization of the DWI signal in the splenium of the corpus callosum (*E*) and dentate nuclei (*F*) and normalization of the FLAIR signal in the splenium of the corpus callosum (*G*) and dentate nuclei (*H*). Findings are consistent with metronidazole toxicity.

increased DWI signal also occurring in the midbrain (tectum, tegmentum, and red nucleus), medulla (vestibular nuclei of the floor of the forth ventricle), pons (vestibular and abducens nuclei, and superior olivary nucleus), and corpus callosum.[38] Of these areas of increased DWI signal, only the lesions within the corpus callosum showed a reduction in the ADC. Increased T2/FLAIR signal with no corresponding enhancement on T1 postgadolinium images has been reported to involve the dentate nuclei, medulla, pons, midbrain, corpus callosum (splenium most commonly), and occasionally the periventricular and subcortical white matter.[34,35,37,38] Overall the most common location for signal abnormality is the dentate nucleus, which is involved in almost every patient, and the splenium is involved in nearly every patient with corpus callosum involvement.[35,38] The signal abnormalities resolve in most patients after stopping the metronidazole, with 83% of patients showing resolution of signal abnormalities on

follow-up scans 3 days to 3 months after discontinuing the medication.[35]

DEMYELINATING DISEASE
Central Pontine Myelinolysis

Central pontine myelinolysis (CPM) is a noninflammatory demyelinating process commonly involving the pons, and less frequently the basal ganglia and cerebral white matter (known as extrapontine myelinolysis).[39] It is characteristically seen in the setting of rapid correction of hyponatremia in alcoholic and malnourished patients, and less frequently in patients with liver and renal failure, transplant patients, and patients with severe burns.[40] The pathologic mechanism is thought to be caused by the osmotic changes induced by the electrolyte disturbances resulting in vacuolization and subsequent myelinolysis of the oligodendrocytes of the myelin sheaths.[41]

Clinically, CPM is characterized initially by seizure and encephalopathy caused by the hyponatremia followed by spastic quadriparesis/ tetraplegia and pseudobulbar palsy, which occurs few days after the rapid correction of the hyponatremia.[42] The affected areas characteristically involve the central part of the pons with sparing of the pontine tegmentum and the corticospinal tracts, which is helpful to differentiate it from pontine infarct, which has a wedge shape[1] (**Fig. 9**). Because of the increased water content, the affected areas show decreased density on CT scan, increased signal intensity on T2 and FLAIR, and decreased T1 signal intensity on MR imaging. There is usually absence of associated mass effect and no abnormal enhancement.[43] These classic imaging findings are usually not evident within the first 2 weeks of the symptoms' onset. However, DWI is more sensitive to the motion of water and it is reported to identify these changes earlier.[42,44]

The mechanism for diffusion restriction in CPM is not fully understood, but it may be caused by the increase of the intracellular osmolality in the setting of hypernatremia and the subsequent shifting of the water from the hypernatremic extracellular space into the intracellular compartment, resulting in cellular swelling and restricted diffusion.[42,44,45] As with acute ischemic changes, the restricted diffusion in CPM eventually evolves to T2 shine-through effects 2 to 3 weeks following the onset of symptoms.[44]

Tumefactive Demyelination

Tumefactive demyelinating lesions describe lesions with atypical imaging characteristics that make them tumorlike, including large size (>2 cm), mass effect, edema, and ring enhancement.[46–48] Tumefactive lesions are rare, with an incidence of about 1 to 2 per 1000 cases of multiple sclerosis.[49] Presentations of patients with tumefactive demyelinating lesions are nonspecific but typically involve multiple symptoms that most commonly include motor, sensory, and cognitive function deficits.[47,48] Early evidence suggested that patients with initial tumefactive lesions may be unlikely to progress to have additional lesions, but more recent studies suggest that new lesions commonly reoccur and progression of disability

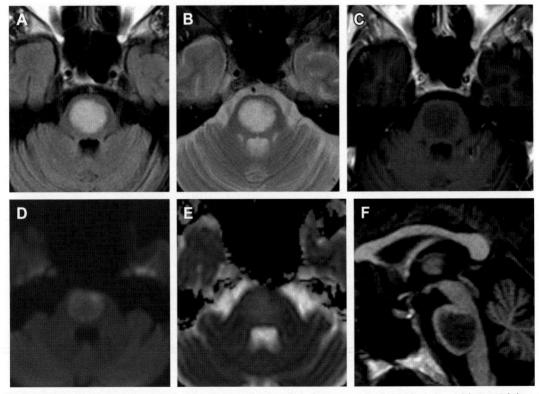

Fig. 9. A 33-year-old man presenting with polyneuropathy of unclear cause. Brain MR imaging with FLAIR (*A*) and T2-weighted (*B*) axial images show abnormal hyperintensity in the central pons, without any enhancement on postcontrast T1-weighted (*C*) axial image. DWI (*D*) and ADC (*E*) axial images show peripheral restricted diffusion. Sagittal T1-weighted (*F*) image shows the lesion diffusely affecting the entire pons. Findings are consistent with CPM.

in patients with tumefactive multiple sclerosis seems to be similar to other forms of multiple sclerosis.[48–50] Treatment of patients with tumefactive demyelinating lesions acutely is usually done with corticosteroids and the addition of plasma exchange (PLEX) therapy if needed.[46] Subsequently, the decision to start disease-modifying medications, such as interferon-beta, is usually contingent on the diagnosis of multiple sclerosis. It is controversial whether the initial tumefactive lesion is enough to establish a diagnosis of multiple sclerosis or whether an additional episode of active demyelination is needed before starting the disease-modifying agents.

Tumefactive lesions are commonly very difficult to distinguish from tumors (such as gliomas and central nervous system lymphoma), abscess, and autoimmune or vasculitic processes.[48,49] The exact definition of tumefactive demyelinating lesions is not standardized, but one previously characterized definition is white matter T2/FLAIR hyperintense lesions greater than 2 cm that may show mass effect and edema.[46] The lesions can show a rim of restricted diffusion on DWI images (Fig. 10). Lesions show significantly lower blood flow on perfusion imaging.[46] Contrast-enhanced T1-weighted images show variable appearances from incomplete or complete ring enhancement, homogeneous enhancement, or punctate enhancement.[46] The open ring pattern of enhancement is more suggestive of a demyelinating lesion than other differential diagnoses.[46] A prior history of multiple sclerosis or multiple additional white matter lesions can help make the diagnosis, but, in the setting of a single lesion with no prior history, biopsy may ultimately be necessary.[46]

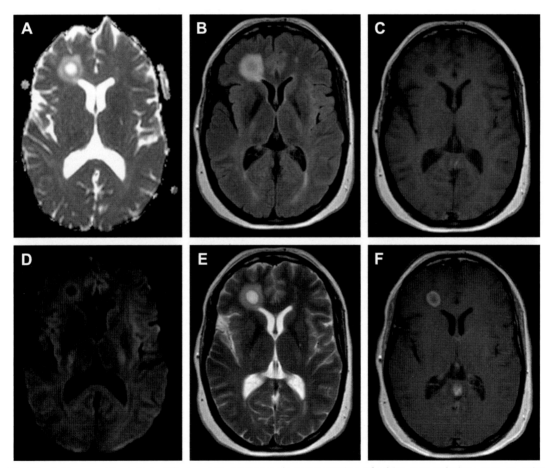

Fig. 10. A 41-year-old woman with no acute symptoms but progression of white matter lesions seen on prior brain MR imaging, being evaluated for possible multiple sclerosis. Brain MR imaging with ADC (*A*), FLAIR (*B*), T1 (*C*) and T2-weighted (*E*) axial images show a hyperintense lesion in the right frontal periventricular white matter, with peripheral restricted diffusion on DWI (*D*) and ring enhancement on postcontrast T1-weighted (*F*) axial images. Findings are consistent with tumefactive demyelinating lesion in the setting of multiple sclerosis.

DEVELOPMENTAL ABNORMALITIES
Epidermoid Cyst

Intracranial epidermoid cysts are congenital lesions resulting from inclusion of ectodermal cells during neural tube closure of embryogenesis,[8,51] comprising up to 1% to 2% of all intracranial neoplasms.[1,51] Acquired intracranial epidermoids are rare but can arise after trauma or surgery. The cerebellopontine angle is the most common location of intracranial epidermoids, followed by the fourth ventricle and sellar region.[1,8,51] Patients are often asymptomatic, with epidermoids detected as an incidental finding. When present, symptoms are usually related to the mass effect exerted by the epidermoid on the adjacent brain.

On MR imaging, epidermoid cysts can appear similar to CSF on all sequences, except for the presence of restricted diffusion (possibly caused by keratinaceous material), a feature that can help differentiate it from arachnoid cysts[1,8,51] (Fig. 11). Enhancement is rare, but can be minimally present; internal FLAIR hyperintensity can also be observed.[51] When large, there can be distortion of the adjacent brain caused by mass effect.

OTHER
Seizure Activity

Seizures correspond with uncontrolled, synchronous neural activity originating in a signal location that can subsequently spread to other regions within the brain.[52] Seizures can be single events or can be recurrent phenomena in the setting of epilepsy.[52] Seizures can arise in abnormal foci of brain tissue or can occur in normal brain tissue when placed under different stressful conditions.[52] Seizures occur commonly, with about 10% of people having a seizure during the course of their lives.[53] Treatment options for seizures range from acute stoppage of a seizure with medications such as benzodiazepines, correction of physiologic abnormalities that lead to seizure development in normal brain, antiepileptic medication to prevent recurrent seizures in abnormal brains, and surgery to remove abnormal tissue sites that trigger seizures.

There are a variety of seizure-related signal abnormalities seen in patients after seizures and these are mostly reversible.[53,54] The most common signal abnormalities are T2/FLAIR increased signal, with the FLAIR sequence being the most

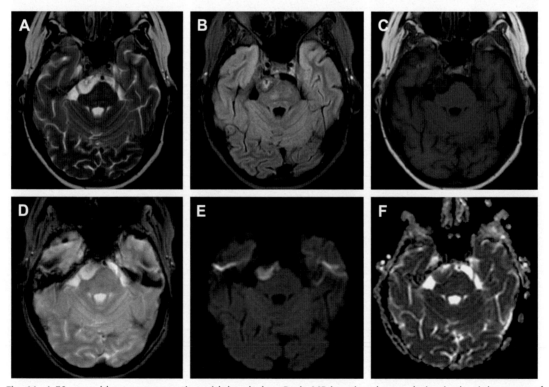

Fig. 11. A 50-year-old woman presenting with headaches. Brain MR imaging shows a lesion in the right aspect of the prepontine cistern that is hyperintense on T2-weighted image (A), heterogeneously isointense to hyperintense on FLAIR (B), hypointense on T1-weighted image (C), without any susceptibility artifact on GRE (D), and with evidence of restricted diffusion on DWI (E) and ADC (F) images. Findings are consistent with an epidermoid cyst.

sensitive. Signal increases range from barely perceptible to intense. There can be mild gadolinium enhancement in areas showing T2/FLAIR hyperintensity.[54] A significant number of areas with T2/FLAIR signal abnormality also show restricted diffusion on DWI (**Fig. 12**). The hippocampus is the most commonly involved brain region with MR signal abnormality; however, related signal abnormality can also be seen in the neocortex, the subcortical white matter, the splenium of the corpus callosum, the basal ganglia, the thalami, and the cerebellum.[53] Signal

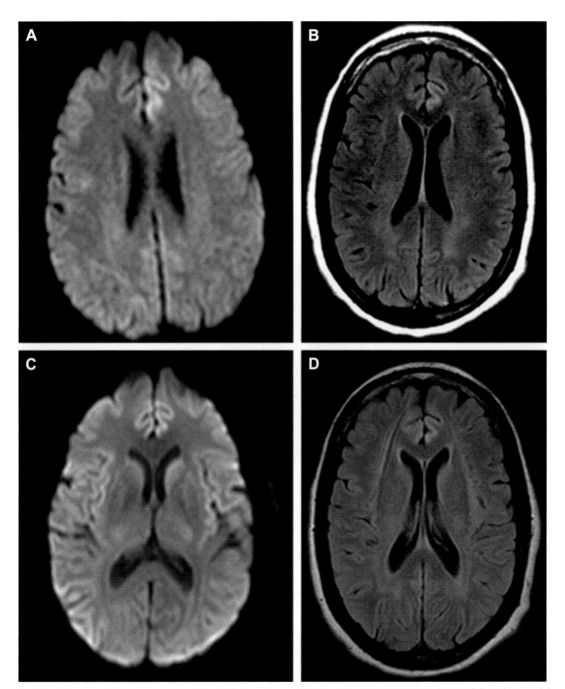

Fig. 12. A 56-year-old woman presenting with recurrent seizures. Brain MR imaging with DWI (*A*) and FLAIR (*B*) axial images show abnormal cortical hyperintensity within the medial aspect of the left frontal lobe and left cingulate gyrus. Follow-up brain MR imaging with DWI (*C*) and FLAIR (*D*) axial images shows resolution of the previously seen signal abnormality. Findings are consistent with seizure-related signal changes.

abnormalities related to seizure activity are usually partially or completely reversible, with residual T2/FLAIR hyperintensity being the most common residual abnormality corresponding with gliosis. Resolution of seizure-related signal abnormalities usually takes months, with one study showing an average time to resolution of about 2 months.[53]

Dural Venous Sinus Thrombosis

Dural venous sinus thrombosis (DVST) is an under-diagnosed entity that can lead to strokes and intra-cranial hemorrhage.[55] DVST can occur in any population, but young women are the most commonly affected, which may be a result of the common risk factors for venous sinus thrombosis being present in this group.[55] The immediate post-partum period, oral hormonal contraception, and coagulation disorders (factor V Leiden most commonly) are the main risk factors for this dis-ease process.[55] Malignancies, hematologic disor-ders, systemic autoimmune diseases, and vasculitides are all lesser risk factors.[55] Headache

is the most common feature in the clinical presen-tation, with nausea, vomiting, altered level of con-sciousness, and less commonly focal neurologic deficits all occurring.[55] The gold standard for diag-nosis is digital subtraction angiography, but MR venogram (MRV) and CT venogram (CTV) have acceptable accuracy to be used as noninvasive means of assessment.[56] In addition, many stan-dard (non-MRV) MR imaging sequences can be useful in diagnosis.[56] The mainstay of treatment is anticoagulation with heparin, and endovascular intervention may be a consideration for high-risk cases or cases that are failing management with just anticoagulation, but the efficacy and role of endovascular intervention are not well established.[56]

At present, the diagnostic imaging studies of choice for DVST are contrast-enhanced MRV and CTV with both showing excellent sensi-tivity and specificity for the diagnosis.[56,57] Stan-dard (non-MRV) sequences on MR imaging, including unenhanced T1-weighted, T2-weighted, DWI, FLAIR, gradient recalled echo (GRE),

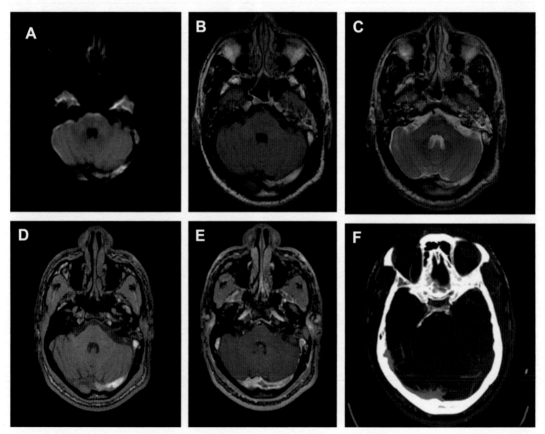

Fig. 13. A 37-year-old man with epilepsy presenting with headaches. Brain MR imaging with DWI (*A*), FLAIR (*B*), and T2-weighted (*C*) axial images shows abnormal hyperintense signal in the left transverse and sigmoid sinuses, with associated hyperintensity on T1-weighted image (*D*), and corresponding filling defect on postcontrast 3D T1-weighted image (*E*). Findings are consistent with acute DVST, confirmed with CT venogram (*F*).

T1-weighted contrast-enhanced, and three-dimensional (3D) T1-weighted contrast-enhanced sequences, can have outstanding sensitivity (99% in 1 study) but low specificity (14%–18%).[57] Another study of the overall suggestion of venous sinus thrombosis based on all imaging sequences except for dedicated venograms showed higher specificity (89.9%) but significantly lower sensitivity (79.2%).[58] Differences between the two studies are likely related to use of abnormal signal on a single imaging sequence resulting in high sensitivity but low specificity, whereas findings of abnormal signal on multiple sequences increase specificity but decrease sensitivity. 3D T1-weighted contrast-enhanced imaging has the highest sensitivity for detection of DVST compared with the other sequences, with a sensitivity of 94% to 97%.[57] GRE sequence has been suggested to have the highest sensitivity for detecting DVST of the nonenhanced sequences by some studies, but this is not a consistent finding.[57] DVST causes an increase in signal in the dural venous sinuses on unenhanced T1-weighted, T2-weighted, DWI, and FLAIR imaging, and decreased signal or blooming on GRE[57] (**Fig. 13**). Filling defects or low signal on T1-weighted contrast-enhanced sequences are suggestive of DVST.[57]

SUMMARY

MR imaging in the emergency setting is most commonly used to diagnose acute stroke, with the DWI sequence playing an important role. There are, however, several other different disorders that can show diffusion abnormality (infection, toxic/metabolic, trauma, seizures), which, in conjunction with other sequences, should be promptly recognized for timely patient management.

REFERENCES

1. O'Connor KM, Barest G, Moritani T, et al. "Dazed and diffused": making sense of diffusion abnormalities in neurologic pathologies. Br J Radiol 2013; 86:20130599.

2. Nathoo N, Nadvi SS, Narotam PK, et al. Brain abscess: management and outcome analysis of a computed tomography era experience with 973 patients. World Neurosurg 2011;75(5–6):716–26 [discussion: 612–7].

3. Villanueva-Meyer JE, Cha S. From shades of gray to microbiologic imaging: a historical review of brain abscess imaging. Radiographics 2015;35(5):1555–62.

4. Hartmann M, Jansen O, Heiland S, et al. Restricted diffusion within ring enhancement is not pathognomonic for brain abscess. AJNR Am J Neuroradiol 2001;22(9):1738–42.

5. Saini J, Gupta RK, Jain KK. Intracranial infections: key neuroimaging findings. Semin Roentgenol 2014;49(1):86–98.

6. Hsu DP. Imaging of infections of the brain and meninges. Semin Roentgenol 2010;45(2):80–91.

7. Raschilas F, Wolff M, Delatour F, et al. Outcome of and prognostic factors for herpes simplex encephalitis in adult patients: results of a multicenter study. Clin Infect Dis 2002;35:254–60.

8. Karaarslan E, Arslan A. Diffusion weighted MR imaging in non-infarct lesions of the brain. Eur J Radiol 2008;65(3):402–16.

9. Hergan K, Schaefer PW, Sorensen AG, et al. Diffusion-weighted MRI in diffuse axonal injury of the brain. Eur Radiol 2002;12(10):2536–41.

10. Parizel PM, Ozsarlak O, Van Goethem JW, et al. Imaging findings in diffuse axonal injury after closed head trauma. Eur Radiol 1998;8(6):960–5.

11. Kinoshita T, Moritani T, Hiwatashi A, et al. Conspicuity of diffuse axonal injury lesions on diffusion-weighted MR imaging. Eur J Radiol 2005;56(1): 5–11.

12. Rose JJ, Wang L, Xu Q, et al. Carbon monoxide poisoning: pathogenesis, management, and future directions of therapy. Am J Respir Crit Care Med 2017;195(5):596–606.

13. Sykes OT, Walker E. The neurotoxicology of carbon monoxide – historical perspective and review. Cortex 2016;74:440–8.

14. O'Donnell P, Buxton PJ, Pitkin A, et al. The magnetic resonance imaging appearances of the brain in acute carbon monoxide poisoning. Clin Radiol 2000;55(4):273–80.

15. Beppu T. The role of MR imaging in assessment of brain damage from carbon monoxide poisoning: a review of the literature. Am J Neuroradiol 2014; 35(4):625–31.

16. Rudd RA, Seth P, David F, et al. Increases in drug and opioid-involved overdose deaths - United States, 2010–2015. MMWR Morb Mortal Wkly Rep 2016;65(5051):1445–52.

17. Hansen N. Drug-induced encephalopathy. In: Tanasescu R, editor. Miscellanea on encephalopathies - a second look. InTech; 2012. p. 39–60.

18. Chen R, Young GB. Metabolic encephalopathies. Baillieres Clin Neurol 1996;5(3):577–98.

19. Leppa M, Korvenoja A, Carlson S, et al. Acute opioid effects on human brain as revealed by functional magnetic resonance imaging. Neuroimage 2006; 31(2):661–9.

20. Ammon-Treiber S, Stolze D, Schroder H, et al. Effects of opioid antagonists and morphine in a hippocampal hypoxia/hypoglycemia model. Neuropharmacology 2005;49(8):1160–9.

21. Chen Q, Lu JY, Lu BX, et al. Roles of cyclooxygenase 2/2', 3'-cyclic nucleotide3' phosphohydrolase in the oligodendrocyte apoptosis in heroin-induced

spongiform leucoencephalopathy. Zhonghua Yi Xue Za Zhi 2008;88(25):1742–5.

22. Offiah C, Hall E. Heroin-induced leukoencephalopathy: characterization using MRI, diffusion-weighted imaging, and MR spectroscopy. Clin Radiol 2008;63(2): 146–52.

23. Morales Odia Y, Jinka M, Ziai WC. Severe leukoencephalopathy following acute oxycodone intoxication. Neurocrit Care 2010;13(1):93–7.

24. Bega DS, McDaniel LM, Jhaveri MD, et al. Diffusion weighted imaging in heroin-associated spongiform leukoencephalopathy. Neurocrit Care 2009;10(3): 352–4.

25. Mantadakis E, Cole PD, Kamen BA. High-dose methotrexate in acute lymphoblastic leukemia: where is the evidence for its continued use? Pharmacotherapy 2005;25(5):748–55.

26. Bhojwani D, Sabin ND, Pei D, et al. Methotrexate-induced neurotoxicity and leukoencephalopathy in childhood acute lymphoblastic leukemia. J Clin Oncol 2014;32(9):949–59.

27. Mahoney DH Jr, Shuster JJ, Nitschke R, et al. Acute neurotoxicity in children with B-precursor acute lymphoid leukemia: an association with intermediate-dose intravenous methotrexate and intrathecal triple therapy: a Pediatric Oncology Group study. J Clin Oncol 1998;16(5):1712–22.

28. Bernini JC, Fort DW, Griener JC, et al. Aminophylline for methotrexate-induced neurotoxicity. Lancet 1995;345(8949):544–7.

29. Rollins N, Winick N, Bash R, et al. Acute methotrexate neurotoxicity: findings on diffusion-weighted imaging and correlation with clinical outcome. AJNR Am J Neuroradiol 2004;25(10):1688–95.

30. Fisher MJ, Khademian ZP, Zimmerman RA, et al. Diffusion-weighted MR imaging of early methotrexate-related neurotoxicity in children. AJNR Am J Neuroradiol 2005;26(7):1686–9.

31. Inaba H, Khan RB, Laningham FH, et al. Clinical and radiological characteristics of methotrexate-induced acute encephalopathy in pediatric patients with cancer. Ann Oncol 2008;19(1):178–84.

32. Baehring JM, Fulbright RK. Delayed leukoencephalopathy with stroke-like presentation in chemotherapy recipients. J Neurol Neurosurg Psychiatry 2008;79(5):535–9.

33. Manousakis G, Hsu D, Diamond CA, et al. Teaching NeuroImages: methotrexate leukoencephalopathy mimicking a transient ischemic attack. Neurology 2010;75(7):e34.

34. Ahmed A, Loes DJ, Bressler EL. Reversible magnetic resonance imaging findings in metronidazole-induced encephalopathy. Neurology 1995;45(3 Pt 1):588–9.

35. Kuriyama A, Jackson JL, Doi A, et al. Metronidazole-induced central nervous system toxicity. Clin Neuropharmacol 2011;34(6):241–7.

36. Hobbs K, Stern-Nezer S, Buckwalter MS, et al. Metronidazole-induced encephalopathy: not always a reversible situation. Neurocrit Care 2015;22(3): 429–36.

37. Heaney CJ, Campeau NG, Lindell EP. MR imaging and diffusion-weighted imaging changes in metronidazole (Flagyl)–induced cerebellar toxicity. AJNR Am J Neuroradiol 2003;24(8):1615–7.

38. Kim E, Na DG, Kim EY, et al. MR imaging of metronidazole-induced encephalopathy: lesion distribution and diffusion-weighted imaging findings. AJNR Am J Neuroradiol 2007;28(9): 1652–8.

39. Lampl C, Yazdi K. Central pontine myelinolysis. Eur Neurol 2002;47(1):3–10.

40. McKee AC, Winkelman MD, Banker BQ. Central pontine myelinolysis in severely burned patients: relationship to serum hyperosmolality. Neurology 1988;38(8):1211–7.

41. Norenberg MD. A hypothesis of osmotic endothelial injury: a pathogenetic mechanism in central pontine myelinolysis. Arch Neurol 1983;40(2):66–9.

42. RuzekK A, Campeau NG, Miller GM. Early diagnosis of central pontine myelinolysis with diffusion weighted imaging. AJNR Am J Neuroradiol 2004; 25(2):210–3.

43. Chua GC, Sitoh YY, Lim CC, et al. MR findings in osmotic myelinolysis. Clin Radiol 2002;57(9):800–6.

44. Cramer SC, Stegbauer KC, Schneider A. Decreased diffusion in central pontine myelinolysis. AJNR Am J Neuroradiol 2001;22(8):1476–9.

45. Chu K, Kang DW, Ko SB. Diffusion-weighted MR findings of central pontine and extrapontine myelinolysis. Acta Neurol Scand 2001;104(6): 385–8.

46. Algahtani H, Shirah B, Alassiri A. Tumefactive demyelinating lesions: a comprehensive review. Mult Scler Relat Disord 2017;14:72–9.

47. Lucchinetti CF, Gavrilova RH, Metz I, et al. Clinical and radiographic spectrum of pathologically confirmed tumefactive multiple sclerosis. Brain 2008;131(7):1759–75.

48. Lin X, Yu W-Y, Liauw L, et al. Clinicoradiologic features distinguish tumefactive multiple sclerosis from CNS neoplasms. Neurol Clin Pract 2017;7(1): 53–64.

49. Tremblaya MA, Villanueva-Meyer JE, Cha S, et al. Clinical and imaging correlation in patients with pathologically confirmed tumefactive demyelinating lesions. J Neurol Sci 2017;381:83–7.

50. Totaro R, Di Carmine C, Splendiani A, et al. Occurrence and long-term outcome of tumefactive demyelinating lesions in multiple sclerosis. Neurol Sci 2016;37(7):1113–7.

51. Osborn AG, Preece MT. Intracranial cysts: radiologic-pathologic correlation and imaging approach. Radiology 2006;239(3):650–64.

52. Jirsa VK, Stacey WC, Quilichini PP, et al. On the nature of seizure dynamics. Brain 2014;137(Pt 8): 2210–30.

53. Cianfoni A, Caulo M, Cerase A, et al. Seizure-induced brain lesions: a wide spectrum of variably reversible MRI abnormalities. Eur J Radiol 2013; 82(11):1964–72.

54. Ong B, Bergin P, Heffernan T, et al. Transient seizure-related MRI abnormalities. J Neuroimaging 2009;19(4):301–10.

55. Weimar C. Diagnosis and treatment of cerebral venous and sinus thrombosis. Curr Neurol Neurosci Rep 2014;14(1):417.

56. Ferro JM, Bousser M-G, Canhão P, et al. European Stroke Organization guideline for the diagnosis and treatment of cerebral venous thrombosis – Endorsed by the European Academy of Neurology. Eur Stroke J 2017;2(3):195–221.

57. Sadigh G, Mullins ME, Saindane AM. Diagnostic performance of MRI sequences for evaluation of dural venous sinus thrombosis. AJR Am J Roentgenol 2016;206(6):1298–306.

58. Patel D, Machnowska M, Symons S, et al. Diagnostic performance of routine brain MRI sequences for dural venous sinus thrombosis. AJNR Am J Neuroradiol 2016;37(11):2026–32.

Emergent Neuroimaging in the Oncologic and Immunosuppressed Patient

Christopher A. Potter, MD[a,b],*, Liangge Hsu, MD[b]

KEYWORDS

- Emergency • Neuroimaging • Oncologic • Immunosuppressed • Infection • HIV • Cerebritis
- Meningitis

KEY POINTS

- Intracranial hemorrhage risk is increased in patients with melanoma, lung, breast, and renal cell carcinoma; high-grade glioma; leukemia; and in hematopoietic stem cell transplant with thrombocytopenia.
- Both intracranial metastases and primary brain tumors increase the risk of cerebral infarction.
- Imaging findings in immunosuppressed patients with infection may be atypical, and significant enhancement and edema may be absent if the patient is unable to mount an appropriate immune response.
- Meningitis is the most frequent intracranial infection in immunosuppressed patients and patients with cancer, and may be complicated by hydrocephalus or subdural empyema.
- Of the many medication-related chemotherapy complications, tacrolimus and cyclosporine A are associated with increased risk of seizure and posterior reversible encephalopathy syndrome.

INTRODUCTION

As the population in North America ages and treatments improve for many malignancies and chronic diseases, the neuroimaging performed in the emergency department increasingly involves patients at increased risk for acute neurologic complications from malignancy and immunosuppression. This includes patients with known malignancy and those who are immunosuppressed because of organ transplantation, chronic disease (eg, diabetes mellitus) or treatment of chronic disease, and human immunodeficiency virus (HIV) positivity. These patients are susceptible to the same infections and emergencies as immunocompetent patients, but may present differently with common illnesses and are susceptible to a variety of other diseases. New drug therapies for these patients introduce new potential neurologic complications or increase their frequency. In addition, the timely availability of important clinical information for the radiologist has often not kept pace with patient disease complexity, although it is essential to imaging interpretation to provide a more accurate and customized diagnosis and treatment. This article reviews important patient risk factors, emergent central nervous system (CNS) abnormalities, and their imaging findings to help optimize imaging in this complex group of patients.

Disclosure Statement: The authors have nothing to disclose.
[a] Emergency Division, Department of Radiology, Brigham and Women's Hospital, 75 Francis Street, Boston, MA 02115, USA; [b] Neuroradiology Division, Department of Radiology, Brigham and Women's Hospital, 75 Francis Street, Boston, MA 02115, USA
* Corresponding author. 75 Francis Street, Boston, MA 02115.
E-mail address: cpotter3@bwh.harvard.edu

neuroimaging.theclinics.com

IMAGING APPROACH

In general, noncontrast head computed tomography (CT) is the initial imaging study for acute intracranial abnormalities because of its sensitivity, rapidity of image acquisition, and availability. Although CT may not be specific enough to definitively diagnose some acute intracranial processes, it remains an excellent triage tool and allows for rapid disposition in the emergency department at a low cost. Noncontrast CT is almost always the initial modality, with intravenous contrast reserved for imaging maxillofacial infections and masses, and for imaging patients unable to undergo MR imaging.

MR imaging is more sensitive and specific for most emergent intracranial abnormalities, although less suited as a first-line imaging modality because of the time required to perform the imaging, MR compatibility, cost, and availability. Increased availability of MR imaging in the emergency department and development of shorter protocols for acute imaging will improve the ease of use of MR imaging as a first-line imaging modality in the near future.

For acute imaging of the spine, radiography and CT are helpful for evaluation of new back pain, especially in the setting of trauma. In patients with suspected cord compression, MR is a much more sensitive and specific modality for epidural masses that can cause spinal canal narrowing obscured on CT.

In patients with known malignancy, MR imaging of the head and spine are performed with intravenous contrast at the authors' institution. The brain MR imaging includes a postcontrast spin echo sequence and thin section axial three-dimensional postcontrast images with coronal and sagittal reformations. In the absence of known malignancy, imaging in patients with altered mental status and back pain are usually performed without intravenous contrast. MR angiography of the circle of Willis is performed without intravenous contrast and MR angiography of the neck with contrast, unless contraindicated.

CEREBRAL HERNIATION AND INTRACRANIAL HEMORRHAGE

Because of limited intracranial volume, many intracranial abnormalities can lead to increased intracranial pressure. When acute, this causes rapid effacement of the extra-axial spaces, midline shift, and cerebral herniation, resulting in altered mental status, cardiovascular collapse, and even death.

There are three cerebral herniation syndromes (subfalcine, uncal, and transtentorial) and all may occur simultaneously depending on the location of the lesion and extent of mass effect. Parafacine herniation can compress the anterior cerebral artery against the falx, causing occlusion and infarction. Uncal herniation typically presents as third nerve palsy and can progress to hemiplegia and respiratory failure as brainstem is compressed. Transtentorial herniation, either downward or less commonly upward from posterior fossa lesions, causes altered mental status, and can progress to coma and death. Initial imaging in these cases is almost always noncontrast CT of the head because of patient instability and altered mental status.[1]

In oncologic patients, increased intracranial pressure and cerebral herniation is most commonly caused by a combination of cerebral edema and tumor enlargement from either primary brain or metastatic malignancy. Symptomatic intracranial metastatic disease occurs in approximately 8% to 10% of all patients with cancer and is more common by an order of magnitude.[2,3] Intracranial metastases are typically seen in lung (16%–19%), renal cell (6%–10%), breast (5%), melanoma (7%), and colorectal carcinomas (2%).[4] With advances in cancer treatment, however, malignancies that were not historically prone to metastasize to the brain, such as prostate cancer, are now occurring more frequently because of improved life expectancy.

In addition to mass effect from underlying disease, hemorrhage in this population can also cause cerebral herniation. Tumor hemorrhage is more common in melanoma, lung and breast cancers, renal cell carcinoma, high-grade glioma, and leukemia. The risk of intracranial hemorrhage is particularly high in patients with acute myeloid leukemia because of hyperleukocytosis, with subdural hemorrhage being one of the most common intracranial complications in this group.[5] Patients undergoing allogenic or autologous stem cell transplantation with prolonged thrombocytopenia are also at increased risk of intracranial hemorrhage. Other causes of intracranial hemorrhage in patients with cancer include vascular injury following radiotherapy and hemorrhage caused by development of secondary cavernomas, often years after whole-brain radiation.

SEIZURE AND POSTERIOR REVERSIBLE ENCEPHALOPATHY SYNDROME

Seizure is common in patients with cancer and has many causes, such as tumor itself, chemotherapy with or without posterior reversible encephalo-pathy syndrome (PRES), acute and long-term sequelae of whole-brain radiation, and brain surgery.[2] Hemorrhagic and nonhemorrhagic infarcts, infection caused by immunosuppression, para-neoplastic syndromes, and systemic metabolic abnormalities are less common causes of seizure. Multiple chemotherapy medications are known to cause seizures, with cyclosporine and tacrolimus being the most common drugs requiring antiepi-leptic therapy.

Status epilepticus is a neurologic emergency that must be treated to prevent permanent neuro-logic injury. The presence of nonconvulsive status epilepticus, however, can be masked by other conditions with altered sensorium and the complexity of the medical condition of many pa-tients with cancer and immunosuppressed pa-tients can lead to delay in diagnosis.[6] Optimal seizure treatment is an important issue in the man-agement of patients with intracranial malignancy because of the frequency of seizures in these pa-tients and its effect on their quality of life, including their end-of-life care.[2]

Imaging findings of seizure are subtle on CT and if evident, appears as subtle gyral expansion with mass effect. They are better seen on MR imaging as increased T2 and fluid-attenuated inversion recovery (FLAIR) signal with or without diffusion-weighted imaging (DWI) abnormality that involves the cortex, the deep gray nuclei, or both. There are often multiple foci of involve-ment and the areas of abnormality may also migrate in the setting of recurrent seizure. In fact, MR imaging abnormalities may be seen at remote sites from the seizure focus. MR imaging findings are transient or permanent depending on the location, duration, and severity of the seizure. Mass effect from seizure is commonly mild, although more mass-like expansion of the gyri can occur and may occasionally be mistaken for tumor. Seizure may also occur in the setting of hypoglycemia caused by neuroendocrine tu-mors or overtreatment of diabetes mellitus, man-ifesting as symmetrically increased FLAIR and DWI signal in the deep gray matter and cortex with occasional white matter involvement. Reduced diffusivity in the setting of hypoglyce-mia can be reversible.

Patients with PRES can present with head-ache, visual symptoms, seizures, and encepha-lopathy, which can occur in patients treated with chemotherapy and immunosuppressive drugs, most commonly calcineurin inhibitors (cyclosporine A, tacrolimus). Transplantation it-self is a possible independent risk factor. The risk of PRES in solid organ transplantation is low, only 0.5%,[7–9] whereas the risk in allogenic stem cell transplantation is much higher, esti-mated at 7% to 9%, with even higher risk in pa-tients undergoing high-dose myeloablative preconditioning. Some studies have reported that the frequency of PRES is greatest in the first 3 months after transplantation, but this is not consistently reported in the literature. The list of drugs associated with PRES is long, including the common medications cytarabine, cisplatin, gemcitabine, bevacizumab, and calcineurin in-hibitors.[8,10] Removal of the offending agent usu-ally reverses the syndrome, although permanent damage can still occur. CT and MR imaging clas-sically show symmetric areas of white matter ab-normality at the parieto-occipital junction, although the findings on CT may also be subtle or absent (Fig. 1). Associated subarachnoid hem-orrhage and less often parenchymal hemorrhage are seen in a minority of cases (10%–17%).[11,12] Untreated PRES can involve the cortex and progress to infarction. Less typical findings in un-treated PRES on MR imaging include associated areas of cytotoxic edema with diffusion restric-tion, and involvement of the deep gray matter, cerebellum, and brainstem. Enhancement is rare, but leptomeningeal and parenchymal enhancement have been reported, although the pattern of enhancement does not reflect known risk factors or patient outcome.[13] A unilateral variant seen in approximately 3% of cases can appear tumefactive and may be mistaken for malignancy.[11]

INFARCT

Stroke is a common problem in the age group of most patients with cancer and the risk of ischemic infarct is increased over baseline in this population. A recent study showed an increased short-term risk of ischemic stroke with a hazard ratio of 1.9 for all patients with cancer compared with control subjects. Stroke risk tends to increase with stage of dis-ease, tumor burden, and type of malignancy, with lung, gastric, and pancreatic cancers hav-ing a higher baseline risk. The odds of death were increased for those with ischemic stroke in the setting of malignancy, carrying a three-fold increased hazard over matched control subjects.[14]

Moreover, it has long been recognized that pa-tients with brain tumors and patients undergoing brain surgery are at increased risk for throm-boembolic events for reasons that remain contro-versial. A recent study demonstrated an elevated recurrent stroke risk in patients with primary brain

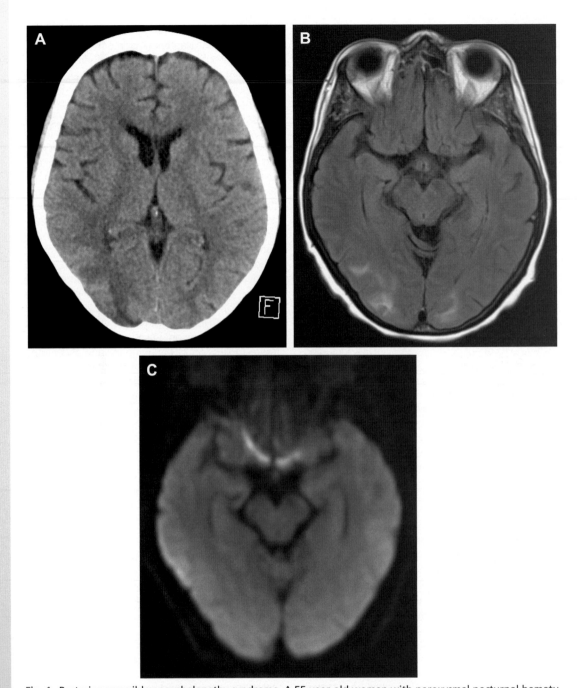

Fig. 1. Posterior reversible encephalopathy syndrome. A 55-year-old woman with paroxysmal nocturnal hematuria treated with eculizumab and allogenic bone marrow transplant, complicated by failure to engraft, pancytopenia, and acute kidney injury presented with altered mental status. Noncontrast CT shows parieto-occipital white matter hypodensities bilaterally (*A*). MR imaging brain demonstrates parieto-occipital lobe white matter hyperintensity on FLAIR (*B*) without corresponding reduced diffusivity (*C*) or abnormal enhancement (not shown), consistent with PRES. Her tacrolimus was changed to sirolimus and her mental status subsequently returned to baseline.

tumors, similar to that with other malignancies.[15] The stroke mechanisms in patients with treated brain tumors may be different than in other malignancies, because radiation vasculopathy and surgical intervention seem to play a larger role (**Fig. 2**).[15]

In patients with malignancy, the increased risk of thromboembolism caused by treatment is difficult

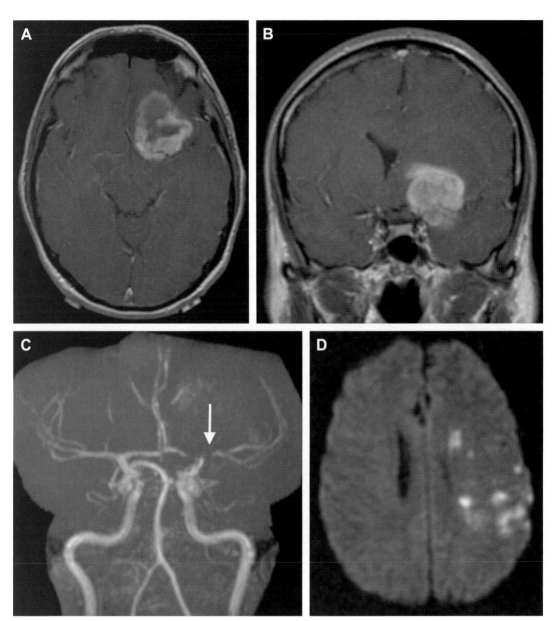

Fig. 2. Glioblastoma multiforme causing infarct. A 47-year-old man with 2 months of frontal headaches who was diagnosed with glioblastoma multiforme and treated with chemoradiation. He developed acute right-sided weakness and aphasia 2 months post-treatment. Axial and coronal postcontrast images show the tumor in the region of the M1 segment of the left middle cerebral artery (MCA) with central necrosis (*A*, *B*). MR angiography three-dimensional MIP images (*C*) show the irregular narrowing throughout the M1 segment of the left MCA caused by tumor encasement (*arrow*). There are multiple foci of reduced diffusivity on DWI in the left MCA distribution caused by embolic infarct from the luminal narrowing (*D*).

to separate from the underlying risk caused by malignancy.[16] Gemcytabine and platinum-based agents, such as cisplatin, thalidomide, and vascular endothelial growth factor receptor–targeted therapies, such as bevacizumab, are associated with increased thromboembolic risk. Risk factors for vascular events on vascular endothelial growth factor treatment include prior thrombotic event and patient age greater than 65 years.[16] In patients treated with newer multi-targeted tyrosine kinase inhibitors (dasatinib, nilotinib, ponatinib), usually for hematologic malignancy, increased risk of arterial cerebrovascular occlusion has also been reported.[17]

Increased stroke risk associated with protease inhibitor use has become an important issue with the aging of HIV-positive patients. HIV positivity itself seems to be an independent risk factor for stroke, particularly in younger HIV-positive patients, although the exact risk is still not well defined.[18–21]

INFECTIOUS AND CARCINOMATOUS MENINGITIS

In patients with cancer the most frequent intracranial infection is bacterial meningitis, with most having undergone neurosurgery for intracranial disease. Bacterial infection is seen in only 0.8% to 1.5% of surgeries.[22] Although meningitis and ventriculitis following ventricular catheter placement occurs more often, in 4% to 17% of patients, most are treated presumptively without imaging evaluation. Corticosteroid treatment, surgical intervention, and radiotherapy all increase the risk of infection (Fig. 3).

Patients undergoing hematopoietic transplant for hematologic malignancy or other causes are susceptible to fungal meningitis, particularly patients with acute myeloid leukemia or myelodysplastic syndrome during induction chemotherapy, and allogenic stem cell transplant patients because of prolonged neutropenia.[22] Patients with indwelling catheters, on long-term corticosteroids, and solid organ transplant patients are also at increased risk for fungal meningitis. Mortality remains high despite modern antifungal treatment.[22] Cryptococcus is the most common fungal agent that causes meningitis in the immunosuppressed patient, with Candida being an important, but less frequent cause of meningitis.

HIV-positive patients are susceptible to a wide range of intracranial infections depending on their state of immunosuppression, with cryptococcal meningitis being the most common infection (Fig. 4).[23] Mycobacterium tuberculosis and neurosyphilis are less common, but important causes of basilar meningitis, which can lead to vasculitis and infarct. Histoplasmosis may cause disseminated disease in HIV-positive patients with uncontrolled disease, but CNS involvement is uncommon, occurring in only 5% to 10% of these patients.[24]

Leptomeningeal carcinomatosis occurs in approximately 5% to 8% of patients with cancer, more frequently in lung and breast cancer, melanoma, B-cell lymphoma, and acute lymphoblastic leukemia. Primary CNS tumors rarely involve the leptomeninges, with glioblastoma multiforme being the most frequent (Fig. 5).[25,26]

Meningitis on CT tends to be subtle and often hydrocephalus is present. MR imaging, however, is much more sensitive and specific for neoplastic and infectious meningitis. Contrast should be administered to increase sensitivity for detecting abnormal leptomeningeal enhancement, especially around the brainstem, cranial nerves, and cerebellar folia. On noncontrast MR imaging, FLAIR hyperintensity may be seen in the sulci, but is dependent on the number of cells and debris in the cerebrospinal fluid (CSF) spaces and evaluation of the basilar cisterns is often limited because of flow artifact. Leptomeningeal carcinomatosis may appear more nodular and irregularly thickened compared with infectious meningitis, but they usually cannot be definitively differentiated on imaging and definitive diagnosis usually requires CSF analysis.

Complications of infectious or carcinomatous meningitis include subdural empyema and hydrocephalus. Subdural empyema can arise de novo or because of surgical intervention, but it is more often caused by spread of infectious meningitis. On imaging, a peripherally enhancing subdural fluid collection is seen with dural and leptomeningeal enhancement. As in bacterial intracranial abscess, decreased diffusivity is present in subdural empyema, but this finding is not as definitive as in cerebral abscess, because subdural hemorrhage may also have abnormal DWI signal caused by blood product decomposition.

Communicating hydrocephalus is a frequent complication of infectious and neoplastic meningitis or sequelae from subarachnoid hemorrhage, leading to impaired CSF absorption. In patients with intracranial malignancy, direct compression by tumor at the cerebral aqueduct or fourth ventricle can also result in noncommunicating hydrocephalus with similar results. Longstanding hydrocephalus tends to cause dilation of the cerebral ventricles without acute effects, whereas acute obstruction leads to altered mental status within hours with only mild increase in ventricular size. CT demonstrates ventricular dilation with or without an obstructing lesion and may show periventricular white matter hypodensity from subependymal leakage of CSF. MR imaging is much more sensitive for subependymal leakage, demonstrating confluent periventricular white matter T2/FLAIR hyperintensity. CT and MR imaging findings in this setting should not be mistaken for chronic microvascular disease of the white matter. Comparison studies are most helpful in either modality to demonstrate the acuity and temporal course of the ventricular dilation (Fig. 6).

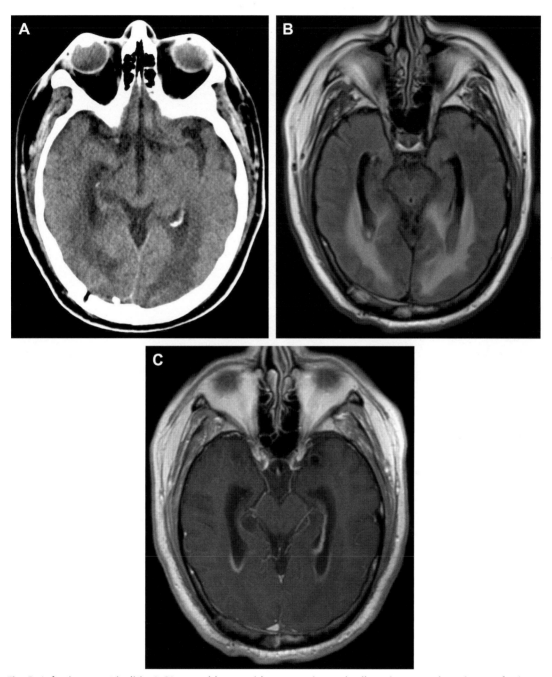

Fig. 3. Infectious ventriculitis. A 61-year-old man with metastatic renal cell carcinoma and craniotomy for intraventricular tumor resection presented after discharge with altered mental status, hypotension, and fever to 101°F. Noncontrast CT shows periventricular white matter hypodensity and indistinct hypodensity in the occipital horns of the lateral ventricles (A). MR imaging better demonstrates the subependymal cerebrospinal fluid leakage on FLAIR (B) with irregular debris in the occipital horns and periventricular subependymal enhancement (C), consistent with ventriculitis.

CEREBRITIS AND ABSCESS

Intracranial infection occurs in oncologic and immunosuppressed patients more often than in immunocompetent patients. Diagnosis is complicated by the fact that the same pathogenic organisms in immunocompetent patients may present with atypical imaging findings in the immunosuppressed and they are moreover susceptible to a broad variety of opportunistic infections,

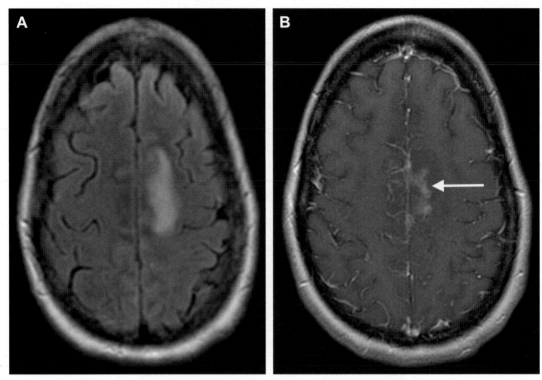

Fig. 4. Cryptococcal meningitis in HIV-positive patient. A 44-year-old woman presented with headache and right upper and lower extremity weakness for 4 days. MR imaging shows increased FLAIR signal in the posterior left frontal lobe and parafalcine sulci (*A*). Postcontrast images show intense leptomeningeal enhancement (*B*) caused by cryptococcal meningitis (*arrow*).

including fungal, bacterial, and viral infections, depending on the level of immunosuppression.

In patients with hematologic malignancy and hematopoietic stem cell transplant (HSCT), the type of underlying malignancy, pretransplant conditioning, donor cell origin, and specific medications used for treatment all have an impact on the patient's level of immunosuppression and potential for complication. The transplanted cell type, either allogenic or autologous, pretransplant conditioning (ie, myeloablative vs nonmyeloablative treatment), and the degree of ablation determine the degree of the immunosuppression. In HSCT patients, although the grafting process may start 2 to 4 months after conditioning, immune reconstitution can last at least 4 months after transplant and full immune system restoration occurs only after 1 year.[5,27] During the neutropenic period, the risk of infection increases, but typical signs of infection are often suppressed, thus complicating diagnosis. Immune reconstitution inflammatory syndrome (IRIS) can also occur in these patients while the immune system reconstitutes.[27]

In patients with solid organ transplants the frequency and severity of infection roughly correlates with the degree of immunosuppression required for maintenance, with lung and heart patients requiring higher degrees of immunosuppression than liver or renal transplant patients. Transplant rejection is a risk in the acute and chronic setting and often needs to be balanced with the risk or treatment of infection.[28] Cerebral abscesses in transplant patients are dominated by fungal infections. In a study of liver transplant patients, all of the cerebral abscesses were fungal in origin and in another study of HSCT patients, 92% of cerebral abscesses were fungal.[29] Aspergillosis is by far the most common CNS fungal source in transplant and immunosuppressed patients. Aspergillus in the CNS is usually angioinvasive and can cause infarct and associated hemorrhage. Invasive candidiasis is less common and almost exclusively seen in the setting of disseminated disease. Invasive candidiasis causes a diffuse pattern of small intracranial microabscesses. Cryptococcus is the most common cause of fungal meningitis in immunosuppressed patients and can cause cryptococcoma in the brain parenchyma, although less commonly. CNS coccidioidomycosis is uncommon even in disseminated disease, usually

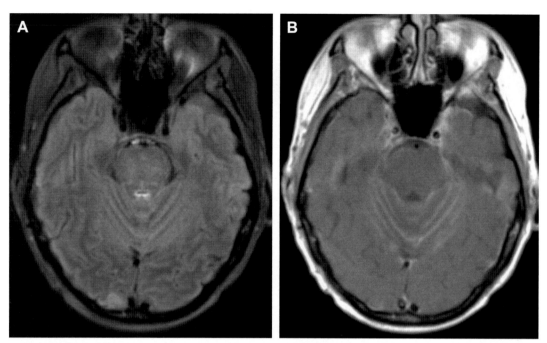

Fig. 5. Leptomeningeal carcinomatosis. A 40-year-old woman with widely metastatic breast cancer presented with mild migraine headaches for 10 days. The symptoms were initially believed to be caused by capecitabine chemotherapy, but they persisted after cessation. Restaging MR imaging revealed increased FLAIR signal in the sulci and cerebellar folia (A) with sulcal enhancement on postcontrast images (B), consistent with leptomeningeal carcinomatosis.

manifesting as meningitis, although granuloma and abscess can rarely occur.

Although imaging findings can be nonspecific, imaging remains an important tool in narrowing the differential diagnosis, identifying potential sites for biopsy and monitoring treatment. Both CT and MR angiography can assist in detecting vascular abnormalities caused by infection and their sequelae. On CT, cerebritis usually shows vasogenic edema with mass effect and sulcal effacement. MR imaging shows increased T2/FLAIR white matter hyperintensity caused by vasogenic edema with variable degrees of gray matter involvement. Diffusion signal abnormality is variable in cerebritis depending on the temporal evolution and may be reversible. Abnormal contrast enhancement may not always occur in immunosuppressed patients, especially those who are profoundly immunocompromised, and the degree of cerebral edema may be less than expected because of the patient's inability to mount an adequate immune response.

Imaging progression of cerebritis to abscess may also be atypical in immunosuppressed patients, because an inadequate immune response may delay or impede the typical appearance of encapsulation. Typical MR imaging findings in abscesses include well-defined T2/FLAIR

hyperintense foci that are isointense/hypointense on T1 with a T2 hypointense rim because of free radicals, although the T2 hypointense rim can be absent in immunosuppressed patients.[24] Internal reduced diffusivity is invariably present in bacterial abscesses, whereas fungal abscesses may appear heterogeneous, with DWI abnormality only associated with nodularity of the abscess wall. Multiplicity and location can at times help distinguish between bacterial and fungal abscesses. Fungal abscess are more often multiple, occur more commonly in the basal ganglia, and are more likely to cause hemorrhagic infarcts (Figs. 7 and 8).

Some fungal diseases have characteristic appearances on MR imaging that can aid in diagnosis. Lesions in invasive candidiasis tend to be small and numerous and many may be too small to identify on T1 images, but can often be seen as foci of T2/FLAIR hyperintensity with associated punctate and nodular foci of enhancement. Cryptococcomas, the parenchymal form of cryptococcal infection, may appear masslike and isointense on T1 and hyperintense on T2 sequences with nodular enhancement.[24] Cryptococcal gelatinous pseudocysts may mimic parenchymal microabscesses, but the characteristic distribution of mucoid material filling the

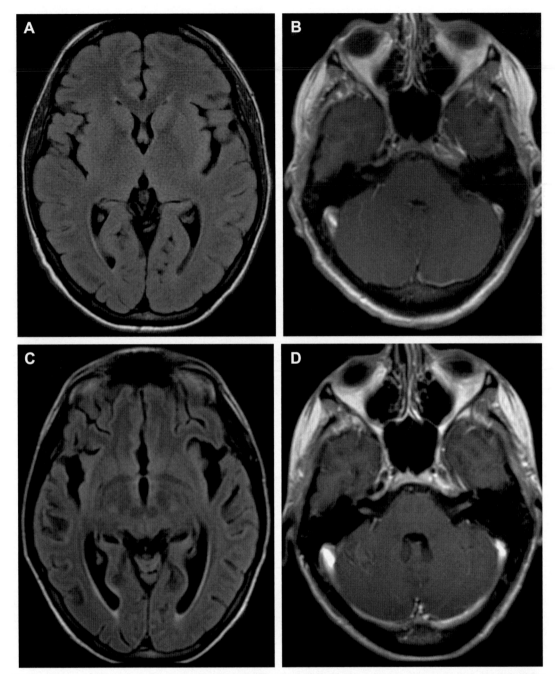

Fig. 6. Hydrocephalus caused by meningitis. A 31-year-old woman with metastatic breast cancer developed leptomeningeal metastases. Initial FLAIR (*A*) and postcontrast (*B*) imaging is normal. She developed worsening nausea, vomiting, and positional headaches. Subsequent MR imaging shows new mild dilation of the lateral ventricles with increased periventricular FLAIR signal caused by subependymal leakage (*C*) and increased enhancement in the bilateral internal auditory canals (*D*) caused by new leptomeningeal metastases.

perivascular spaces in the basal ganglia without peripheral enhancement helps lead to the correct diagnosis.

Parenchymal tuberculosis is much less common than meningitis, but presents in the form of tuberculomas or rarely abscesses, which are more common in HIV-positive patients. On CT, tuberculomas may be low or high in density and usually enhance peripherally with surrounding vasogenic edema. On MR imaging tuberculomas

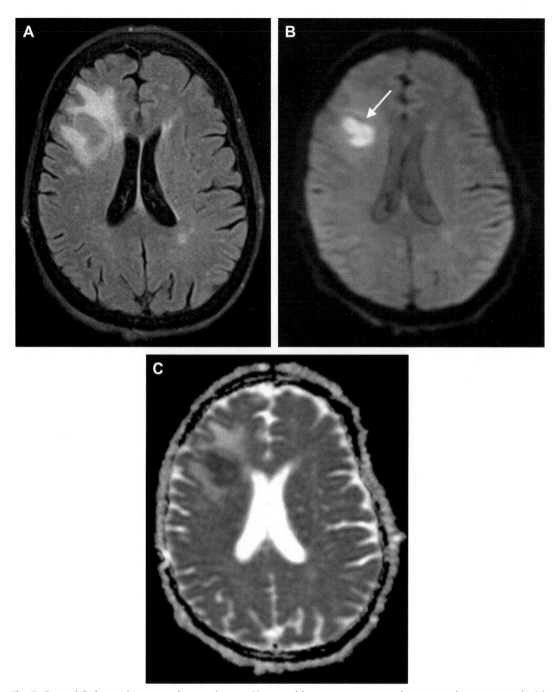

Fig. 7. Bacterial abscess in a transplant patient. A 69-year-old woman status post lung transplant presented with somnolence and subtle left weakness 2 days after dialysis fistula thrombectomy. FLAIR (*A*) shows the vasogenic edema and gyral expansion in the right frontal lobe with central reduced diffusivity on DWI (*arrow*) and ADC map (*B, C*), consistent with abscess. *Nocardia* was found to be the causative organism on biopsy.

are variable in signal and contrast enhancement depending on whether they are caseating, noncaseating, or necrotic.[30]

Intracranial viral infections are rare, but important to recognize. The most common

neuroinvasive arboviral infection in North America is West Nile virus, which is prevalent throughout the United States with most cases reported in California and Texas. Several studies have suggested that neuroinvasive disease and neurologic

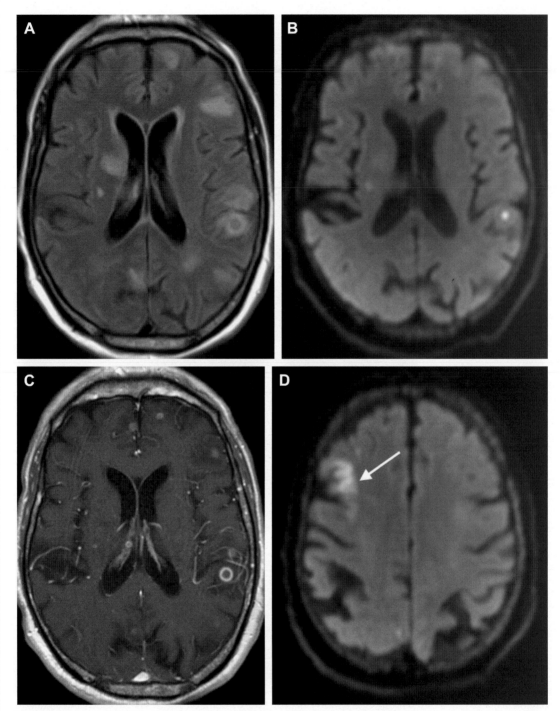

Fig. 8. Disseminated fungal infection with infarction. A 78-year-old man with a history of mantle cell lymphoma presented with headache, waxing and waning confusion, and slowed speech. FLAIR shows multiple target-like lesions throughout the brain with vasogenic edema (*A*), variable reduced diffusivity on DWI (*B*), and increased peripheral enhancement (*C*). These were presumed to be fungal abscesses and the patient responded to antifungal treatment. A focal gyriform area of reduced diffusivity on DWI (*D*) in the right anterior frontal cortex (*arrow*) caused by acute infarction is likely embolic or caused by invasive fungal infection.

complications may be more frequent in immunosuppressed patients, including transplant patients, but the evidence is largely observational.[31,32] Other arboviruses, such as La Crosse virus, St. Louis encephalitis virus, Jamestown Canyon virus, Powassan virus, and eastern equine encephalitis, are known to cause neuroinvasive disease, but all are rarer. Zika virus has been reported to cause meningoencephalitis in adults. A case of severe Zika encephalitis in a transplant patient has been described with an appearance similar to that of West Nile virus, but it is not yet known whether immunosuppressed patients are more susceptible or develop universally worse neuroinvasive disease compared with immunocompetent patients.[33,34] Imaging findings of neuroinvasive arboviral diseases are similar, with T2/FLAIR hyperintensity in the basal ganglia and thalamus with variable cortical and white matter involvement. Associated DWI abnormality and leptomeningeal enhancement may or may not be present (**Fig. 9**).[35,36]

HIV-positive patients with uncontrolled disease are susceptible to a wide range of opportunistic infections that occur more often in this subgroup than in other immunosuppressed populations. The spectrum of acute neurologic complications in HIV patients has evolved in the past decades in North America. Opportunistic infections are still present in the era of highly active antiretroviral therapy, but more often affect patients who receive delayed care or are unable to maintain antiretroviral treatment.[37,38] The imaging findings and correlation with CD4 count have been described in other reviews. In particular, cerebral toxoplasmosis and cytomegalovirus (CMV) remain common causes of intracranial infection in HIV-positive patients. Cerebral toxoplasmosis often presents with focal neurologic symptoms, altered mental status, and seizures. On MR imaging, small to large T2 hyperintense lesions are seen with a predilection for the corticomedullary junction, basal ganglia, thalamus, and less commonly the brainstem. Lesions are usually associated with extensive edema and some even with daughter lesions. Peripheral enhancement increases proportionately to the CD4 count, typically with lack of enhancement with a CD4 count of less than 50 cells/mm³.[39] CMV ventriculitis and encephalitis typically occurs with a CD4 count of less than 100 cells/mm³ and often causes ependymal DWI signal abnormality and enhancement (**Figs. 10** and **11**).

IRIS can occur in the CNS, usually after initiation of antiretroviral therapy in HIV-positive patients with low CD4 count. Other immunosuppressed patients are also susceptible, such as those on immune modulation therapy (eg, natalizumab) for chronic diseases (eg, multiple sclerosis and Crohn disease); patients with B-cell malignancy, rheumatoid arthritis, or systemic lupus erythematosis treated with rituximab; patients with psoriasis treated with efalizumab; and allogenic stem cell transplant patients. CNS-IRIS may occur in patients with a known opportunistic infection, subclinical infection, or even previously resolved infection. Most cases are caused by cryptococcal meningeal disease or progressive multifocal leukoencephalopathy from JC virus infection, although other infectious agents have been implicated, including varicella zoster virus, CMV, HIV, *Candida*, *M tuberculosis*, and *Toxoplasma gondii*. Most CNS-IRIS is self-limiting and symptoms are often mild, but uncommonly the response is severe and fulminant, leading to herniation and death in a short period of time. A high index of suspicion is therefore important because medical management may need to be changed drastically for these patients. In patients with paradoxically new or progressive symptoms despite medical therapy, suspicious imaging findings suggesting CNS-IRIS on MR imaging include new edema, mass effect, enhancement, or restricted diffusion.[40]

Paraneoplastic limbic encephalitis is a rare cause of encephalitis that typically presents with seizure, anterograde memory loss, and even psychiatric symptoms. Paraneoplastic disease is associated more commonly with lung, breast, testicular and ovarian cancer, and thymoma.[41] CT is usually negative, whereas findings on MR imaging may be confused with other etiologies of temporal lobe encephalitis, such as herpes simplex virus. Limbic encephalitis tends to involve the medial temporal lobes symmetrically, whereas herpes tends to be asymmetric and involve the insular and cingulate cortex. Infarct and hemorrhage also commonly occurs with later stages of herpes encephalitis, but is extremely rare in paraneoplastic limbic encephalitis.[42] Post-transplant acute limbic encephalitis is an uncommon, but serious complication, thought to be caused by human herpesvirus 6.[43] In one series, the incidence was 1.5% in transplant patients, but the reported incidence ranges from 0% to 11.6%.[44] Patients often present with memory loss, seizure, and loss of consciousness. MR imaging findings are similar to paraneoplastic limbic encephalitis, although data are limited because of rarity. The mortality is high and survivors may have serious sequelae, such as epilepsy and memory loss. To

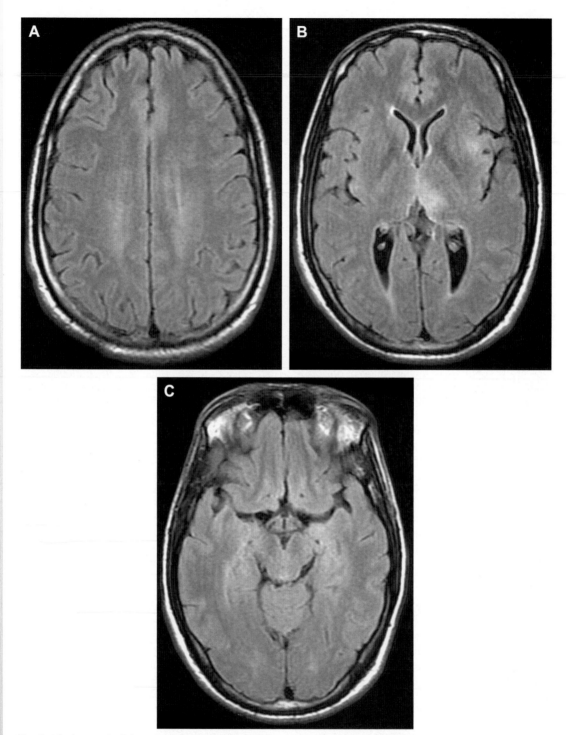

Fig. 9. Viral encephalitis. A 51-year-old HIV-positive man with hemophilia presented with persistent head-aches. FLAIR images demonstrate hyperintensity in the corona radiata (*A*), left insula and thalamus (*B*), and hippocampi (*C*). There was no reduced diffusivity or abnormal enhancement. The initial diagnosis was broad, including viral encephalitis, progressive multifocal leukoencephalopathy, HIV encephalitis, lymphoma, and acute demyelinating encephalomyelitis. MR imaging 2 weeks later showed near resolution, consistent with viral encephalitis.

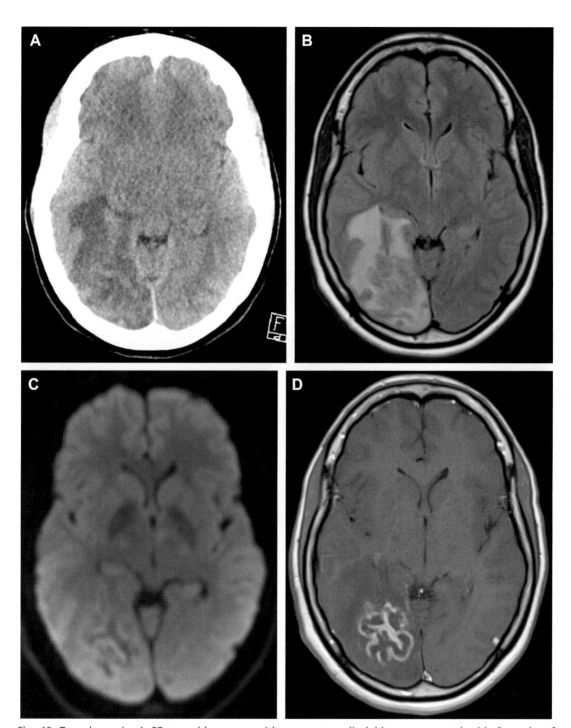

Fig. 10. Toxoplasmosis. A 27-year-old woman with no past medical history presented with 2 weeks of severe headache. CT shows vasogenic edema in the right temporal and occipital lobes with an irregular hypodense lesion (*A*). MR imaging demonstrates the extensive vasogenic edema on FLAIR images (*B*) without reduced diffusivity on DWI (*C*). Postcontrast images show an irregular, peripherally enhancing lesion (*D*). The patient was found to be HIV-positive with a CD4 count of 40 cells/mm^3 and biopsy identified toxoplasmosis.

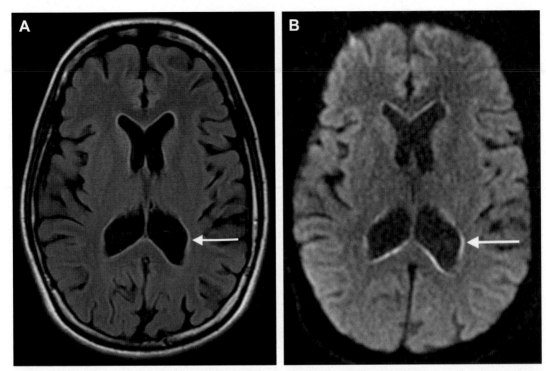

Fig. 11. CMV ventriculitis in HIV patient. A 31-year-old woman with no past medical history presented with confusion and altered mental status. Noncontrast head CT was negative (not shown). On MR imaging, there is increased ependymal FLAIR (*A*) and DWI signal (*B*) (*arrows*) with subtly increased ependymal enhancement (not shown). On further work-up, the patient was found to be HIV-positive with elevated CMV on CSF polymerase chain reaction and findings were consistent with CMV ventriculitis. Periventricular hyperintensity on FLAIR and DWI resolved with treatment.

date, no validated prophylaxis or treatment has been established.[44]

MEDICATION COMPLICATIONS

Among an expanding list of oncologic drugs, several common medications and their complications are important for radiologists to recognize. In solid organ transplant patients, cyclosporine A is commonly used for immunosuppression and is known to cause seizure, cerebellar ataxia, motor weakness, and PRES. Some degree of neurotoxicity is seen in 10% to 28% of treated patients.[45] Tacrolimus has a similar neurotoxicity profile. Mycophenalate mofetil and rituximab increase CMV reactivation risk and conversion from cyclosporine and tacrolimus to mycophenalate mofetil is in itself a risk factor for infection.[5]

For patients receiving HSCT, metabolic- and drug-related toxicities actually represent most neurologic complications. Both busulfan and ifosfamide can cause encephalopathy and seizure that can progress to coma, cytarabine can cause

a pancerebellar syndrome, and cytarabine and carmustine can lead to severe encephlaopathy.[27] In addition, carboplatin, cyclosporine, etoposide, linezolid, tacrolimus, and sirolimus have all been associated with PRES, and the cephalosporins used for prophylactic antibiosis in these patients during neutropenia can precipitate status epilepticus.[2,27]

In HIV-positive patients, neuropsychiatric effects of HIV medications are common. Although they are rarely life threatening, they may prompt emergent imaging to exclude other causes, such as infection.

FACE/SINUS INFECTIONS

Invasive sinusitis, often fungal, usually affects patients with diabetes mellitus and severely immunosuppressed patients. The risk is substantially higher in patients with hematologic malignancy, particularly in patients with neutropenia with acute leukemia or post-myeloablative treatment, although the number of affected patients is smaller because of the much larger diabetic population. Invasive sinusitis is devastating with a high mortality, reported as up to 100% in some studies. The pathogens are usually *Aspergillus* or *Zygomycetes* causing invasive aspergillosis and mucormycosis, respectively.[46,47] Infection generally begins in the ethmoid sinuses, causing nonspecific nasal mucosal thickening. Early CT findings are usually nonspecific and benign appearing. From the sinuses, infection can spread to the orbits, meninges, and brain. The angioinvasive nature of these pathogens can result in carotid arteritis and stenosis, and cavernous sinus thrombosis in some patients. MR imaging is much more sensitive than CT and should be performed as early as possible when there is any clinical suspicion. Decreased T1 and increased T2 and FLAIR signal in the periantral fat posterior to the maxillary sinus is seen in early invasive infection, with T2/FLAIR hyperintensity and increased enhancement in the soft tissues as infection spreads. Intracranial extension can occur without bony erosion because of the angioinvasive nature of the organisms. Bony erosion is best seen on CT, but is usually a late finding when intracranial extension has already occurred. Intracranial extension generally portends a poor prognosis. Rapid surgical debridement and antifungal therapy are the mainstays of treatment and the disease is uniformly fatal without treatment (**Fig. 12**).

SPINE

Epidural spread of disease and pathologic fracture caused by bony metastases are the most common spinal complications of malignancy, putting the patient at risk for cord compression

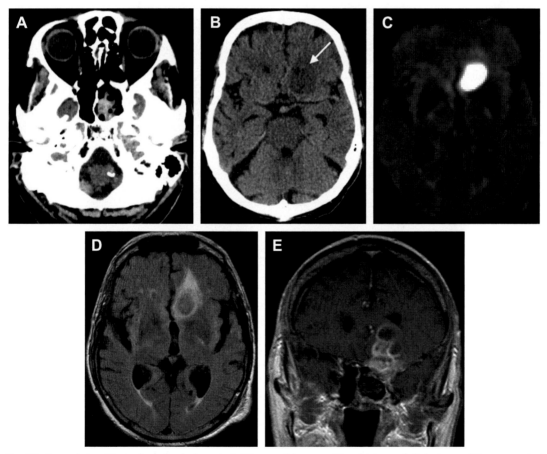

Fig. 12. Fungal sinusitis and cerebral abscess. A 79-year-old man with a history of diabetes mellitus presented with worsening headache over 1 week and onset of left-sided vision loss for 1 day. CT shows frothy debris in the left sphenoid sinus (*A*) and a parenchymal hypodensity (*arrow*) in the anterior inferior frontal lobe (*B*). The parenchymal hypodensity on CT corresponds with reduced diffusivity on DWI (*C*), consistent with abscess. Surrounding vasogenic edema is seen on FLAIR images (*D*). The extent of the peripherally enhancing abscess is seen on the coronal postcontrast image (*E*).

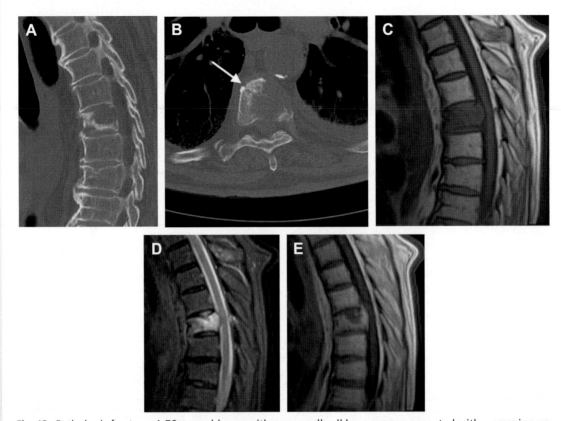

Fig. 13. Pathologic fracture. A 76-year-old man with non–small cell lung cancer presented with worsening upper back pain for several days. Sagittal and axial noncontrast CT images of the thoracic spine show a lytic lesion in the T6 vertebral body with subtle linear lucency (*arrow* in *B*) and mild height loss, consistent with acute pathologic fracture (*A*, *B*). T1 (*C*) and STIR (*D*) sagittal images demonstrate the degree of vertebral body involvement and associated mild cord deformity. Epidural extension of tumor is seen on the postcontrast image (*E*).

and occurring most frequently in prostate, lung, and breast cancer. Cord compression occurs in about 5% to 10% of patients with cancer with weakness being the presenting symptom in 35% to 75%.[48] Cord compression is considered a neurosurgical emergency, because the ability for a patient to walk following treatment of spinal cord compression is most closely correlated with their pretreatment neurologic status.[48] The most frequent sites of involvement in order are the thoracic spine, lumbar spine, and cervical spine because of epidural extension. MR imaging is the best study for evaluation of cord compression and the sensitivity has been reported up to 100% (**Fig. 13**). Contrast administration is preferred, but in the setting of contrast contraindication, noncontrast MR imaging is still the study of choice. Circumferential tumor resection and subsequent radiotherapy for radiosensitive tumors is the most common treatment pathway and surgical fixation can help restore neurologic integrity.[49,50]

In addition to the risk of pathologic fracture, the risk of osteoporotic fracture is also increased because of many chemotherapy drugs, such

as glucocorticoids, cyclophosphamide, methotrexate, ifosfamide, alkylating agents, aromatase inhibitors, and selective estrogen-receptor modulators. Moreover, radiation therapy, orchiectomy, and oophorectomy all may cause bone loss that increases the risk of osteoporotic fracture.

Other spinal cord complications are much less frequent, but are nonetheless important for radiologists to recognize. In immunosuppressed patients, acute myelopathy can occur and often the causative source is not identified. In transplant patients, cytarabine and methotrexate are known to cause subacute combined degeneration.[51] Stavudine, an antiretroviral medication, is associated with an ascending paralysis that usually resolves with medication cessation. HIV itself can cause an acute demyelinating polyneuropathy with an appearance similar to Guillain-Barre syndrome on imaging and must be recognized and aggressively treated. On MR imaging, acute cord myelopathy usually presents with cord expansion and central T2 hyperintensity without associated contrast enhancement (**Fig. 14**).

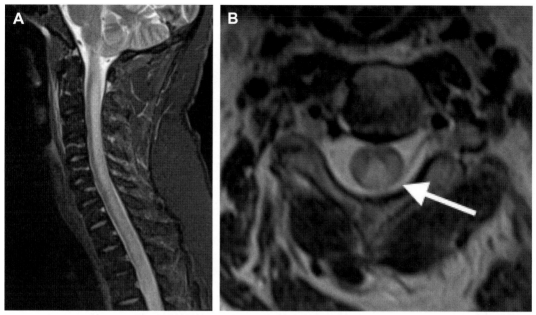

Fig. 14. Transverse myelitis in bone marrow transplant patient. A 28-year-old man with acute lymphoblastic T-cell leukemia and pancytopenia following chemoradiation therapy and allogenic bone marrow transplant developed quadriplegia and autonomic dysfunction. MR imaging of the cervical spine with and without contrast showed diffuse hyperintensity of the dorsal columns on sagittal STIR and axial T2 images (*arrow*) with cord enlargement (*A*, *B*), but without abnormal enhancement (not shown). No definite cause was identified following extensive work-up.

SUMMARY

Oncologic and immunosuppressed patients are susceptible to numerous emergent neurologic complications depending on their degree of immune suppression, medication, underlying malignancy or type of transplantation, or chronic disease. Detailed knowledge of patient risk factors and specific complications is essential for optimal image acquisition, interpretation, diagnosis, and treatment.

REFERENCES

1. Laine FJ, Shedden AI, Dunn MM, et al. Acquired intracranial herniations: MR imaging findings. AJR Am J Roentgenol 1995;165(4):967–73.

2. Baldwin KJ, Zivkovic SA, Lieberman FS. Neurologic emergencies in patients who have cancer: diagnosis and management. Neurol Clin 2012;30(1):101–28.

3. Lin AL, Avila EK. Neurologic emergencies in the patients with cancer. J Intensive Care Med 2016;32(2):99–115.

4. Katabathina VS, Restrepo CS, Betancourt Cuellar SL, et al. Imaging of oncologic emergencies: what every radiologist should know. Radiographics 2013;33(6):1533–53.

5. Pruitt AA, Graus F, Rosenfeld MR. Neurological complications of transplantation. Neurohospitalist 2012;3(1):24–38.

6. Cole AJ. Status epilepticus and periictal imaging. Epilepsia 2004;45(Suppl 4):72–7.

7. Bartynski WS, Boardman JF. Catheter angiography, MR angiography, and MR perfusion in posterior reversible encephalopathy syndrome. AJNR Am J Neuroradiol 2008;29(3):447–55.

8. Bartynski WS. Posterior reversible encephalopathy syndrome, part 1: fundamental imaging and clinical features. Am J Neuroradiology 2008;29(6):1036–42.

9. Bartynski WS, Tan HP, Boardman JF, et al. Posterior reversible encephalopathy syndrome after solid organ transplantation. Am J Neuroradiology 2008;29(5):924–30.

10. Chen S, Hu J, Xu L, et al. Posterior reversible encephalopathy syndrome after transplantation: a review. Mol Neurobiol 2016;53(10):6897–909.

11. McKinney AM, Short J, Truwit CL, et al. Posterior reversible encephalopathy syndrome: incidence of atypical regions of involvement and imaging findings. AJR Am J Roentgenol 2007;189(4):904–12.

12. Hefzy HM, Bartynski WS, Boardman JF, et al. Hemorrhage in posterior reversible encephalopathy syndrome: imaging and clinical features. Am J Neuroradiology 2009;30(7):1371–9.

13. Karia SJ, Rykken JB, McKinney ZJ, et al. Utility and significance of gadolinium-based contrast enhancement

in posterior reversible encephalopathy syndrome. Am J Neuroradiology 2016;37(3):415–22.

14. Navi BB, Reiner AS, Kamel H, et al. Risk of arterial thromboembolism in patients with cancer. J Am Coll Cardiol 2017;70(8):926–38.

15. Parikh NS, Burch JE, Kamel H, et al. Recurrent thromboembolic events after ischemic stroke in patients with primary brain tumors. J Stroke Cerebrovasc Dis 2017;26(10):2396–403.

16. Torrisi JM, Schwartz LH, Gollub MJ, et al. CT findings of chemotherapy-induced toxicity: what radiologists need to know about the clinical and radiologic manifestations of chemotherapy toxicity. Radiology 2011;258(1):41–56.

17. Moslehi JJ. Cardiovascular toxic effects of targeted cancer therapies. Longo DL, ed. N Engl J Med 2016;375(15):1457–67.

18. Benjamin LA, Bryer A, Emsley HC, et al. HIV infection and stroke: current perspectives and future directions. Lancet Neurol 2012;11(10):878–90.

19. Ovbiagele B, Nath A. Increasing incidence of ischemic stroke in patients with HIV infection. Neurology 2011;76(5):444–50.

20. Singer S, Grommes C, Reiner AS, et al. Posterior reversible encephalopathy syndrome in patients with cancer. Oncologist 2015;20(7):806–11.

21. Lorenz MW, Stephan C, Harmjanz A, et al. Both long-term HIV infection and highly active antiretroviral therapy are independent risk factors for early carotid atherosclerosis. Atherosclerosis 2008;196(2):720–6.

22. Pruitt A. Central nervous system infections in cancer patients. Semin Neurol 2010;30(03):296–310.

23. Katchanov J, Branding G, Jefferys L, et al. Neuroimaging of HIV-associated cryptococcal meningitis: comparison of magnetic resonance imaging findings in patients with and without immune reconstitution. Int J STD AIDS 2015;27(2):110–7.

24. Mathur M, Johnson CE, Sze G. Fungal infections of the central nervous system. Neuroimaging Clin N Am 2012;22(4):609–32.

25. Prömmel P, Pilgram-Pastor S, Sitter H, et al. Neoplastic meningitis: how MRI and CSF cytology are influenced by CSF cell count and tumor type. ScientificWorldJournal 2013;2013(4):1–5.

26. Chamberlain MC. Neoplastic meningitis. Oncologist 2008;13(9):967–77.

27. Mathew RM, Rosenfeld MR. Neurologic complications of bone marrow and stem-cell transplantation in patients with cancer. Curr Treat Options Neurol 2007;9(4):308–14.

28. Dineen RA, Sibtain N, Karani JB, et al. Cerebral manifestations in liver disease and transplantation. Clin Radiol 2008;63(5):586–99.

29. Singh N, Husain S. Infections of the central nervous system in transplant recipients. Transpl Infect Dis 2000;2(3):101–11.

30. Harisinghani MG, McLoud TC, Shepard JA, et al. Tuberculosis from head to toe. Radiographics 1909;20(2):449–70 [quiz: 528–9, 532].

31. Yango AF, Fischbach BV, Levy M, et al. West Nile virus infection in kidney and pancreas transplant recipients in the Dallas-Fort Worth Metroplex during the 2012 Texas epidemic. Transplantation 2014;97(9):953–7.

32. Gomez AJ, Waggoner JJ, Itoh M, et al. Fatal West Nile virus encephalitis in a heart transplant recipient. J Clin Microbiol 2015;53(8):2749–52.

33. Patel A, Small JE, Pradhan F, et al. Case report: Zika virus meningoencephalitis and myelitis and associated magnetic resonance imaging findings. Am J Trop Med Hyg 2017;97(2):340–3.

34. Schwartzmann PV, Ramalho LNZ, Neder L, et al. Zika virus meningoencephalitis in an immunocompromised Patient. Mayo Clin Proc 2017;92(3):460–6.

35. Ali M, Safriel Y, Sohi J, et al. West Nile virus infection: MR imaging findings in the nervous system. AJNR Am J Neuroradiol 2005;26(2):289–97.

36. Kleinschmidt-DeMasters BK, Marder BA, Levi ME, et al. Naturally acquired West Nile virus encephalomyelitis in transplant recipients: clinical, laboratory, diagnostic, and neuropathological features. Arch Neurol 2004;61(8):1210–20.

37. Spudich SS, Ances BM. Neurologic complications of HIV infection: highlights from the 2013 conference on retroviruses and opportunistic infections. Top Antivir Med 2013;21:100–8.

38. Ho EL, Jay CA. Altered mental status in HIV-infected patients. Emerg Med Clin North Am 2010;28(2):311–23.

39. Offiah CE, Turnbull IW. The imaging appearances of intracranial CNS infections in adult HIV and AIDS patients. Clin Radiol 2006;61(5):393–401.

40. Post MJD, Thurnher MM, Clifford DB, et al. CNS–immune reconstitution inflammatory syndrome in the setting of HIV infection, part 1: overview and discussion of progressive multifocal leukoencephalopathy–immune reconstitution inflammatory syndrome and cryptococcal–immune reconstitution inflammatory syndrome. Am J Neuroradiology 2013;34(7):1297–307.

41. Hess CP, Barkovich AJ. Seizures: emergency neuroimaging. Neuroimaging Clin N Am 2010;20(4):619–37.

42. Saket RR, Geschwind MD, Josephson SA, et al. Autoimmune-mediated encephalopathy: classification, evaluation, and MR imaging patterns of disease. Neurograph 2011;1(1):2–16.

43. Guzmán-De-Villoria JA, Fernández-García P, Borrego-Ruiz PJ. Neurologic emergencies in HIV-negative immunosuppressed patients. Radiologia 2017;59(1):2–16.

44. Ogata M, Fukuda T, Teshima T. Human herpesvirus-6 encephalitis after allogeneichematopoietic cell transplantation: what we do and do not know. Bone Marrow Transplant 2015;50(8):1030–6.

45. Marco S, Cecilia F, Patrizia B. Neurologic complications after solid organ transplantation. Transpl Int 2009;22(3):269–78.

46. Pagano L, Offidani M, Fianchi L, et al. Mucormycosis in hematologic patients. Haematologica 2004;89(2):207–14.

47. Velayudhan V, Chaudhry ZA, Smoker WRK, et al. Imaging of intracranial and orbital complications of sinusitis and atypical sinus infection: what the radiologist needs to know. Curr Probl Diagn Radiol 2017;46(6):441–51.

48. Cole JS, Patchell RA. Metastatic epidural spinal cord compression. Lancet Neurol 2008;7(5):459–66.

49. Ropper AE, Ropper AH. Acute spinal cord compression. Longo DL, ed. N Engl J Med 2017;376(14):1358–69.

50. Guimaraes MD, Bitencourt AG, Marchiori E, et al. Imaging acute complications in cancer patients: what should be evaluated in the emergency setting? Cancer Imaging 2014;14(1):1–12.

51. Flanagan EP, Pittock SJ. Diagnosis and management of spinal cord emergencies. Handb Clin Neurol 2017;140:319–35.

Emergent Neuroimaging During Pregnancy and the Postpartum Period

Guangzu Gao, MD[a], Rebecca L. Zucconi, MD[b],
William B. Zucconi, DO[a],*

KEYWORDS

- Patient-centered imaging • Pregnancy • Postpartum • Emergency neuroradiology

KEY POINTS

- Patient-centered neuroimaging in pregnancy and the postpartum period requires the radiologist to be well versed in latest imaging recommendations, while considering the needs and preferences of the individual patient and her family.
- A diagnostic challenge inherent to acute neurologic conditions during pregnancy and the postpartum period is that the presenting symptoms of several distinct pathologic conditions often overlap, and the conditions themselves are not mutually exclusive.
- The radiologist and imaging care providers must be effective and proactive members of the multidisciplinary care team commonly assembled in support of these patients.

INTRODUCTION

Acute neurologic symptoms during pregnancy can herald life-threatening disease processes and are anxiety provoking to both patients and clinicians. Implementation of a patient-centered care model in radiology can alleviate a patient's stress, reinforce appropriate imaging workup, improve patient satisfaction, and lead to improved outcomes.[1–5] The optimal approach entails seamless communication between the referring clinical teams, radiologic care providers, and the patient and relevant family members.[1,5,6] Exemplary patient-centered care includes a discussion of the goals, expectations and potential limitations of the imaging studies, duration of the examination, risks and benefits, monitoring of the examination, and providing timely results. To deliver on this promise, the radiologist must be a proactive member of the multidisciplinary care team, which may include consultants in obstetrics, and often emergency medicine, neurology, interventional neuroradiology, critical care, neonatology, and medical physics.[7,8] The radiologist must also be able to use the latest imaging recommendations with regard to appropriateness criteria, use of contrast, and radiation safety with consideration for the needs and preferences of the individual patient and her family.

A diagnostic challenge inherent to acute neurologic conditions during pregnancy and the postpartum period is that the presenting symptoms of several distinct pathologic conditions often overlap, and the conditions themselves are not mutually exclusive.[7–10] With a focus on patient-centered care, the authors present the evaluation, differential diagnosis, and recommended imaging protocols for the three most common acute neurologic symptoms in pregnancy and the postpartum

Disclosure Statement: The authors have nothing to disclose.
[a] Department of Radiology and Biomedical Imaging, Yale Diagnostic Radiology, Yale School of Medicine, 20 York Street, PO Box 208042, New Haven, CT 06520-8042, USA; [b] Department of Medical Sciences, Frank H Netter MD School of Medicine, Quinnipiac University, 275 Mount Carmel Avenue, Hamden, CT 06518-1905, USA
* Corresponding author.
E-mail address: william.zucconi@yale.edu

Neuroimag Clin N Am 28 (2018) 419–433
https://doi.org/10.1016/j.nic.2018.03.005

period: headache, seizure, and focal neurologic deficit. With the patient's symptoms as a reference point, the referring physician in consultation with the radiologist can effectively implement the optimal imaging procedures and expedite effective therapies.

PHYSIOLOGIC CHANGES OF PREGNANCY

The radiologist should be familiar with the physiologic changes of pregnancy that increase the risk for neurologic complications. Because of the elevation of estrogen, changes in the coagulation and fibrinolytic pathways place pregnant women in a hypercoagulable state. Pregnant women have an increased risk of thromboembolism, which persists 6 weeks into the postpartum period[11,12] because of an increase in several clotting factors, decreased inhibition of clotting mechanisms, and inhibition of fibrinolysis.[13,14] Total blood volume increases by 40% at term, leading to an increased risk of hypertension,[14,15] and rising progesterone levels in the third trimester contribute to increased venous compliance, capillary leakage, and vasogenic edema.[16] Hypercoagulability, hypertension, and increased vascular permeability help explain many of the imaging features seen in acute neurologic disease of pregnant and postpartum patients.

HEADACHE

An estimated 40% of postpartum women experience headaches.[17] Primary headache disorders, such as tension-type headache and migraine, are the most common cause.[18] Migraines are often improved in pregnancy, however, and should be diagnosed with caution so as not to miss a secondary cause.[19–21] Signs or symptoms that warrant additional workup include new, severe, or thunderclap headache, change in preexisting headache character or pattern, accompanying hypertension, or history of previous cerebrovascular disease.[7] Similarly, visual disturbance, altered mental status, or focal neurologic deficits warrant imaging.[18] MR imaging without contrast is the most appropriate imaging study for pregnant women with new headache when available, followed by computed tomography (CT) without intravenous contrast.[22]

Preeclampsia/Eclampsia

A common cause of new headaches in pregnancy is preeclampsia/eclampsia. Preeclampsia is characterized by new-onset hypertension (blood pressure >140/90 mm Hg) and proteinuria (24-hour urine collection >300 mg) that develops after 20 weeks' gestation.[23] It is a condition unique to pregnancy and the postpartum period, affecting an estimated 2% to 8% of pregnancies. Patients with preeclampsia often complain of headache and visual disturbances such as scintillating scotoma and may exhibit hyperreflexia.[24] Eclampsia is characterized by the addition of generalized tonic-clonic seizures and affects approximately 0.3% to 0.5% of all pregnancies,[23,24] most commonly during the third trimester, but can also occur postpartum.[23]

There are no specific imaging findings of preeclampsia, and brain imaging is not recommended in classic, uncomplicated cases.[25] Nonspecific signal hyperintensity on T2/fluid-attenuated inversion recovery (FLAIR) sequences can be seen in the brain parenchyma (Fig. 1), attributable to a hypertensive encephalopathy syndrome, or posterior reversible encephalopathy syndrome (PRES), a clinical and radiologic diagnosis with the neuroimaging findings of vasogenic edema, classically involving the posterior circulation territories.[26] PRES is, of course, not unique to preeclampsia/eclampsia patients. Severe hypertension, renal failure, and certain medications are among the many conditions predisposing to PRES.[27] The precise pathophysiology of PRES remains poorly understood, but likely relates to endothelial dysfunction, acute fluctuations of blood pressure, and impairment of cerebral auto-regulation resulting in brain edema, and in severe cases, infarction and hemorrhage.[26]

Head CT scan is abnormal in approximately 45% of patients with PRES,[26] with vasogenic edema most commonly visualized in the posterior cerebral hemispheres. MR imaging findings of PRES are best seen on T2-weighted and FLAIR images as hyperintensity (Fig. 2) and are more sensitive to involvement of the brainstem and cerebellum. The lesions less commonly demonstrate contrast enhancement, hemorrhage, or restricted diffusion, which portend a worse prognosis.[26] Eclampsia-specific PRES tends to involve the thalamus, midbrain, and pons less frequently than other PRES associations.[10] Preeclamptic or eclamptic patients with PRES also have less edema, hemorrhage, and contrast enhancement and tend to have more frequent complete resolution of imaging findings than other causes of PRES.[28] Most patients will respond to treatment at the vasogenic edema stage and achieve complete neurologic recovery within several weeks.[29] Although pharmacologic therapy with magnesium sulfate is given routinely for seizure treatment and

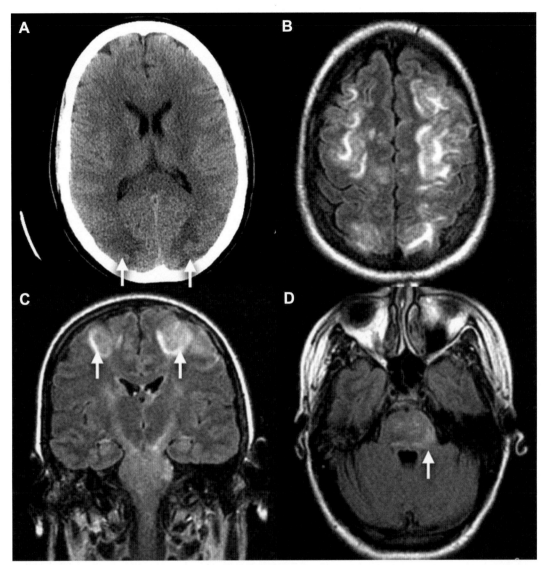

Fig. 1. White matter changes in preeclampsia complicated by HELLP. A 29-year-old G2P1 patient with preeclampsia complicated by HELLP syndrome who had induced delivery at 32 weeks for a viable vaginal delivery. She developed seizures immediately after the delivery. (*A*): Noncontrast CT shows nonspecific subcortical white matter hypoattenuation in the posterior hemispheres (*arrows*). (*B–D*) FLAIR image shows hyperintense signal predominantly within the white matter (*B, C; arrows*). Note involvement of the pons (*D; arrow*).

prophylaxis, and antihypertensives can be used to control blood pressure in severe cases, the definitive treatment of preeclampsia and eclampsia is delivery.[30]

Subarachnoid Hemorrhage

Patients with abrupt onset of thunderclap headache should receive a thorough evaluation to exclude subarachnoid hemorrhage (SAH), including lumbar puncture in equivocal or high suspicion cases.[7] In the pregnant patient, MR

imaging without contrast should be considered the test of choice, if available on an emergent basis. Otherwise, CT without contrast should be performed. In young patients with SAH, underlying structural lesions such as vascular malformations and aneurysms must be excluded. SAH that occurs adjacent to the circle of Willis raises the suspicion of an underlying aneurysm, whereas high-convexity SAH may indicate postpartum angiopathy, or venous thrombosis.[7] In these cases, noncontrast MR angiography (MRA), MR venography (MRV), or a contrast-enhanced

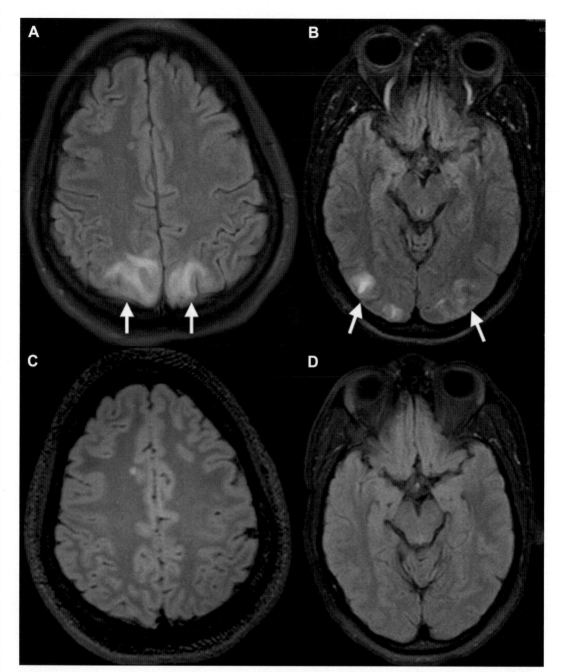

Fig. 2. PRES. Postpartum MR imaging in a15-year-old patient with eclampsia, axial FLAIR imaging. (*A, B*) Hyperintense signal is seen bilaterally in the posterior cerebral hemispheres, primarily involving subcortical white matter (*arrows*). (*C, D*) Resolution of pathologic signal 1 year later, consistent with PRES.

CT angiography (CTA)/CT venography should be pursued as needed.

Postdural Puncture Headache

An important consideration for the postpartum woman with a headache is intracranial hypotension following spinal anesthesia, or after a misguided dural puncture during the administration of epidural anesthesia. Iatrogenic cerebrospinal fluid (CSF) leaks often lead to nuchal and occipital headaches that commonly begin 1 to 7 days postpartum, worsen upon standing, and are relieved by lying supine.[31] Tinnitus and diplopia can also occur.[31] Approximately 0.5% to 1.5% women who have received neuroaxial anesthetics will develop this condition.[32] A blood patch procedure is usually an effective treatment, after which the symptoms typically resolve within 48 hours.[32] Complications such as subdural hematoma and cerebral venous thrombosis (CVT) may arise. Subdural hematoma related to intracranial hypotension is presumably due to the tearing of bridging veins in a slack brain.[7] Noncontrast CT can demonstrate subdural collections and tonsillar ectopia/descent of brain structures (brainstem, hypothalamus, and tonsillar ectopia). In additionally, MR imaging findings include dural venous engorgement, pachymeningeal enhancement, pituitary enlargement, subdural effusions, reduced CSF volume, and diffuse brain swelling[33] (**Fig. 3**).

Cerebral Venous Thrombosis

CVT risk is highest in the first 2 weeks after delivery.[34] There is also an increased incidence in the first trimester, which may be related to women who become pregnant with an underlying thrombophilia.[35] Women with hypertension, advanced maternal age, cesarean delivery, infection, and hyperemesis are at increased risk of CVT.[36] Depending on the severity and location of the thrombosis, the clinical presentation of CVT includes progressively worsening headache, seizure, focal neurologic deficit, and coma.[37]

Noncontrast CT may demonstrate hyperattenuation of the thrombosed vein and regional vasogenic edema with or without the complications of venous infarction and/or hemorrhage[9] (**Fig. 4**). MR imaging is more sensitive than CT in early detection of thrombosis and more accurate in depicting the extent and complications of CVT. Filling defects and lack of intraluminal venous enhancement can be seen on postcontrast MR or CT. Although pregnant, noncontrast MRV is the recommended study of choice, associated parenchymal findings of CVT are edema, mass effect, sulcal effacement, infarcts, and hemorrhage, which may not conform to the arterial territories.[38]

Rare causes of headache in pregnancy and the postpartum period are pituitary hemorrhage, and mass lesions from primary or metastatic neoplasms. The aforementioned conditions often present with seizures and are discussed later.

Postpartum Cerebral Angiopathy/Reversible Cerebral Vasoconstriction Syndrome

Postpartum cerebral angiopathy (PCA), a form of reversible cerebral vasoconstriction syndrome

(RCVS), is another disease unique to pregnancy and typically occurs within 1 to 4 weeks of delivery in normotensive women.[39] PCA is poorly understood, and this term has been used to describe any form of cerebral arteriopathy in the postpartum period.[9]

Idiopathic PCA, also known as Call-Fleming postpartum angiopathy, classically presents in a postpartum patient with severe recurrent thunderclap headache with or without seizures, focal neurologic deficits, and intracranial hemorrhage.[40] PCA can also occur secondary to vasoactive medications, such as bromocriptine to suppress lactation, ergot alkaloids to control postpartum hemorrhage, or sympathomimetics for cold and nasal congestion.[9]

PCA should be considered in a postpartum patient with newly diagnosed parenchymal or SAH. On routine imaging, reversible signal hyperintensity on T2-weighted sequences within the cortex and white matter has been described.[40] CTA and MRA are first-line examinations in patients with suspected PCA; however, they may be insensitive in the first few days of symptom onset. With persistent concern, repeat imaging should be performed. Catheter angiography is the most sensitive modality and will demonstrate multifocal stenoses and dilations of the medium- and small-caliber cerebral arteries[41] (**Fig. 5**). Transcranial Doppler ultrasound has been described as a useful modality in monitoring the disease process and treatment.[42]

SEIZURES

Seizures in the pregnant and postpartum patient may be due to underlying medical conditions that predate the pregnancy, such as a seizure disorder or brain tumor (**Fig. 6**). New seizures in a previously healthy patient are worrisome and not uncommon in patients with PRES.[8] They usually occur in the absence of preceding symptoms, whereas seizures associated with CVT nearly always follow headache.[7] Generalized tonic-clonic seizures are the defining feature of eclampsia, but may also accompany PRES and PCA/RCVS.[7]

Brain Tumors

Pregnancy appears to enhance the growth of meningiomas.[43] About 70% of meningiomas express progesterone receptors and 30% express estrogen receptors,[43,44] and are known to regress after delivery.[9] Pregnancy is not known to increase the incidence or alter the behavior of gliomas[9] (see **Fig. 6**).

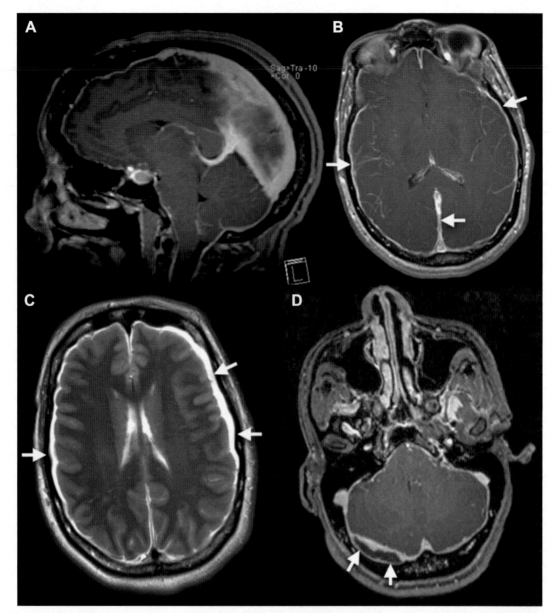

Fig. 3. Intracranial hypotension and CVT after epidural anesthesia. A 35-year-old woman with history of migraines and epidural anesthesia who developed intense positional headaches. All postcontrast images (*A, B, D*) demonstrate abnormal pachymeningeal enhancement. (*A*) Sagittal postcontrast MR image demonstrates prominence the pituitary gland with caudal descent of cerebellar tonsils, effacement of ambient, suprasellar, and prepontine cisterns. (*B*) Axial postcontrast MR imaging illustrates diffuse pachymeningeal enhancement (*arrows*). (*C*) Bilateral thin subdural collections are seen on axial T2-weighted MR imaging (*arrows*). (*D*) Filling defect (*arrows*) compatible with transverse dural venous sinus thrombus on axial postcontrast MR imaging. The patient was diagnosed with intracranial hypotension. She was treated with anticoagulation and a blood patch with good outcome. (*Courtesy of* Diego Nunez, MD.)

Breast cancer and choriocarcinoma are the two most common cancers that metastasize to the brain during pregnancy and may cause seizure or focal deficit. Choriocarcinoma (**Fig. 7**) is a malignant form of gestational trophoblastic disease (gestational trophoblastic neoplasia) and is highly

sensitive to chemotherapy. Metastases from both breast cancer and choriocarcinoma have a propensity to bleed.[9]

Noncontrast MR imaging is the preferred imaging modality if available for the workup of new onset focal seizures, incorporating hemorrhage sensitive

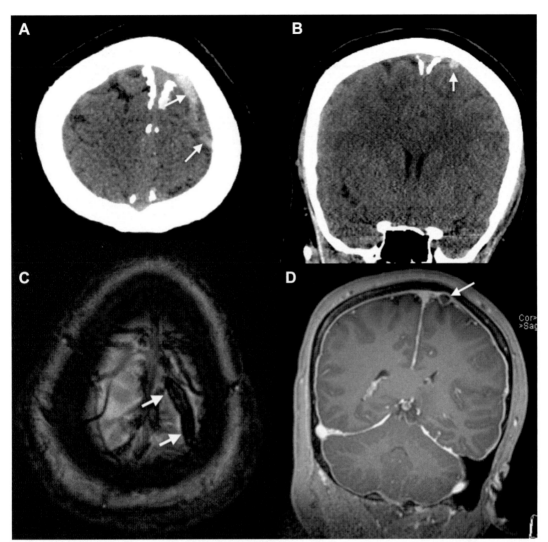

Fig. 4. CVT. A 21-year-old woman with worsening headaches and focal seizures 5 days after giving birth. (*A*, *B*) Noncontrast CT shows tubular hyperdensity (*arrows*) over the left upper convexity. (*C*) MR imaging SWI blooming supports left-sided cortical venous thrombosis (*arrows*). (*D*) Postcontrast axial MR imaging confirms filling defect (*arrow*). The superior sagittal sinus was not involved. The patient had a negative workup for coagulopathy. She was treated with anticoagulation with no long-term sequelae.

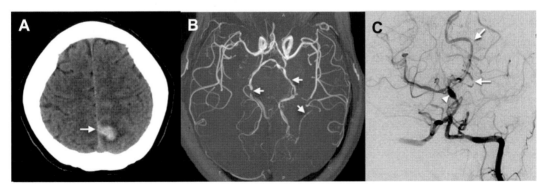

Fig. 5. PCA. A 32-year-old woman with a history of migraines who experienced sudden onset of blurry vision and severe headache 8 days postpartum. (*A*) Noncontrast CT shows acute left parietal intraparenchymal hemorrhage (*arrow*). (*B*) MRA maximum intensity projection image demonstrates multifocal stenosis (*arrows*) affecting the posterior cerebral arteries. (*C*) Angiography, frontal injection of the left vertebral artery shows areas of arterial irregularity with dilation (*arrowhead*) and narrowing (*arrows*) within the posterior circulation. The patient was medically managed and had no residual neurologic deficits.

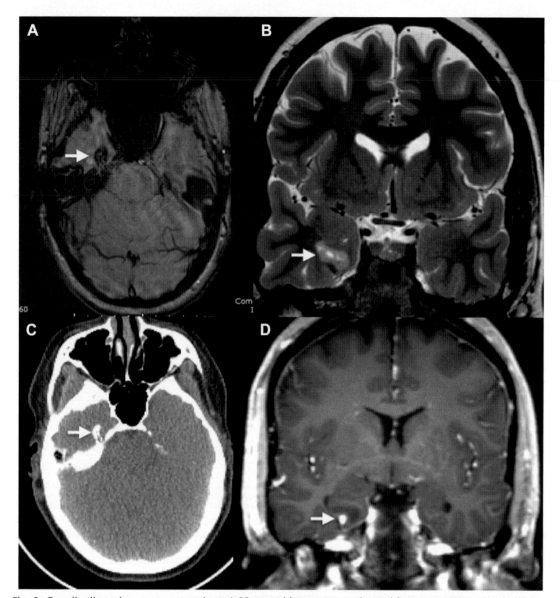

Fig. 6. Ganglioglioma in a pregnant patient. A 33-year-old pregnant patient with new onset nocturnal seizures. (*A*) SWI imaging demonstrates focal susceptibility artifact in the medial aspect of the right temporal lobe (*arrow*). (*B*) Hyperintense and cystic components of the lesion are seen on the coronal T2-weighted MR imaging (*arrow*). (*C*) Noncontrast CT (acquired as part of PET/CT in postpartum workup) shows a calcification corresponding to the SWI abnormality in the right temporal lobe (*arrow*). (*D*) Coronal postcontrast T1-weighted image, obtained after delivery, demonstrates a small focus of intense enhancement (*arrow*). After delivery, surgical pathology from resection revealed a ganglioglioma. (*Courtesy of* Richard Bronen, MD.)

sequences (gradient-recalled echo [GRE]/susceptibility-weighted imaging [SWI]). The authors recommend a low threshold for adding MRV.

FOCAL NEUROLOGIC DEFICIT

Visual symptoms can occur in the setting of pathologic pituitary enlargement through mass effect on the optic chiasm or cavernous sinus. They may also occur in conditions affecting the visual cortex, such as PRES, preeclampsia, ischemic arterial stroke, and CVT. Sensorimotor dysfunction and/or speech and language deficits may indicate ischemic stroke or hemorrhage.

Pituitary Disorders

The adenohypophysis increases in volume by 30% during pregnancy, as a consequence of estrogen's stimulatory effect on lactotroph cells.[45]

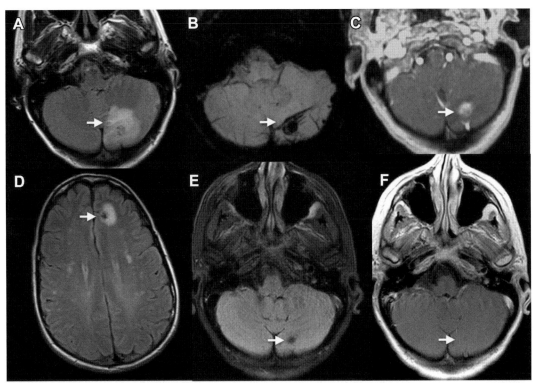

Fig. 7. Postpartum woman with metastatic choriocarcinoma. (*A, D*) Axial FLAIR images show representative left frontal and cerebellar lesions with accompanying vasogenic edema and central loss of signal (*arrows*). (*B*) Axial SWI image demonstrates susceptibility artifact compatible with hemorrhage corresponding to the cerebellar lesion (*arrow*). (*C*) Axial postcontrast T1 showed avid enhancement (*arrow*). (*E, F*) Axial FLAIR and postcontrast T1, respectively, show resolution of edema and enhancement following treatment (*arrows*).

Prolactinomas are the most common pituitary tumors occurring during pregnancy, although only 1.6% of patients with microadenomas show signs and symptoms of tumor enlargement.[46] In contrast, 23.3% patients with macroadenomas develop symptomatic tumor enlargement.[46] In pregnancy, evaluation of pituitary tumors poses a significant challenge because of rising prolactin levels, and a reluctance to administer gadolinium contrast material.[47] A pituitary adenoma is suspected if the pituitary height exceeds 12 mm on high-resolution MR without contrast material, in the appropriate clinical context[46] (**Fig. 8**).

Lymphocytic hypophysitis is a rare inflammatory autoimmune disorder of the anterior lobe of the pituitary gland, which can occur in the postpartum period.[9] It has been associated with other autoimmune diseases, such as pernicious anemia and autoimmune thyroiditis, and certain medications. MR is the imaging modality of choice and demonstrates enlargement of the pituitary gland with suprasellar extension in 60% to 80% of patients.[9] In most patients, there is early and homogeneous enhancement of the gland (**Fig. 9**), and hemorrhage is not associated with this condition.[9] Lymphocytic hypophysitis and nonhemorrhagic pituitary adenomas cannot be distinguished on imaging.[46]

Pituitary apoplexy presents with headache and visual deficits in a patient with an acutely enlarging hemorrhagic or infarcting pituitary adenoma. Neurosurgical and endocrine consultations for potential suprasellar decompression and hormonal support are required. CT and MR imaging show hemorrhage in a prominent pituitary gland.[9]

Ischemic Arterial Stroke

Ischemic arterial stroke in pregnancy and the postpartum period is rare, but the risk is increased compared with nonpregnant aged-matched controls, especially in late pregnancy and early postpartum,[48] possibly because of relative hypercoagulability just before delivery.[49] Additional risk factors for stroke are older maternal age, African American race, preexisting hypertension, heart disease, cesarean delivery, thrombocytopenia, anemia, and hyperemesis.[50]

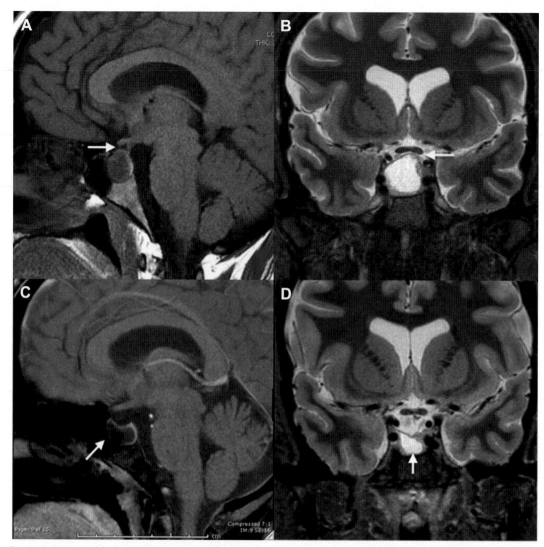

Fig. 8. A 26-year-old woman with cystic prolactinoma who experienced bilateral visual field defects during her pregnancy. (*A*) Sagittal noncontrast T1 image obtained during the initial weeks of the pregnancy shows a cystic sellar and suprasellar mass. The suprasellar cistern (*arrow, in A*) is partially preserved under the chiasm. (*B*) Coronal T2-weighted MR images obtained later in the pregnancy show the enlarging cystic prolactinoma contacting the optic chiasm (*arrow*). (*C, D*) 3 months after delivery, sagittal T1 postcontrast and coronal T2 MR images, respectively, show the lesion had decreased in size (*arrows*). The patient's visual field defects were resolved.

The greatest risk of ischemic events is reported in the 2 days before and first day following delivery.[51] Thrombocytopenia is also associated with HELLP syndrome (see **Fig. 1**), a severe form of preeclampsia with features of hemolysis, elevated liver enzymes, and low platelets, which can present with strokelike symptoms, cerebral ischemia, and hemorrhage.[52] Cervicocranial arterial dissection is another cause of stroke in pregnancy and the postpartum period. The incidence of dissection does not appear to be increased in pregnancy but may be related to strenuous labor.[53] Patients with dissection may develop

isolated headache without neurologic deficit, but they can also have brain infarctions.[54,55] Stroke should always be considered when a pregnant woman is affected by acute neurologic deficits (**Fig. 10**).

Rare Conditions

Amniotic fluid embolism occurs when amniotic fluid, fetal cells, hair, or other debris enter the maternal circulation via ruptured membranes or blood vessels.[56] The reported incidence ranges from 1 in 8000 to 1 in 80,000 deliveries.[57] Most

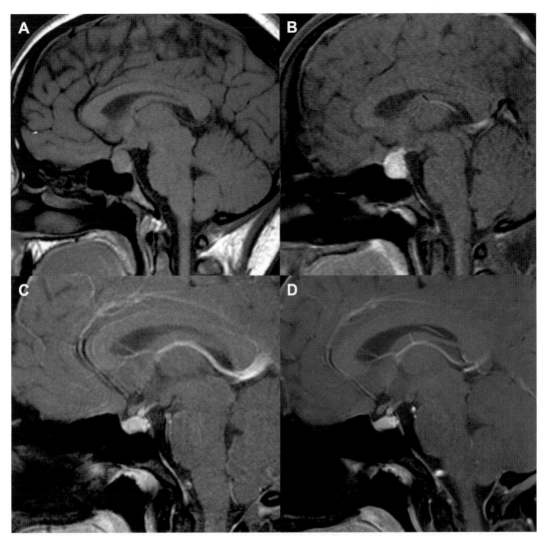

Fig. 9. Lymphocytic hypophysitis in pregnancy. A 24-year-old woman, 36 weeks' pregnant, presented with blurred vision, ultimately diagnosed with lymphocytic hypophysitis. (*A*) Sagittal noncontrast T1 shows enlargement of the pituitary versus sellar/suprasellar mass. She underwent cesarean section, (*B*) and a postcontrast MR imaging showed a homogenous enhancing pituitary and thickened/enhancing infundibulum. (*C, D*) One-year and 7-year MR follow-up images, respectively, showed the pituitary gland eventually returned to normal size.

cases occur during labor and are characterized by the rapid onset of confusion, seizures, and encephalopathy in the context of cardiovascular and respiratory collapse.[56] Ischemic stroke related to an amniotic fluid embolism can occur in the setting of a right-to-left shunt.

Air embolism occurs when air enters the uterine myometrium, travels through the venous circulation to the right ventricle, reducing cardiac output. Air embolism may result in seizures and abnormal cognition during or immediately following delivery.[58] Air may also cause stroke symptoms in the context of a right-to-left shunt.[58]

IMAGING SAFETY CONCERNS
Computed Tomography-Related Safety Concerns

For head and neck imaging, the estimated radiation exposure is very low for the fetus, and exposure from scatter is negligible from a deterministic point of view.[59] No well-controlled prospective studies in pregnant women have investigated the effect of iodinated intravenous contrast material; however, animal studies have failed to show adverse effects.[60] The US Food and Drug Administration classifies iodinated

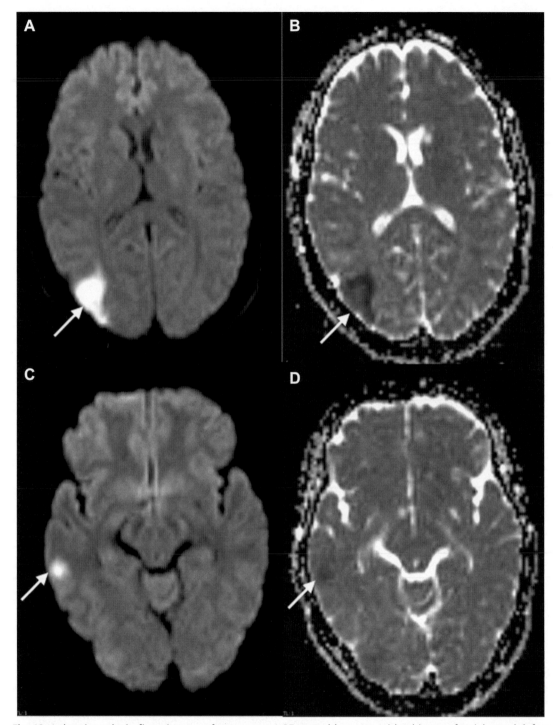

Fig. 10. Ischemic stroke in first trimester of pregnancy. A 27-year-old woman with a history of atrial septal defect presented with right retro-orbital headache and blurred vision. MR imaging diffusion-weighted imaging and apparent diffusion coefficient showed acute right parietal (*A, B, arrows*) and temporal (*C, D, arrows*) infarcts. The patient opted to terminate the pregnancy and underwent atrial septal defect closure.

contrast as pregnancy category B,[7] and informed consent is recommended before use. It has been shown that intravenous iodinated contrast does not affect short-term neonatal thyroid-stimulating hormone,[61] but long-term effects are unknown. No cases of neonatal hypothyroidism from maternal intravascular injection of water-soluble iodinated contrast agents are reported.[62]

Assessing fetal thyroid function in the first few weeks after birth following iodinated contrast administration in pregnancy is thought to be unnecessary.[61] No special precaution or cessation of breastfeeding is recommended for breastfeeding women who receive iodinated contrast.[7,61]

MR Imaging Safety

Gadolinium compounds cross the placenta and are excreted into the amniotic fluid by fetal urine, which is then swallowed by the fetus. Gadolinium-based compounds have been shown to cause abortion and developmental abnormalities in animal studies[60] in the setting of repeated high doses, but there are no data to suggest adverse effects in humans with administration of routine diagnostic doses.[61,63] Gadolinium is classified as pregnancy category C.[7] The current recommendation is to avoid the use of gadolinium contrast material in pregnant women unless there is a clear benefit expected to the mother and/or fetus, the administration cannot reasonably wait until after delivery, and that no alternative diagnostic test can provide the required information.[7,61] When gadolinium-based contrast material is used, informed consent is recommended with documentation of the above, after consulting the referring clinician.[7,61] Similar to iodinated contrast, only a very low amount of gadolinium-based contrast material is delivered from the mother to the infant via breast milk, and less still is absorbed in the infant's gastrointestinal tract. As such, breastfeeding precautions are not recommended, but could be adopted based on the patient's preferences.[61]

CONCLUSION

In a patient-centered model of care, the radiologist is an integral member of the multidisciplinary team caring for the pregnant and postpartum patient with acute neurologic disease. The collective goals are to ensure optimal imaging, provide a timely and accurate diagnosis, and minimize the risks of radiation and contrast exposure.

REFERENCES

1. Gunderman RB, Davilla J, Shetty S, et al. Visibility matters. J Am Coll Radiol 2005;2(12):971–4.
2. Brandt-Zawadski M, Kerlan RK Jr. Patient-centered radiology: use it or lose it! Acad Radiol 2009;16(5):521–3.
3. Basu PA, Ruiz-Wibbelsmann JA, Spielman SB, et al. Creating a patient-centered imaging service: determining what patients want. AJR Am J Roentgenol 2011;196(3):605–10.
4. Miller LS, Shelby RA, Balmadrid MH, et al. Patient anxiety before and immediately after imaging-guided breast biopsy procedures: impact of radiologist-patient communication. J Am Coll Radiol 2013;10(6):423–31.
5. Kanzaria HK, Hall MK, Moore CL, et al. Emergency department diagnostic imaging: the journey to quality. Acad Emerg Med 2015;22(12):1380–4.
6. Mangano MD, Rahman A, Choy G, et al. Radiologists' role in the communication of imaging examination results to patients: perceptions and preferences of patients. AJR Am J Roentgenol 2014;203(5):1034–9.
7. Edlow JA, Caplan LR, O'Brien K, et al. Diagnosis of acute neurological emergencies in pregnant and post-partum women. Lancet Neurol 2013;12(2):175–85.
8. Shainker SA, Edlow JA, O'Brien K. Cerebrovascular emergencies in pregnancy. Best Pract Res Clin Obstet Gynaecol 2015;29(5):721–31.
9. Zak IT, Dulai HS, Kish KK. Imaging of neurologic disorders associated with pregnancy and the post-partum period. Radiographics 2007;27(1):95–108.
10. Mortimer AM, Bradley MD, Likeman M, et al. Cranial neuroimaging in pregnancy and the post-partum period. Clin Radiol 2013;68(5):500–8.
11. Cipolla MJ. Cerebrovascular function in pregnancy and eclampsia. Hypertension 2007;50(1):14–24.
12. Sidorov EV, Feng W, Caplan LR. Stroke in pregnant and postpartum women. Expert Rev Cardiovasc Ther 2011;9(9):1235–47.
13. Chandra S, Tripathi AK, Mishra S, et al. Physiological changes in hematological parameters during pregnancy. Indian J Hematol Blood Transfus 2012;28(3):144–6.
14. Soma-Pillay P, Nelson-Piercy C, Tolppanen H, et al. Physiological changes in pregnancy. Cardiovasc J Afr 2016;27(2):89–94.
15. Costantine MM. Physiologic and pharmacokinetic changes in pregnancy. Front Pharmacol 2014;5:65.
16. Bremme KA. Haemostatic changes in pregnancy. Best Pract Res Clin Haematol 2003;16(2):153–68.
17. Goldszmidt E, Kern R, Chaput A, et al. The incidence and etiology of postpartum headaches: a prospective cohort study. Can J Anaesth 2005;52(9):971–7.
18. Robbins MS, Farmakidis C, Dayal AK, et al. Acute headache diagnosis in pregnant women: a hospital-based study. Neurology 2015;85(12):1024–30.
19. Sances G, Granella F, Nappi RE, et al. Course of migraine during pregnancy and postpartum: a prospective study. Cephalalgia 2003;23(3):197–205.
20. Melhado E, Maciel JA Jr, Guerreiro CA. Headaches during pregnancy in women with a prior history of menstrual headaches. Arq Neuropsiquiatr 2005;63(4):934–40.
21. Goadsby PJ, Goldberg J, Silberstein SD. Migraine in pregnancy. BMJ 2008;336(7659):1502–4.

22. Douglas AC, Wippold FJ 2nd, Broderick DF, et al. ACR appropriateness criteria headache. J Am Coll Radiol 2014;11(7):657–67. Available at: https://acsearch.acr.org/docs/69482/Narrative/. [Accessed 30 September 2017].

23. Duley L, Meher S, Abalos E. Management of pre-eclampsia. BMJ 2006;332(7539):463–8.

24. Sibai BM. Diagnosis, prevention, and management of eclampsia. Obstet Gynecol 2005;105(2):402–10.

25. Aukes AM, De Groot JC, Wiegman MJ, et al. Long-term cerebral imaging after pre-eclampsia. BJOG 2012;119(9):1117–22.

26. Bartynski WS, Boardman JF. Distinct imaging patterns and lesion distribution in posterior reversible encephalopathy syndrome. AJNR Am J Neuroradiol 2007;28(7):1320–7.

27. Hinchey J, Chaves C, Appignani B, et al. A reversible posterior leukoencephalopathy syndrome. N Engl J Med 1996;334(8):494–500.

28. Liman TG, Bohner G, Heuschmann PU, et al. Clinical and radiological differences in posterior reversible encephalopathy syndrome between patients with preeclampsia-eclampsia and other predisposing diseases. Eur J Neurol 2012;19(7):935–43.

29. Covarrubias DJ, Luetmer PH, Campeau NG. Posterior reversible encephalopathy syndrome: prognostic utility of quantitative diffusion-weighted MR images. AJNR Am J Neuroradiol 2002;23(6):1038–48.

30. Sawle GV, Ramsay MM. The neurology of pregnancy. J Neurol Neurosurg Psychiatry 1998;64(6):711–25.

31. Klein AM, Loder E. Postpartum headache. Int J Obstet Anesth 2010;19(4):422–30.

32. Van de Velde M, Schepers R, Berends N, et al. Ten years of experience with accidental dural puncture and post-dural puncture headache in a tertiary obstetric anaesthesia department. Int J Obstet Anesth 2008;17(4):329–35.

33. Farb RI, Forghani R, Lee SK, et al. The venous distension sign: a diagnostic sign of intracranial hypotension at MR imaging of the brain. AJNR Am J Neuroradiol 2007;28(8):1489–93.

34. Mas JL, Lamy C. Stroke in pregnancy and the puerperium. J Neurol 1998;245(6–7):305–13.

35. Cantu-Brito C, Arauz A, Aburto Y, et al. Cerebrovascular complications during pregnancy and postpartum: clinical and prognosis observations in 240 Hispanic women. Eur J Neurol 2011;18(6):819–25.

36. Lanska DJ, Kryscio RJ. Stroke and intracranial venous thrombosis during pregnancy and puerperium. Neurology 1998;51(6):1622–8.

37. Estella A, Payares JL. Postpartum headache: sinus venous thrombosis. BMJ Case Rep 2010;2010 [pii: bcr0620091936].

38. Connor SE, Jarosz JM. Magnetic resonance imaging of cerebral venous sinus thrombosis. Clin Radiol 2002;57(6):449–61.

39. Ducros A. Reversible cerebral vasoconstriction syndrome. Lancet Neurol 2012;11(10):906–17.

40. Neudecker S, Stock K, Krasnianski M. Call-Fleming postpartum angiopathy in the puerperium: a reversible cerebral vasoconstriction syndrome. Obstet Gynecol 2006;107(2 Pt 2):446–9.

41. Marder CP, Donohue MM, Weinstein JR, et al. Multi-modal imaging of reversible cerebral vasoconstriction syndrome: a series of 6 cases. AJNR Am J Neuroradiol 2012;33(7):1403–10.

42. Bogousslavsky J, Despland PA, Regli F, et al. Postpartum cerebral angiopathy: reversible vasoconstriction assessed by transcranial Doppler ultrasounds. Eur Neurol 1989;29(2):102–5.

43. Wahab M, Al-Azzawi F. Meningioma and hormonal influences. Climacteric 2003;6(4):285–92.

44. Smith JS, Quiñones-Hinojosa A, Harmon-Smith M, et al. Sex steroid and growth factor profile of a meningioma associated with pregnancy. Can J Neurol Sci 2005;32(1):122–7.

45. Dinc H, Esen F, Demirci A, et al. Pituitary dimensions and volume measurements in pregnancy and post partum. MR assessment. Acta Radiol 1998;39(1):64–9.

46. Molitch ME. Pituitary disorders during pregnancy. Endocrinol Metab Clin North Am 2006;35(1):99–116, vi.

47. Molitch ME. Evaluation and management of pituitary tumors during pregnancy. Endocr Pract 1996;2(4):287–95.

48. Salonen Ros H, Lichtenstein P, Bellocco R, et al. Increased risks of circulatory diseases in late pregnancy and puerperium. Epidemiology 2001;12(4):456–60.

49. Jaigobin C, Silver FL. Stroke and pregnancy. Stroke 2000;31(12):2948–51.

50. Tate J, Bushnell C. Pregnancy and stroke risk in women. Womens Health (Lond) 2011;7(3):363–74.

51. Bateman BT, Schumacher HC, Bushnell CD, et al. Intracerebral hemorrhage in pregnancy: frequency, risk factors, and outcome. Neurology 2006;67(3):424–9.

52. McCrae KR. Thrombocytopenia in pregnancy. Hematology Am Soc Hematol Educ Program 2010;2010:397–402.

53. Tettenborn B. Stroke and pregnancy. Neurol Clin 2012;30(3):913–24.

54. Arnold M, Camus-Jacqmin M, Stapf C, et al. Postpartum cervicocephalic artery dissection. Stroke 2008;39(8):2377–9.

55. McKinney JS, Messé SR, Pukenas BA, et al. Intracranial vertebrobasilar artery dissection associated with postpartum angiopathy. Stroke Res Treat 2010;2010 [pii:320627].

56. Rudra A, Chatterjee S, Sengupta S, et al. Amniotic fluid embolism. Indian J Crit Care Med 2009;13(3):129–35.

57. Morgan M. Amniotic fluid embolism. Anaesthesia 1979;34(1):20–32.

58. Muth CM, Shank ES. Gas embolism. N Engl J Med 2000;342(7):476–82.

59. Tremblay E, Thérasse E, Thomassin-Naggara I, et al. Quality initiatives: guidelines for use of medical imaging during pregnancy and lactation. Radiographics 2012;32(3):897–911.

60. Nelson JA, Livingston GK, Moon RG. Mutagenic evaluation of radiographic contrast media. Invest Radiol 1982;17(2):183–5.

61. American College of Radiology Committee on Drugs and Contrast Media. ACR manual on contrast media. Vol. Version 10.3. Reston (Virginia): American College of Radiology; 2017.

62. Kochi MH, Kaloudis EV, Ahmed W, et al. Effect of in utero exposure of iodinated intravenous contrast on neonatal thyroid function. J Comput Assist Tomogr 2012;36(2):165–9.

63. Webb JA, Thomsen HS, Morcos SK, et al. The use of iodinated and gadolinium contrast media during pregnancy and lactation. Eur Radiol 2005;15(6): 1234–40.

Imaging the Unconscious "Found Down" Patient in the Emergency Department

Carlos Torres, MD, FRCPC[a,b,*], Nader Zakhari, MD, FRCPC[c],
Sean Symons, BASc, MPH, MD, FRCPC, DABR, MBA[d],
Thanh B. Nguyen, MD, FRCPC[c]

KEYWORDS

- Coma • Unconscious • Found down • Emergency department • Encephalitis
- Metabolic encephalopathy • Toxic encephalopathy • Diffuse axonal injury

KEY POINTS

- Unconsciousness may be due to severe brain damage or to potentially treatable or reversible causes.
- The ascending reticular activating system plays a crucial role in maintaining behavioral arousal and consciousness.
- Unwitnessed seizures are among the most common neurologic causes of an unconscious patient.
- Carbon monoxide toxicity represents the most common cause of accidental poisoning in North America and Europe, and is a major cause of suicide.
- Noncontrast head CT is the imaging modality of choice in the assessment of the unconscious patient in the emergency department.
- MR imaging plays an important role in the assessment of acutely encephalopathic patients that may show no significant abnormality on CT.

INTRODUCTION

Unconsciousness is the condition of being in a mental state that involves complete or markedly reduced responsiveness to people and other environmental stimuli. It occurs when we lose the ability to maintain awareness of self and the environment.

The ascending reticular activating system (ARAS) plays a crucial role in maintaining behavioral arousal and consciousness. It is a complex pathway that connects several neuronal circuits from the pons and dorsal aspect of the midbrain to the cerebral cortex via pathways that project through the thalamus and hypothalamus.[1]

Single structural lesions, such as a tumor or an ischemic infarct, may produce coma by direct disruption of this pathway in the upper brainstem. Unilateral cerebral hemispheric lesions do not produce coma unless there is enough mass effect and

Disclosure: The authors have nothing to disclose.
[a] Department of Radiology, University of Ottawa, 1053 Carling Avenue, Ottawa, ON K1Y 4E9, Canada;
[b] Department of Medical Imaging, The Ottawa Hospital, Civic Campus, 1053 Carling Avenue, Ottawa, ON K1Y 4E9, Canada; [c] Department of Radiology, University of Ottawa, The Ottawa Hospital, Civic and General Campus, 1053 Carling Avenue, Ottawa, ON K1Y 4E9, Canada; [d] Neuroradiology, Department of Medical Imaging, University of Toronto, Sunnybrook Health Sciences Centre, 2075 Bayview Avenue, Toronto, ON M4N 3M5, Canada
* Corresponding author. The Ottawa Hospital, Civic Campus, 1053 Carling Avenue, Ottawa, ON K1Y 4E9, Canada.
E-mail address: catorres@toh.ca

Neuroimag Clin N Am 28 (2018) 435–451
https://doi.org/10.1016/j.nic.2018.03.006
1052-5149/18/© 2018 Elsevier Inc. All rights reserved.

midline shift adversely affecting the ARAS bilaterally, typically at the thalamic level. Coma, however, also may occur from extensive, severe bilateral cortical lesions (ie, multiple hemorrhages) or from metabolic processes that suppress cortical function in a global way, such as drug intoxication or hypoglycemia.[2]

Unconsciousness may be due to severe brain damage or to potentially treatable or reversible causes. Prompt evaluation of an unconscious patient is therefore required to proceed with appropriate therapeutic intervention. Any patient suffering loss of consciousness should be assessed in hospital, as the patient may likely require a computed tomography (CT) scan of the head, in accordance with the National Institute for Health and Care Excellence head injury guidelines.[3] Depending on the clinical history and the CT findings, MR imaging of the brain may be necessary. Not uncommonly, the MR imaging reveals key information that often leads to a definite diagnosis. The purpose of this article was to describe common and important disorders that may lead to unconsciousness, including vascular, metabolic, and toxic entities, as well as traumatic brain injury and epilepsy. The emergency department (ED) radiologist must be familiarized with these entities to develop a patient-centered approach that may allow for a prompt diagnosis and management.

HEAD INJURY: TRAUMA

Traumatic brain injury affects 1.7 million people annually in the United States,[4] and can cause intracranial bleed or diffuse cerebral edema. Intracranial hemorrhage alone does not usually lead to a comatose state unless there is increased intracranial pressure or if the ARAS is affected. Diffuse brain edema, however, can lead to transtentorial herniation with secondary compression of the brain stem, which can damage the ARAS pathway (**Fig. 1**). Diffuse axonal injury (DAI) in the context of high-velocity accidents may lead to unconsciousness.

Diffuse Axonal Injury

DAI is one of the most common primary traumatic neuronal injuries. It results from shearing of the brain parenchyma due to rotational acceleration and deceleration forces. Transient loss or severe impairment of the level of consciousness at the moment of impact is characteristic of DAI.[5] DAI is classified based on anatomic location: grade I lesions at the gray-white matter interface and more common in the frontotemporal regions; grade II lesions in the corpus callosum (most common in the splenium) and lobar white matter; grade III lesions along the dorsolateral aspect of the mesencephalon in addition to the involvement of the cortical-subcortical junctions and of the corpus callosum (**Fig. 2**). The severity of the injury increases, and the prognosis worsens, as the deeper structures are involved.[4,5]

DAI manifests on CT as punctate hyperdense hemorrhagic foci at the aforementioned typical locations. However, CT underestimates the extent of DAI, as most of the lesions are very small and initially nonhemorrhagic. Only 20%

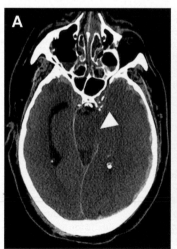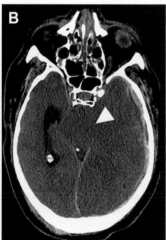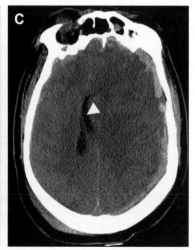

Fig. 1. Unenhanced head CT in the axial plane (*A–C*) in a patient involved in a motor vehicle accident, demonstrates an acute left holohemispheric SDH with associated mass effect causing effacement of the perimesencephalic cisterns (*arrowheads A, B*) with secondary compression of the brain stem, which can damage the ARAS pathway. In addition, there is significant subfalcine herniation (*arrowhead in C*).

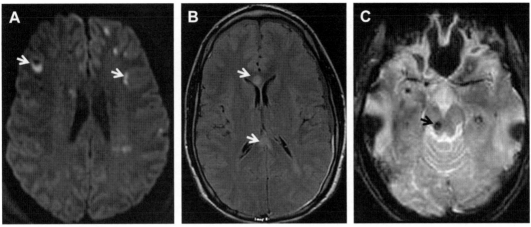

Fig. 2. Axial DWI sequence (*A*) shows multiple nonhemorrhagic shearing injuries involving the U fibers in both frontal lobes (*white arrows*) consistent with Grade I DAI. Axial FLAIR sequence (*B*) demonstrates additional shearing injuries (*white arrows*) in the genu and splenium of the corpus callosum (Grade II DAI). Axial GRE sequence (*C*) in a different patient, shows blooming artifact in the right dorsolateral aspect of the mesencephalon (*black arrow*), in keeping with Grade III DAI.

of DAI lesions contain sufficient hemorrhage to be seen on CT.[5] Hence, DAI should be suspected when there is discrepancy between the initial CT findings and the clinical symptoms. The presence of intraventricular hemorrhage on the initial CT after trauma has been shown to be a marker of DAI detected on subsequent MR imaging.[6]

MR imaging is superior to CT for DAI detection; therefore, it provides a better explanation for neurologic deficits after trauma. Nonhemorrhagic DAI is seen as multifocal T2 and fluid attenuation inversion recovery (FLAIR) hyperintense foci. Gradient-echo T2* sequences (GRE) sensitive to blood products demonstrate more DAI lesions than CT. Susceptibility-weighted imaging (SWI) is even more sensitive in detecting hemorrhagic DAI than conventional GRE.[7,8] On diffusion-weighted imaging (DWI), acute DAI lesions show foci of high signal on B1000 and low signal on apparent diffusion coefficient (ADC) map, in keeping with diffusion restriction secondary to cellular death. DWI can identify additional DAI lesions not detectable on T2/FLAIR or T2* sequences.[7,9]

Epidural Hematoma

An epidural hematoma (EDH) is the collection of blood in the potential space between the dura and the inner calvarial table. It can be arterial or venous in origin but more commonly arterial in nature due to laceration of meningeal arteries.[4] On CT, acute EDH appears as a biconvex usually hyperdense extra-axial collection, not crossing suture lines, commonly associated with an overlying skull fracture. Acute EDH tends to expand rapidly in the presence of internal lower density components, known as "the swirl sign," which indicates active extravasation of unclotted blood.[10] EDH causing mass effect and brain herniation can lead to altered level of consciousness or coma. EDH may require surgery when its volume is greater than 30 mL, its thickness more than 15 mm or when it causes more than 5 mm of midline shift.[11,12]

Subdural Hematoma

A subdural hematoma (SDH) is the collection of blood in the subdural space. It is usually venous in origin due to laceration of bridging veins during sudden head deceleration. The incidence of SDH is higher in elderly patients, as prominent extra-axial spaces allow increased motion between the brain and the calvarium. On CT, SDH appears as a crescentic collection overlying the cerebral convexity.[5] The clinical presentation depends on the degree of mass effect and the presence of brain herniation. Different degrees of altered level of consciousness could be observed, ranging from confusion to coma (**Fig. 3**).

Subarachnoid Hemorrhage

Loss of consciousness (LOC) is common in the context of subarachnoid hemorrhage (SAH) secondary to increased intracranial pressure and

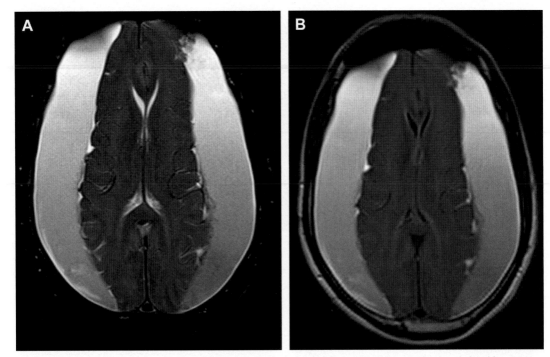

Fig. 3. Axial T2-weighted (*A*) and FLAIR (*B*) sequences show large bilateral holohemispheric subdural hematomas causing severe compression of the brain parenchyma, with almost complete effacement of the lateral ventricles.

reduced cerebral perfusion pressure. LOC at onset of SAH is usually associated with severe bleeding, larger SAH, global cerebral edema, and early brain injury. It carries a 2.8-fold increased risk of poor outcome after SAH.[13]

The most common cause of spontaneous non-traumatic SAH is by far saccular aneurysm rupture (85%). Patients present with sudden severe "thunderclap" headache with SAH predominantly seen in the suprasellar and central basal cisterns with peripheral extension (**Fig. 4**A). Perimesencephalic nonaneurysmal hemorrhage is the second most common cause (10%), and is mostly venous in

origin with a more favorable clinical course.[14,15] On imaging, the SAH is centered anterior to the midbrain or pons involving the perimesence-phalic and low basal cisterns with no peripheral extension or frank intraventricular hemorrhage (**Fig. 4**B).[16]

The third and least common pattern of SAH is the convexal SAH (**Fig. 4**C), in which blood is localized within a few cerebral convexity sulci. This a heterogeneous group with multiple etiologies that can present with altered mental status. The most common underlying etiology is reversible cerebral vasoconstriction syndrome in patients younger

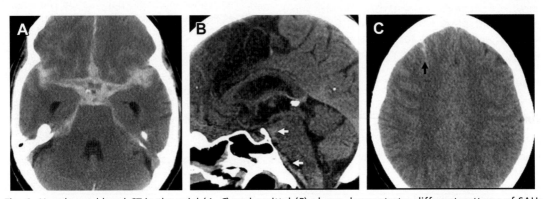

Fig. 4. Unenhanced head CT in the axial (*A, C*) and sagittal (*B*) planes demonstrates different patterns of SAH: diffuse aneurysmal SAH (*A*), perimesencephalic SAH (*white arrows* in *B*), and convexal SAH (*black arrow* in *C*).

than 60 years and cerebral amyloid angiopathy in patients older than 60. Other diagnoses associated with this pattern include posterior reversible encephalopathy syndrome, cortical venous thrombosis, vasculitis, and coagulation disorders, among others.[16,17]

Unenhanced head CT is the modality of choice to rule-in or to rule-out SAH with sufficient accuracy when obtained within 6 hours of headache onset (sensitivity 100% within 6 hours and 89% beyond that).[18] Depending on the CT findings and the clinical suspicion, further workup includes lumbar puncture, CT angiography (CTA), and digital subtraction angiography. MR imaging can be especially useful to identify the underlying etiology of isolated convexal SAH.[16] As the CT attenuation of SAH decreases with time, subacute SAH can be best seen on MR imaging using double inversion recovery (DIR), FLAIR, T2*, and SWI sequences.[19] T2*/SWI are the best sequences to identify location of remote SAH.[20]

EPILEPSY AND STATUS EPILEPTICUS

Unwitnessed seizures are among the most common neurologic causes of an unconscious patient. Epileptic seizures are very common. It is estimated that approximately 10% of the population in developed countries will experience a seizure during their lifetimes.[21] Epileptic seizures can be classified into generalized and partial seizure, the latter could be simple or complex. Generalized and complex partial seizures are associated with LOC.[22] Status epilepticus is a life-threatening condition defined as more than 30 minutes of continuous seizure activity or 2 or more sequential seizures without full recovery of consciousness between seizures.[23]

MR imaging is the imaging modality of choice in epilepsy.[22] Peri-ictal changes on MR imaging present as diffusion restriction, T2/FLAIR hyperintensity, and mild swelling of the cortical gray matter and subcortical white matter not confined to a vascular territory (**Fig. 5**). Mild associated leptomeningeal contrast enhancement can be seen, as well as focally increased perfusion.[21,24–27] Although status epilepticus is not a prerequisite for developing these findings, a longer seizure duration increases the chance of detecting these abnormalities. These peri-ictal changes are most commonly seen in the mesial temporal lobe/hippocampus. However, they also can be detected in the cerebral cortex involved in seizure generation, in the thalamus (pulvinar), and in the corpus callosum, especially in the splenium.[21,24] It has been suggested that the changes in the white matter are secondary to vasogenic edema induced by focally increased perfusion and vascular permeability, whereas the gray matter change is related to cytotoxic edema induced by focal ischemia or other metabolic abnormalities. The reversibility and characteristic locations of the signal changes may help exclude the possibility of epileptogenic structural lesions.[27] However, in some cases, the regions of peri-ictal signal abnormality may progress into atrophy and laminar necrosis, potentially becoming a new epileptic focus.[26]

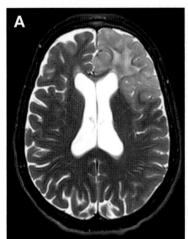 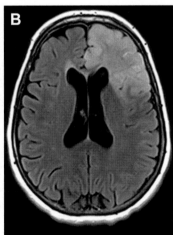 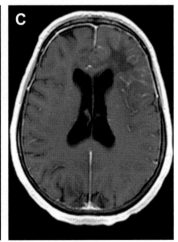

Fig. 5. A 58-year-old patient, unconscious, with history of tonic-clonic seizure. Axial T2-weighted (*A*) and axial FLAIR (*B*) sequences demonstrate focal cortical swelling in the left frontal lobe, with associated increased signal intensity of the cortex and subcortical white matter. The axial T1-weighted sequence postcontrast (*C*) shows mild leptomeningeal enhancement likely related to hyperemia.

TOXIC ENCEPHALOPATHIES

The brain is susceptible to damage from various toxins. MR imaging often may demonstrate imaging abnormalities that could explain the sudden onset of neurologic dysfunction. Therefore, in the setting of acute encephalopathy, recognition of the different imaging patterns of toxic injury to the brain may help narrow the differential diagnosis. We review herein the characteristic MR imaging features of several toxic encephalopathies, including carbon monoxide, methanol, cocaine, and heroin intoxication.[28]

Carbon Monoxide

Carbon monoxide (CO) is a highly toxic tasteless and odorless gas produced by incomplete combustion of hydrocarbons. It represents the most common cause of accidental poisoning in North America and Europe, and is a major cause of suicide. Bilateral and symmetric necrosis of the globus pallidus is the most common brain injury found in patients with carbon monoxide poisoning. These lesions are hypodense on CT and show low T1 and high T2/FLAIR signal intensity on MR imaging. Involvement of the cerebral white matter, predominantly in the centrum semiovale, could be seen[28,29] (Fig. 6).

Methanol

Acute methanol intoxication may be deliberate or accidental, and can be fatal unless treatment is rapidly instituted. Following ingestion, there is a clinically silent period of 12 to 24 hours, that corresponds to the time required for methanol to be metabolized into formaldehyde and formic acid, which ultimately results in severe metabolic acidosis.[30,31] The most characteristic finding is bilateral necrosis of the putamen[32] (Fig. 7); however, the visual pathway tends to be affected as well. Hemorrhage could be seen in 7% to 14% of cases[30,32] and is associated with a poor prognosis. On CT, bilateral putaminal hypodensity due to edema or, less often, hyperdensity related to petechial hemorrhage may be seen. MR imaging shows T2 hyperintensity of the lateral putamen that may extend into the globus pallidus, corona radiata, and the centrum semiovale.[30,33] T1 hyperintensity could be seen in the presence of hemorrhage.

Cocaine

Cocaine can produce toxic encephalopathy from direct toxic effects after intravenous (IV) use or inhalation. Cocaine abuse also can cause vasospasm and vasculitis leading to ischemic and hemorrhagic infarcts. On MR imaging, lesions with increased T2 signal have been reported in the globi pallidi, splenium of the corpus callosum, and cerebral white matter, with the affected regions often showing diffusion restriction (Fig. 8).[28,34]

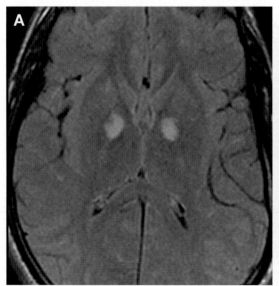
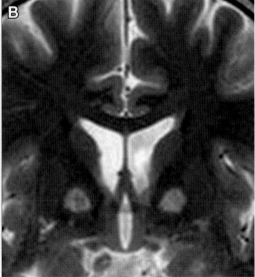

Fig. 6. Axial FLAIR (A) and coronal T2W (B) sequences show focal symmetric increased signal intensity in the bilateral globus pallidus in a patient with CO intoxication.

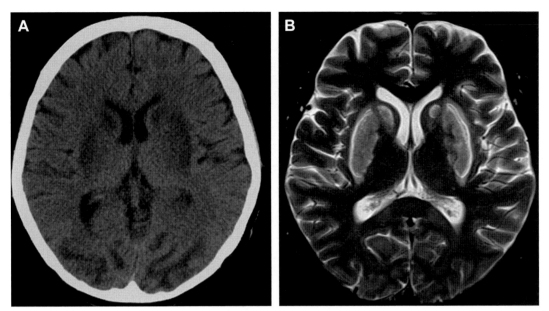

Fig. 7. Methanol intoxication. Axial head CT (*A*) shows symmetric hypodensity of the basal ganglia and of the subcortical white matter in both occipital lobes. Axial T2-weighted sequence (*B*) at the same level shows increase signal intensity of the bilateral putamen and head of the caudate nuclei secondary to necrosis.

Heroin

Ischemia is the most common acute neurovascular complication. The proposed pathomechanisms include the following: (1) direct heroin toxicity leading to reversible vasospasm from stimulation of the vascular smooth muscles, (2) vasculitis from immune-mediated response, or (3) embolic events from impure additives.[35,36] Ischemia is more common after IV injection compared with

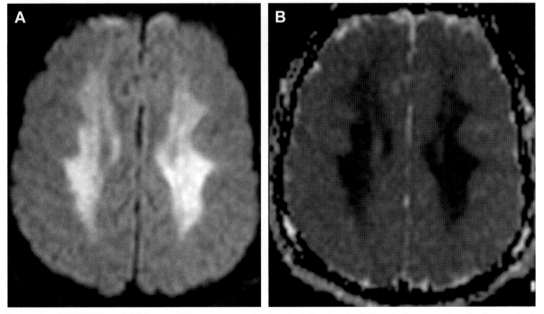

Fig. 8. Axial DWI (*A*) and ADC map (*B*) sequences obtained at the level of the centrum semiovale demonstrate restricted diffusion in a patient with cocaine toxicity. (*Courtesy of* Dr Marlise P. dos Santos, University of Ottawa, Ottawa, ON, Canada.)

other routes, such as oral ingestion or inhalation,[36] and the brain structure more commonly affected is the globus pallidus.

Heroin-induced leukoencephalopathy, also known as "chasing the dragon," is exclusively seen after heroin inhalation.[37–39] The drug is heated over tinfoil and the emerging fumes are inhaled. Acute leukoencephalopathy may occur, presumably due to activation of unknown substances or additives, leading to generalized brain edema.[40] Key imaging findings include symmetric involvement of the cerebellar white matter, cerebellar peduncles, brainstem, posterior cerebral white matter, and posterior limbs of the internal capsules. CT demonstrates low density of these structures, and MR imaging shows increased signal intensity on T2-weighted sequences (**Fig. 9**). Of note, DWI shows increased signal intensity in the affected regions of the brain, but there is no associated diffusion restriction.[37–39]

ENCEPHALITIS

Patients with encephalitis typically present with altered level of consciousness, fever, headache, seizures, and focal deficits. In patients with herpes simplex encephalitis, the most common viral etiology, MR imaging usually shows asymmetric T2/FLAIR signal abnormality, with or without diffusion restriction, in the inferomedial aspect of the temporal lobes with extension to the insular cortex. Involvement of the inferior frontal lobes, cingulate gyrus, and thalamus also can be seen.[41] Although temporal lobe involvement also can be seen in patients with Japanese encephalitis or West Nile encephalitis, it is less common. In Japanese encephalitis, a more prevalent entity in India and East Asia, the hippocampus could be involved, but the rest of the temporal lobe is typically spared.[42] Characteristic imaging findings of Japanese encephalitis include increased T2/FLAIR signal of the thalami and substantia nigra bilaterally, usually with associated restricted diffusion. The basal ganglia, pons, cerebellum, cerebral cortex, and spinal cord also may be involved. Definite confirmation of the diagnosis is made through detection of virus-specific immunoglobulin M antibodies through enzyme-linked immunosorbent assay test done on serum or cerebrospinal fluid.[42,43] In West Nile meningoencephalitis, areas of signal abnormality on T2/FLAIR images are often present in the brainstem, thalami, cerebral white matter, and anterior horns of the spinal cord. High signal abnormality can be seen on the trace images on DWI even when FLAIR abnormalities are absent or subtle (**Fig. 10**).[44]

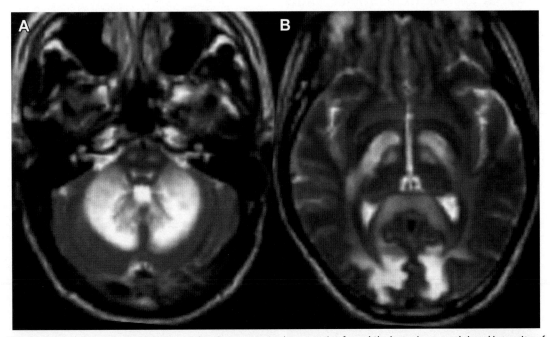

Fig. 9. Chasing the dragon. Axial T2-weighted sequence in the posterior fossa (*A*), shows increased signal intensity of the cerebellar white matter, middle cerebellar peduncles, and pons. The axial T2-weighted sequence at the level of the third ventricle (*B*) demonstrates hypersignal in the subcortical white matter of both occipital lobes and in the posterior limbs of the internal capsules. (*Courtesy of* Dr Marlise P. dos Santos, University of Ottawa, Ottawa, ON, Canada.)

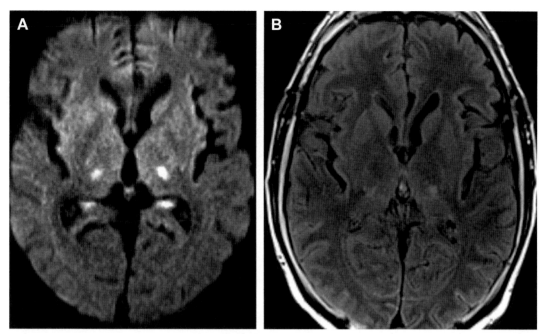

Fig. 10. West Nile encephalitis. Axial DWI (*A*) sequence demonstrates focal symmetric increased signal intensity of the thalami, a finding that is subtler in the FLAIR (*B*) sequence. (*Courtesy of* Dr Girish M. Fatterpekar, MD, NYU Langone Medical Center, New York, NY.)

AUTOIMMUNE ENCEPHALITIS

Autoimmune encephalitis was first described as a paraneoplastic syndrome typically associated with small-cell lung cancer; however, non-paraneoplastic encephalitides have been recognized more recently.[45] In paraneoplastic limbic encephalitis, there is increased T2/FLAIR signal in the mesial temporal lobes bilaterally, with variable involvement of the cerebellum and brainstem (Fig. 11). This is most frequently associated with the presence of Anti-Hu (anti-neuronal nuclear antibody 1) antibodies. In anti-CV2 (collapsin response mediator protein 5) encephalitis, which is a rare form of paraneoplastic syndrome associated with small-cell lung cancer or malignant thymoma, there is increased signal on T2/FLAIR in the striatum, similar to other diseases, such as hypoglycemia, CO poisoning, and hyperammonemia. In N-methyl D-aspartate receptor (NMDAR) encephalitis, mild cortical hyperintense T2 signal

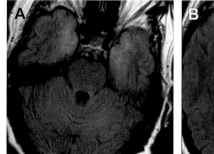
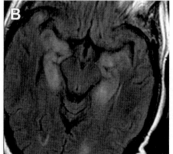
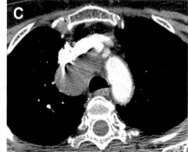

Fig. 11. A 68-year-old woman presenting with a rapid cognitive decline. Axial FLAIR images (*A*, *B*) show bilateral symmetric hyperintense signal in the mesial temporal lobes in keeping with limbic encephalitis. Testing for Purkinje cell cytoplasmic type 2 (PCA-2) antibody was positive. Initial workup for malignancy was negative. CT of the chest (*C*) performed 1 year later revealed a mediastinal adenopathy. Mediastinal biopsy revealed small-cell lung carcinoma.

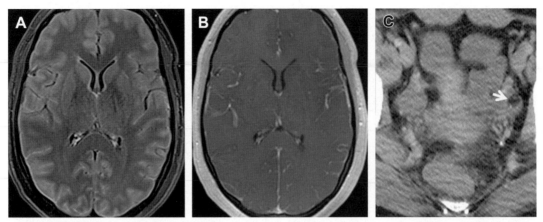

Fig. 12. A 28-year-old woman with anti-NMDA receptor encephalitis presenting with prolonged stupor requiring prolonged intensive care unit admission. Axial FLAIR (A) and T1-weighted sequence postcontrast (B) show diffuse meningeal enhancement. CT scan of the abdomen (C) revealed a fat-containing adnexal mass (arrow), which was histopathologically proven to be a teratoma.

can be seen without restricted diffusion or enhancement, although imaging has been reported to be normal in most patients. Although rare, NMDAR encephalitis can present with meningitis; hence, leptomeningeal enhancement could be the only abnormality on MR imaging (Fig. 12)[45,46]

METABOLIC DISORDERS
Hypoglycemia

Although unenhanced head CT may show white matter hypodensities or diffuse cerebral edema in the acute setting, MR imaging is a better modality to demonstrate parenchymal changes related to hypoglycemia. Using DWI, patients

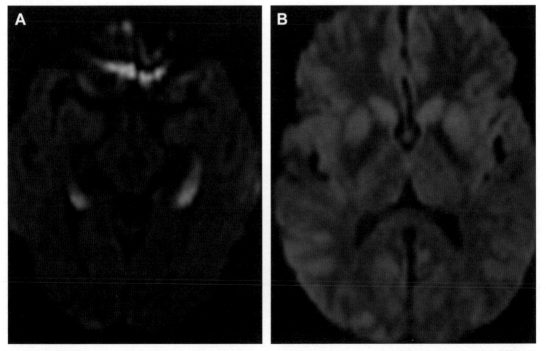

Fig. 13. Axial DWI sequence (A, B) in 2 different patients with hypoglycemic coma. (A) shows restricted diffusion, along the posterior aspect of the hippocampi, whereas (B) demonstrates restricted diffusion in the cortex of both cerebral hemispheres and in the bilateral basal ganglia.

with hypoglycemic coma can be classified into 3 categories at initial presentation: (1) normal examination; (2) focal lesion in a white matter tract, such as the internal capsule, cerebellar peduncle, and splenium; or (3) diffuse lesions involving the hemispheric white matter, basal ganglia, and cerebral cortex.[47] The hippocampus is also a frequently affected area[48] (**Fig. 13**). Abnormal restricted diffusion is thought to represent cytotoxic edema and may be reversible.[49] Patients with diffuse involvement of the cortex or cerebral white matter have a poorer outcome, compared with those with a focal white matter lesion.[47,50] Involvement of the thalamus, brainstem, and cerebellum is not usually seen with hypoglycemic coma and is more suggestive of a hypoxic-ischemic injury due to cardiac arrest.[51]

Hepatic Encephalopathy

Patients with acute hyperammonemic encephalopathy present with progressive drowsiness, seizures, and coma due to primary toxic effects of ammonia on the brain parenchyma.[52] In adults, this condition is usually seen in very ill patients in the intensive care unit. Acute hepatic dysfunction is usually the underlying cause,

but other etiologies include portosystemic shunt surgery, infection, hypothyroidism, multiple myeloma, and after lung or bone marrow transplantation.[53]

MR imaging demonstrates bilateral and symmetric increased T2/FLAIR signal intensity of the insular cortex and cingulate gyrus, with corresponding areas of restricted diffusion (**Fig. 14**). Diffusion restriction in the thalamus, cortex, and white matter is indicative of acute hepatic encephalopathy secondary to liver failure and may be reversible. The extent of restricted diffusion is associated with plasma ammonia levels. Involvement of the cortex in the frontal, temporal, parietal, or occipital lobes could be seen, but is more asymmetric and variable in extent. Postcontrast enhancement is not usually seen.[53] In hyperammonemic coma, brain glutamine level is elevated and can be measured with MR spectroscopy.[54]

Osmotic Demyelination Syndrome

Unenhanced head CT is usually normal in the first week and then typically shows a hypodensity within the central pons. Extrapontine involvement of the thalamus, basal ganglia, and cerebral white matter also may be present. MR

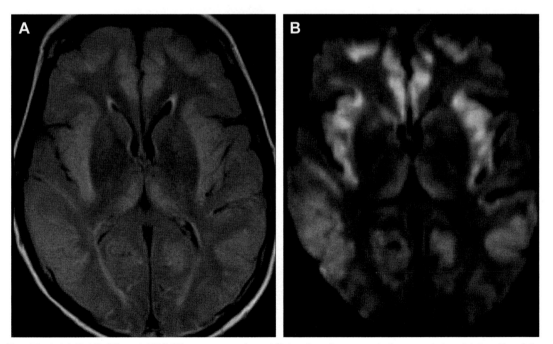

Fig. 14. Axial FLAIR (*A*) and DWI (*B*) sequences show bilateral and symmetric increased signal intensity of the insular and posterior temporal cortex, cingulate gyri, and of the mesial aspect of the thalami corresponding to restricted diffusion in a patient with acute hyperammonemia.

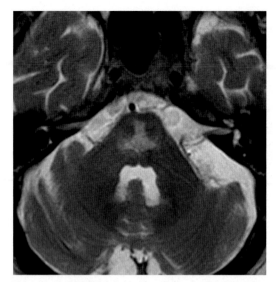

Fig. 15. Axial T2-weighted sequence demonstrates a characteristic symmetric triangular hyperintense lesion in the pons, sparing the corticospinal tracts, in the setting of osmotic myelinolysis.

imaging is more sensitive and may show the pontine abnormality as early as day 2.[55] A symmetric triangular pontine lesion of low signal intensity on T1 and high signal on T2 is a characteristic finding that has been coined as the "trident" sign (Fig. 15). There is no mass effect or enhancement. Typically, the descending corticospinal tracts are preserved. DWI shows variable signal depending on the stage of the disease.[56]

Vascular Causes

A hyperdense basilar artery on the noncontrast head CT is suggestive of acute thrombosis (Fig. 16). This sign had 71% sensitivity

and 98% specificity for basilar artery occlusion in patients with suspected acute posterior circulation stroke.[57] Prompt confirmation of the diagnosis should be performed with CTA (see Fig. 16) or time-of-flight MR angiography, given the patient might be a candidate for recanalization. Extensive ischemic changes in the posterior circulation territory (thalamus, brainstem, cerebellum, occipital lobes) on the initial CT or MR imaging is associated with a poor clinical outcome, even in patients who underwent successful recanalization[58]

In patients with thalamic hypodensity secondary to ischemic change, it is important to determine if the infarction is arterial or venous in origin. Occlusion of the top of the basilar artery or of the artery of Percheron can lead to bilateral arterial thalamic infarction (Fig. 17). The artery of Percheron is a rare anatomic variant that arises from the P1 segment of the posterior cerebral artery and supplies the paramedian thalamus and midbrain bilaterally.

Venous thalamic infarcts are due to thrombosis of the internal cerebral veins, which appear hyperdense on noncontrast CT. Dural venous thrombosis can be confirmed with CT venogram or MR venogram (Fig. 18). Treatment with anticoagulation or endovascular therapy can reverse neurologic deficits.

Anoxic-Ischemic Injury

Adult patients with cardiac ischemia/arrhythmia or asphyxia develop secondary hypoxemia, which can involve the thalamus, basal ganglia, hippocampi, and cerebral cortex. Immediate head CT performed after the injury often fails to reveal the extent of ischemic changes. Subtle loss of the gray-white matter differentiation and decreased density of the deep gray matter can be seen. A more evident finding is the presence

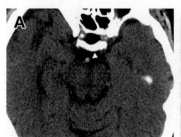
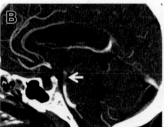
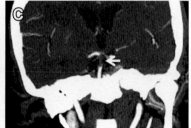

Fig. 16. Unenhanced head CT (A) demonstrates a hyperdense distal basilar artery (arrowhead), in keeping with acute thrombosis. CT angiogram of the same patient in the sagittal (B) and coronal (C) planes shows a filling defect in the distal basilar artery confirming the presence of thrombus (arrows).

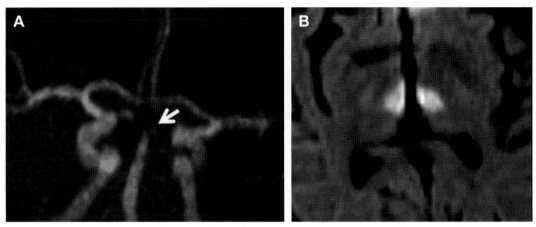

Fig. 17. Time-of-flight MR angiogram (*A*) demonstrates a filling defect at the basilar tip (*arrow*). Axial DWI (*B*) demonstrates acute bithalamic infarcts, within the artery of Percheron vascular territory.

of bilateral sulcal effacement due to diffuse edema. The "reversal sign" is seen on CT when the cerebral white matter or cerebellar cortex appears denser than the cerebral cortex, and is indicative of a poor clinical outcome[59] MR imaging with DWI is more sensitive to early ischemic changes. Areas of restricted diffusion in the cortex/deep gray matter can be seen within the first few hours after the event (**Fig. 19**). Acute infarctions can be seen in the cortex and centrum semiovale at the border zone between vascular territories.

Decompression Illness

Decompression illness related to diving is induced by a fast decrease of environmental pressure leading to rapid gas bubble formation in tissues and the bloodstream during the ascent. These bubbles can affect the central nervous system via different

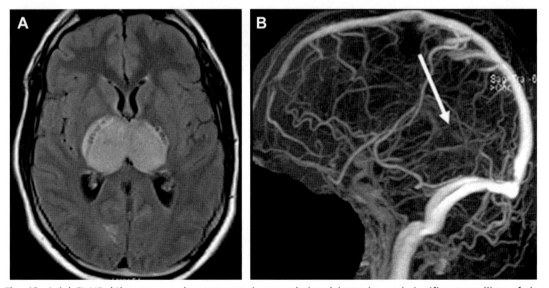

Fig. 18. Axial FLAIR (*A*) sequence demonstrates increased signal intensity and significant swelling of the bilateral thalami. The maximum intensity projection image of a contrast-enhanced MR venogram (*B*) in the sagittal plane shows lack of contrast opacification of the straight sinus (*arrow*) in keeping with thrombosis.

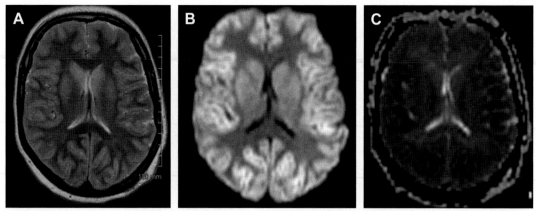

Fig. 19. Unconscious patient after cardiac arrest. Axial T2-weighted sequence (A) demonstrates mild diffuse thickening and increased signal intensity of the cortex in both cerebral hemispheres. Similar changes are seen in the bilateral basal ganglia. Associated restricted diffusion in DWI (B) and ADC map (C), secondary to anoxic brain injury.

mechanisms, including arterial occlusion, venous obstruction, or direct nitrogen toxicity. It can occur in circumstances such as ascent from diving, flying, or climbing mountains immediately after a dive.[60,61] Diving-related decompression illness is usually divided into 2 main categories: arterial gas embolism due to pulmonary decompression barotrauma and decompression sickness.[61]

Symptoms range from mild to life-threatening. Severe decompression sickness after rapid ascent from significant depth is deadly. Postmortem CT and MR imaging of the brain and spinal cord has shown extensive amount of gas in cerebral and spinal arteries as well as in cerebrospinal fluid spaces, whereas the intracranial venous sinuses remained unaffected (Fig. 20).[62]

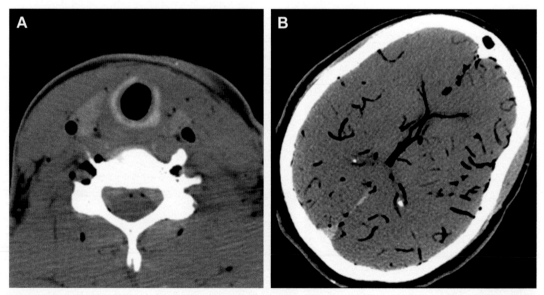

Fig. 20. Decompression illness in patient found down in the shores of Lake Ontario. Axial image of a CT scan of the neck (A) shows air within multiple vessels, including carotid and vertebral arteries. Axial CT scan of the head (B) demonstrates extensive amount of gas in cerebral and cerebrospinal fluid spaces, whereas the intracranial venous sinuses seem preserved. (Courtesy of Dr Omar Islam, Queen's University, Kingston, ON, Canada.)

SUMMARY

The unconscious patient represents a challenge to the emergency physician and also a dilemma to the ED radiologist given the lack of clinical information. Both the ED physician and the ED radiologist rely heavily on imaging to establish the correct diagnosis. Noncontrast head CT is the imaging modality of choice, as it is useful and readily available. It may help identify acute ischemic and hemorrhagic lesions as well as certain patterns of toxic or metabolic encephalopathy. MR imaging plays an important role in the assessment of acutely encephalopathic patients who may show only subtle or negative findings on CT.[63] The ED radiologist must be aware of the potential causes of unconsciousness to develop a patient-centered approach that allows for a prompt diagnosis and treatment of these entities.

REFERENCES

1. Steriade M. Neuromodulatory systems of thalamus and neocortex. Semin Neurosci 1995;7(5): 361–70.

2. Merchut MP. Approach to the comatose patient. In: Biller J, editor. Practical neurology. 4th edition. Philadelphia: Lippincott Williams & Wilkins; 2012. p. 45–50.

3. National Collaborating Centre for Acute Care. Head injury. Triage, assessment, investigation and early management of head injury in infants, children and adults. London (UK): National Institute for Health and Clinical Excellence (NICE); 2007. p. 54.

4. Mutch CA, Talbott JF, Gean A. Imaging evaluation of acute traumatic brain injury. Neurosurg Clin N Am 2016;27(4):409–39.

5. Le TH, Gean AD. Imaging of head trauma. Semin Roentgenol 2006;41(3):177–89.

6. Mata-Mbemba D, Mugikura S, Nakagawa A, et al. Intraventricular hemorrhage on initial computed tomography as marker of diffuse axonal injury after traumatic brain injury. J Neurotrauma 2015;32(5): 359–65.

7. Huisman TA, Sorensen AG, Hergan K, et al. Diffusion-weighted imaging for the evaluation of diffuse axonal injury in closed head injury. J Comput Assist Tomogr 2003;27(1):5–11.

8. Liu J, Kou Z, Tian Y. Diffuse axonal injury after traumatic cerebral microbleeds: an evaluation of imaging techniques. Neural Regen Res 2014;9(12):1222–30.

9. Provenzale JM. Imaging of traumatic brain injury: a review of the recent medical literature. AJR Am J Roentgenol 2010;194(1):16–9.

10. Al-Nakshabandi NA. The swirl sign. Radiology 2001; 218(2):433.

11. Dubey A, Pillai SV, Kolluri SV. Does volume of extra-dural hematoma influence management strategy and outcome? Neurol India 2004;52(4):443–5.

12. Chen TY, Wong CW, Chang CN, et al. The expectant treatment of "asymptomatic" supratentorial epidural hematomas. Neurosurgery 1993;32(2):176–9 [discussion: 179].

13. Suwatcharangkoon S, Meyers E, Falo C, et al. Loss of consciousness at onset of subarachnoid hemorrhage as an important marker of early brain injury. JAMA Neurol 2016;73(1):28–35.

14. Van der Schaaf IC, Velthuis BK, Gouw A, et al. Venous drainage in perimesencephalic hemorrhage. Stroke 2004;35(7):1614–8.

15. Van Gijn J, Rinkel GJ. Subarachnoid haemorrhage: diagnosis, causes and management. Brain 2001; 124(Pt 2):249–78.

16. Marder CP, Narla V, Fink JR, et al. Subarachnoid hemorrhage: beyond aneurysms. AJR Am J Roentgenol 2014;202(1):25–37.

17. Kumar S, Goddeau RP Jr, Selim MH, et al. Atraumatic convexal subarachnoid hemorrhage: clinical presentation, imaging patterns, and etiologies. Neurology 2010;74(11):893–9.

18. Carpenter CR, Hussain AM, Ward MJ, et al. Spontaneous subarachnoid hemorrhage: a systematic review and meta-analysis describing the diagnostic accuracy of history, physical examination, imaging, and lumbar puncture with an exploration of test thresholds. Acad Emerg Med 2016;23(9): 963–1003.

19. Hodel J, Aboukais R, Dutouquet B, et al. Double inversion recovery MR sequence for the detection of subacute subarachnoid hemorrhage. AJNR Am J Neuroradiol 2015;36(2):251–8.

20. Mule S, Soize S, Benaissa A, et al. Detection of aneurysmal subarachnoid hemorrhage 3 months after initial bleeding: evaluation of T2* and FLAIR MR sequences at 3 T in comparison with initial non-enhanced CT as a gold standard. J Neurointerv Surg 2016;8(8):813–8.

21. Cianfoni A, Caulo M, Cerase A, et al. Seizure-induced brain lesions: a wide spectrum of variably reversible MRI abnormalities. Eur J Radiol 2013; 82(11):1964–72.

22. Karis JP. Epilepsy. AJNR Am J Neuroradiol 2008; 29(6):1222–4.

23. Treatment of convulsive status epilepticus. Recommendations of the epilepsy foundation of America's working group on status epilepticus. JAMA 1993; 270(7):854–9.

24. Williams JA, Bede P, Doherty CP. An exploration of the spectrum of peri-ictal MRI change; a comprehensive literature review. Seizure 2017; 50:19–32.

25. Nair PP, Kalita J, Misra UK. Status epilepticus: why, what, and how. J Postgrad Med 2011;57(3):242–52.

26. Mendes A, Sampaio L. Brain magnetic resonance in status epilepticus: a focused review. Seizure 2016; 38:63–7.

27. Kim JA, Chung JI, Yoon PH, et al. Transient MR signal changes in patients with generalized tonico-clonic seizure or status epilepticus: periictal diffusion-weighted imaging. AJNR Am J Neuroradiol 2001;22(6):1149–60.

28. Sharma P, Eesa M, Scott JN. Toxic and acquired metabolic encephalopathies: MRI appearance. AJR Am J Roentgenol 2009;193:879–86.

29. O'Donnell P, Buxton PJ, Pitkin A, et al. The magnetic resonance imaging appearances of the brain in acute carbon monoxide poisoning. Clin Radiol 2000;55:273–80.

30. Geibprasert S, Gallucci M, Krings T. Alcohol-induced changes in the brain as assessed by MRI and CT. Eur Radiol 2010;20:1492–501.

31. McMartin KE, Ambre JJ, Tephly TR. Methanol poisoning in human subjects. Role for formic acid accumulation in the metabolic acidosis. Am J Med 1980;68:414–8.

32. Sefidbakht S, Rasekhi AR, Kamali K. Methanol poisoning: acute MR and CT findings in nine patients. Neuroradiology 2007;49:427–35.

33. Kuteifan K, Oesterle H, Tajahmady T, et al. Necrosis and haemorrhage of the putamen in methanol poisoning shown on MRI. Neuroradiology 1998;40: 158–60.

34. De Roock S, Hantson P, Laterre PF, et al. Extensive pallidal and white matter injury following cocaine overdose. Intensive Care Med 2007;33:2030–1.

35. Brust JC, Richter RW. Stroke associated with addiction to heroin. J Neurol Neurosurg Psychiatry 1976; 39:194–9.

36. Volkow ND, Valentine A, Kulkarni M. Radiological and neurological changes in the drug abuse patient: a study with MRI. J Neuroradiol 1988;15: 288–93.

37. Bartlett E, Mikulis DJ. Chasing "chasing the dragon" with MRI: leukoencephalopathy in drug abuse. Br J Radiol 2005;78:997–1004.

38. Keogh CF, Andrews GT, Spacey SD, et al. Neuroimaging features of heroin inhalation toxicity: "chasing the dragon." AJR Am J Roentgenol 2003; 180:847–50.

39. Offiah C, Hall E. Heroin-induced leukoencephalopathy: characterization using MRI, diffusion-weighted imaging, and MR spectroscopy. Clin Radiol 2008; 63:146–52.

40. Geibprasert S, Gallucci M, Krings T. Addictive illegal drugs: structural neuroimaging. AJNR Am J Neuroradiol 2010;31:803–8.

41. Küker W, Nägele T, Schmidt F, et al. Diffusion-weighted MRI in herpes simplex encephalitis: a report of three cases. Neuroradiology 2004;46(2): 122–5.

42. Handique SK, Das RR, Barman K, et al. Temporal lobe involvement in Japanese encephalitis: problems in differential diagnosis. AJNR Am J Neuroradiol 2006;27(5):1027–31.

43. Prakash M, Kumar S, Gupta RK. Diffusion-weighted MR imaging in Japanese encephalitis. J Comput Assist Tomogr 2004;28(6):756–61.

44. Ali M, Safriel Y, Sohi J, et al. West Nile virus infection: MR imaging findings in the nervous system. AJNR Am J Neuroradiol 2005;26(2): 289–97.

45. Kelley BP, Patel SC, Marin HL, et al. Autoimmune encephalitis: pathophysiology and imaging review of an overlooked diagnosis. AJNR Am J Neuroradiol 2017;38(6):1070–8.

46. Sirichai K, Metha A. Meningitis as early manifestation of anti-NMDAR encephalitis. Neurol Asia 2014; 19(4):413–5.

47. Bathla G, Policeni B, Agarwal A. Neuroimaging in patients with abnormal blood glucose levels. Am J Neuroradiol 2014;35(5):833–40.

48. Lim CC, Gan R, Chan CL, et al. Severe hypoglycemia associated with an illegal sexual enhancement product adulterated with glibenclamide: MR imaging findings. Radiology 2009;250(1): 193–201.

49. Johkura K, Nakae Y, Kudo Y, et al. Early diffusion MR imaging findings and short-term outcome in comatose patients with hypoglycemia. AJNR Am J Neuroradiol 2012;33:904–9.

50. Kang EG, Jeon SJ, Choi SS, et al. MR imaging of hypoglycemic encephalopathy. AJNR Am J Neuroradiol 2010;31(3):559–64.

51. Fujioka M, Okuchi K, Hiramatsu KI, et al. Specific changes in human brain after hypoglycemic injury. Stroke 1997;28(3):584–7.

52. Clay AS, Hainline BE. Hyperammonemia in the ICU. Chest 2007;132:1368–78.

53. U-King-Im JM, Yu E, Bartlett E. Acute hyperammonemic encephalopathy in adults: imaging findings. AJNR 2011;32:413–8.

54. O'Donnell-Luria AH, Lin AP, Merugumala SK, et al. Brain MRS glutamine as a biomarker to guide therapy of hyperammonemic coma. Mol Genet Metab 2017;121(1):9–15.

55. Chua GC, Sitoh YY, Lim CC, et al. MRI findings in osmotic myelinolysis. Clin Radiol 2002;57(9): 800–6.

56. Guo Y1, Hu JH, Lin W, et al. Central pontine myelinolysis after liver transplantation: MR diffusion, spectroscopy and perfusion findings. Magn Reson Imaging 2006;24(10):1395–8.

57. Goldmakher GV, Camargo EC, Furie KL, et al. Hyperdense basilar artery sign on unenhanced CT predicts thrombus and outcome in acute posterior circulation stroke. Stroke 2009;40(1): 134–9.

58. Strbian D, Tiina S, Silvennoinen H, et al. Thrombolysis of basilar artery occlusion: impact of baseline ischemia and time. Ann Neurol 2013; 73(6):688–94.

59. Huang BY, Castillo M. Hypoxic-ischemic brain injury: imaging findings from birth to adulthood. Radiographics 2008;28(2):417–39.

60. Oriani G, Marroni A, Wattel F, et al. Decompression illness. In: Oriani G, Marroni A, Wattel F, editors. Handbook on hyperbaric medicine. Berlin: Springer-Verlag; 1996. p. 135–82.

61. Kamtchum Tatuene J, Pignel R, Pollak P, et al. Neuroimaging of diving-related decompression illness: current knowledge and perspectives. AJNR Am J Neuroradiol 2014;35(11):2039–44.

62. Ozdoba C, Weis J, Plattner T, et al. Fatal scuba diving incident with massive gas embolism in cerebral and spinal arteries. Neuroradiology 2005;47:411–6.

63. Torres C, Nguyen T. The unconscious patient. In: Kruskal JB, Menias C, editors. Categorical course syllabus: the dark side of radiology: multispecilaty after-hours imaging. American Roentgen Ray Society (ARRS); 2015. p. 1–8.

Neurologic Emergencies in Pediatric Patients Including Accidental and Nonaccidental Trauma

Gaurav Saigal, MD*, Nisreen S. Ezuddin, MD, Gabriela de la Vega, MD

KEYWORDS

- Accidental injury • Calvarial fractures • Nonaccidental injury • Meningitis • Encephalitis
- Subdural empyema • Cerebral venous sinus thrombosis • Arterial stroke

KEY POINTS

- Traumatic and non-traumatic neurologic emergencies can be seen in children.
- Imaging is determined by the level of neurologic status and suspected etiology.
- Pearls, pitfalls and variants in imaging in various conditions are highlighted in this article.

INTRODUCTION

In neurologic emergencies in children, neuroimaging is very often needed because of the limitations in gathering an accurate history as well as difficulties with performing the neurologic examination. In such a situation, the challenge for the physician is in deciding (1) if an imaging test is required emergently and (2) what is the most appropriate imaging test. The causes of neurologic emergencies in pediatric patients are numerous (**Box 1**). Specific entities that are common and unique to pediatric patients are discussed, with an emphasis on pearls and pitfalls for the radiologist as well as the referring physician.

GUIDELINES FOR IMAGING

There are differences that characterize optimal imaging in pediatric patients in comparison with adults. Part of this due to different disease processes that occur in children, some of which can be congenital. Age is often a factor when deciding the appropriateness of an imaging test. Children are more sensitive to the harmful effects of radiation; therefore, MR imaging is the preferred modality for imaging in older children when sedation does not need to be administered. Longer scanning times for MR imaging are generally required for sedation in younger children, generally younger than 6 years. Computed tomography (CT) may be considered as a first choice of imaging, rather than magnetic resonance (MR), if it can provide the necessary information.

INDICATIONS FOR CHOICE OF MODALITY

CT is considered the modality of choice in situations when determination of etiology needs to be done emergently, because of deteriorating neurologic status secondary to suspected hemorrhage during trauma, and in uncooperative patients. CT is also very useful for detection of calcifications, bony structures, and before a lumbar puncture to rule out a mass or bleeding. MR imaging is superior to CT in the evaluation of epilepsy, known tumors, white matter pathology, and infection/inflammation in the brain. MR imaging is generally

Financial Disclosure: The authors have not received funding in the preparation of this article.
Department of Radiology, University of Miami Miller School of Medicine, Jackson Memorial Hospital, 1611 Northwest 12th Avenue, Suite WW279, Miami, FL 33136, USA
* Corresponding author.
E-mail address: gsaigal@med.miami.edu

Neuroimag Clin N Am 28 (2018) 453–470
https://doi.org/10.1016/j.nic.2018.03.007
1052-5149/18/© 2018 Elsevier Inc. All rights reserved.

neuroimaging.theclinics.com

Box 1
Causes of neurologic emergencies in the pediatric population

Nontraumatic

  Infection

    Meningitis

    Encephalitis (HSV)

    Subdural empyema

  Acute hydrocephalus

  Stroke

    CVST

    Arterial stroke

    HIE

  Metabolic

    Amino acid/urea cycle disorders

  Toxic

    Methotrexate-induced encephalopathy

    Cyclosporine-induced PRES

  Neoplastic

  Epilepsy

  Others: ADEM

Traumatic

  Accidental

  Nonaccidental

Abbreviations: ADEM, acute disseminated encephalomyelitis; CVST, cerebral venous sinus thrombosis; HIE, hypoxic ischemic encephalopathy; HSV, herpes simplex virus; PRES, posterior reversible encephalopathy syndrome.

---

performed without contrast, except in cases of a known brain tumor or when suspicion for a tumor is very high, ataxia, and when suspecting infection. When evaluating for vascular pathology, MR angiography is preferred in children to avoid radiation exposure; but CT may be indicated in specific conditions, such as vasculitis. A fast MR imaging scan, consisting of 1 or 2 sequences, is now used, instead of CT, in many institutions for the evaluation and follow-up of hydrocephalus. Most children who present with headaches do not require any advanced neuroimaging. Neuroimaging should be reserved for children who have an abnormal neurologic examination (eg, ataxia, papilledema, or diplopia), new-onset thunderclap headache, associated with morning vomiting or failure in improvement after 4 weeks of symptomatic treatment.

NONTRAUMATIC
Infection

Meningitis

Meningitis is an infectious/inflammatory infiltration of the leptomeninges (pia and arachnoid mater), which can be acute (bacterial or viral) or chronic (tuberculosis or fungal).[1] The infection can be spread hematogenously, via local infection (eg, sinusitis, mastoiditis, or orbital cellulitis) or directly via implantation.[2] Patients may present with a severe headache, neck stiffness, fever, photophobia, and altered mental status.[3]

Meningitis is associated with leptomeningeal enhancement. Although dural enhancement can be seen normally, leptomeningeal enhancement is considered abnormal.[4] Normal enhancement of the dura is thin, markedly discontinuous, and most prominent in the parasagittal regions. It appears symmetric and does not usually extend into the sulci. Meningeal enhancement due to meningitis is seen extending to the base of the sulci and is asymmetric.[5] The pattern of leptomeningeal enhancement in bacterial and viral meningitis is thin and linear, whereas it is thick, lumpy, and nodular in fungal meningitis.[6] Acute meningitis will manifest with pathologic enhancement over the cerebral convexity, whereas chronic meningitis enhances most prominently in the basal cisterns.[2]

Only 50% of patients show imaging features consistent with meningitis and the diagnosis of meningitis is made clinically with cerebrospinal fluid (CSF) cultures. The primary role of imaging is to exclude increased intracranial pressure before lumbar puncture, to rule out meningitis mimickers, and to evaluate for any complications of meningitis.[7,8]

An initial CT or MR imaging early in the disease process may appear normal; progression of the disease may reveal mild hydrocephalus and loss of the gray-white matter differentiation, suggesting cerebral edema on a noncontrast CT. In severe cases, obliteration of the CSF spaces and basal cisterns with exudate can be seen. MR imaging has the advantage of increased sensitivity for the detection of enhancement in the subarachnoid spaces.[9] The exudate will appear isointense on T1 and hyperintense on T2/fluid-attenuated inversion recovery (FLAIR) images and may demonstrate restricted diffusion.[9] Postcontrast MR imaging is best for observing leptomeningeal involvement[10,11] (**Fig. 1**A, B). Postcontrast FLAIR imaging is superior in sensitivity to postcontrast T1-weighted imaging in the detection of early abnormal meningeal enhancement.[11] T1 postcontrast images, on the other hand, are more sensitive in the detection of parenchymal enhancement.[10]

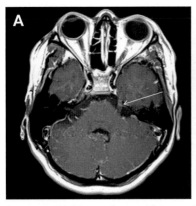
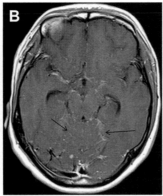
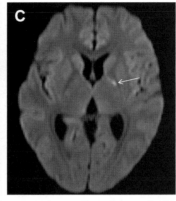

Fig. 1. Meningitis: A 15 year old presenting with fever and multiple cranial neuropathy, confirmed as meningitis. Postcontrast axial (*A, B*) and diffusion (*C*) MR images of the brain demonstrating leptomeningeal enhancement in the basilar cisterns and along the cerebellar folia (*black arrows*). Enhancement of the left trigeminal nerve is noted (*long white arrow*). Enhancement of multiple other cranial nerves at the base of the skull were noted (not shown). Small focus of restricted diffusion suggestive of an acute lacunar infarct is noted in the left globus pallidus (*short white arrow*).

Diffusion-weighted imaging (DWI) is extremely useful in differentiating between vasogenic and cytotoxic edema and helps in identifying early cerebritis and in detecting infected material within extra-axial collections.

It is important to note that meningeal enhancement alone is a nonspecific finding and can result from infectious or noninfectious causes, such as inflammatory, chemical, drug induced, neoplastic, and collagen vascular disorders.[12] Involvement of the dura can help distinguish carcinomatous meningitis from infectious meningitis. Although the former most commonly involves the dura and the leptomeninges, the latter most commonly involves the leptomeninges alone.[13] MR imaging is also valuable in evaluating for the complications of meningitis, such as hydrocephalus, cerebritis, brain abscess, ventriculitis and choroid plexitis, and vascular complications, such as vasculopathy and infarction (**Fig. 1C**), and involvement of the cranial nerves (see **Fig. 1A**).[14]

Pearls, pitfalls, and variants
- Meningitis is a clinical diagnosis; imaging is used to check for increased intracranial pressure before lumbar puncture and to evaluate for the complications of meningitis.
- Delayed contrast-enhanced FLAIR is best to evaluate for subtle findings.
- DWI is the most sensitive MR sequence to evaluate for the complications of meningitis, such as cerebritis, infarction, and abscess.

What the referring physician needs to know
Because clinical findings are unreliable, the diagnosis of meningitis relies on the examination of CSF obtained from lumbar puncture. Although

neuroimaging does not have a very high sensitivity in the diagnosis, it may help in suggesting it and may also help in diagnosing complications. Delayed initiation of antibiotics can worsen mortality; therefore, treatment should be started promptly, as soon as the diagnosis is suspected.

Encephalitis: herpes simplex virus
Herpes simplex virus (HSV) encephalitis is the most common cause of fatal, fulminant necrotizing encephalitis and has characteristic imaging findings.[15] Unfortunately, the symptoms are nonspecific consisting of fever, headaches, focal neurologic deficits, seizure, and decreased level of consciousness. The gold standard for diagnosis is by polymerase chain reaction or viral culture.[16]

HSV infection predominantly affects the limbic system, targeting the medial temporal and inferior frontal lobes.[17] This effect is thought to result from the spread of infection intracranially along the small meningeal branches of the trigeminal nerve from the trigeminal ganglion, where it resides latently.[18] On initial imaging, CT or MR imaging may demonstrate edema involving the limbic system, medial temporal lobes, insular cortices, and the inferolateral frontal lobes. MR imaging is superior to CT, given that it is more sensitive in the detection of subtle edema involving the limbic system and more readily detects petechial hemorrhages, which is a sign of necrotizing encephalitis (**Fig. 2A**).[18] In the later stages of the infection, gyriform enhancement may be seen.[19] The DWI sequence is the most sensitive sequence and is helpful in detecting cytotoxic edema in the involved regions (**Fig. 2B**).[20] It is important to note that restricted diffusion may disappear within 2 weeks, whereas the hyperintensities present on T2/FLAIR sequences may last longer.[19]

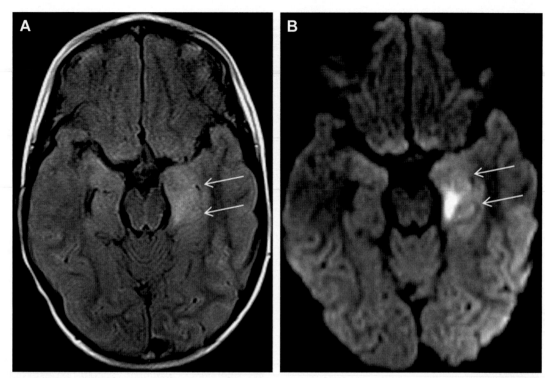

Fig. 2. Herpes simplex encephalitis: A 6 year old presenting with focal seizures, headache, and fever. Axial FLAIR (*A*) and diffusion (*B*) MR images demonstrating areas of abnormal signal with corresponding restricted diffusion involving the medial aspect of the left temporal lobe with associated mass effect on the temporal horn of the left lateral ventricle (*white arrows*). Slightly less intense signal abnormality is noted involving the medial aspect of the right temporal lobe. These findings were highly suspicious for herpes encephalitis, and patient was immediately started on acyclovir therapy.

The imaging appearance of neonatal HSV type 2 encephalitis is different in that changes are typically diffuse and involve the cerebral cortex, deep white matter and the thalami. Hemorrhage is less common compared with HSV-1 encephalitis.[21]

Pearls, pitfalls, and variants Herpes encephalitis should be considered as a presumptive diagnosis, given the appropriate clinical setting, whenever involvement of the limbic system is noted. The DWI sequence is critical, with restricted diffusion seen in involved regions of the brain.

What the referring physician needs to know Presumptive diagnosis can be made based on clinical features supported by imaging findings. Mortality and morbidity differ drastically, depending on the timing of treatment; early intravenous antiviral therapy should be instituted as soon as a diagnosis is made.

Subdural empyema

A subdural empyema (SDE) is an infected collection that occurs between the dura and arachnoid, most commonly caused by direct spread of infection from the posterior wall of the frontal sinus or middle ear,[22] or indirect spread secondary to thrombophlebitis. It is thought to be a complication of bacterial sinusitis and meningitis in children. SDE is a neurologic emergency that can progress rapidly and cause increased intracranial pressure, leading to coma and death within 24 to 48 hours if untreated. It presents as a headache, fever, focal neurologic deficits, meningismus, and/or seizures.[23] It can be complicated by abscess and CVST in about 10% of cases.

SDEs do not cross the midline and are crescentic shaped. On CT, SDEs appear as isodense to low-density extra-axial collections with rim enhancement (**Fig. 3**A).[22] On MR imaging, SDEs show high signal on T2-weighted imaging, are isointense to brain on T1-weighted imaging, and show peripheral enhancement. DWI is extremely useful in determining the cause and the presence, extent, and complications of SDE (**Fig. 3**B, C).

Differential diagnosis

- Chronic subdural hematoma: MR imaging will show signal changes of blood products. Enhancement of the periphery and underlying membranes may be seen. There is no restricted diffusion.

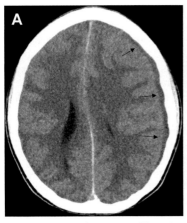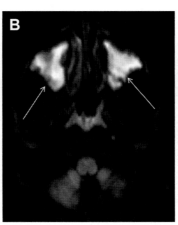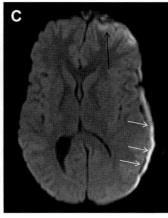

Fig. 3. SDE secondary to maxillary sinusitis: Child presenting to the emergency department with headache, fever, and speech difficulty. Axial CT scan of the brain (*A*) done in an outside institution was read as a left subdural hygroma (*short black arrows*). There was pan sinus opacification (not shown). Axial diffusion MR images (*B, C*) of the brain done a few hours later demonstrate restricted diffusion in both completely opacified maxillary sinuses (*long white arrows*), consistent with acute sinusitis, as well as restricted diffusion in the left subdural space (*short white arrows*), consistent with a subdural empyema. Subtle restricted diffusion was noted in the left frontal lobe cortex (*long black arrow*), suggestive of focal cerebritis.

- Subdural effusion: It is a nonenhancing, nonrestricting collection associated with meningitis.
- Subdural hygroma: It is a nonenhancing, CSF equivalent collection with a trauma history.

Pearls, pitfalls, and variants
- Most sensitive test: MR with contrast and DWI; if not possible → get CT
- DWI useful for differentiating between SDE and subdural effusions and chronic subdural hematomas
- To monitor treatment response → use MR with DWI

What the referring physician should know
Emergency physicians should be aware of the risks of SDE and the need for emergency neurosurgical intervention because they carry a seriously increased morbidity and mortality risk if not recognized early. SDEs are relatively rare and a difficult diagnosis because the symptoms are vague. Any child with a sinus infection, progressive headaches, or any neurologic deficits should be evaluated with CT or MR imaging to rule out SDE.

Acute Hydrocephalus

Hydrocephalus can occur either due to overproduction of CSF, such as in the case of a choroid plexus papilloma, or obstruction to the flow of CSF, or decreased absorption of CSF.[24] Obstructive hydrocephalus can be further divided into 2 types: communicating and noncommunicating hydrocephalus. Noncommunicating hydrocephalus is when there is an obstruction to CSF flow in any part of the ventricular system, which results in ventricular dilation proximal to the obstruction. The communicating type occurs when the obstruction is distal to the ventricular system (ie, in the basilar cisterns, subarachnoid space, and arachnoid villi).

Pediatric patients with hydrocephalus present to the emergency department (ED) in 3 scenarios: (1) shunted hydrocephalus, (2) noncommunicating hydrocephalus, and (3) communicating hydrocephalus.

Shunted hydrocephalus
CSF shunts consist of 3 parts: (1) ventricular catheter tubing that passes from the ventricle through the skull to connect to the (2) valve (used to prevent excessive CSF drainage; valves have reservoirs that can be punctured percutaneously for diagnostic purposes) and (3) distal tubing connecting the valve to a distal body site (eg, peritoneal cavity, right atrium, pleural cavity, and so forth), where CSF can be absorbed into the venous circulation.

Children with shunted hydrocephalus present to the ED for 2 main reasons: infection or shunt malfunction.

1. Infection: Children present with altered mental status, fever, nausea, and vomiting. The diagnosis can be made in almost 95% of cases by cultures of the CSF obtained from the reservoir.[25] The role of imaging is limited to cases whereby the infection spreads intracranially and causes meningitis.

2. Shunt malfunction: This complication is the most common complication of ventricular shunts. Children present with headache, nausea, vomiting, and altered mental status. Malfunctions can occur secondary to obstruction of the shunt, infection, overdrainage or underdrainage, mechanical breakdown, or migration of shunt.[26]

The initial evaluation of a shunt malfunction is done with a shunt survey, which includes multiple radiographs of the skull, neck, chest, and abdomen. The length of the shunt can be assessed; common causes of obstruction, such as a shunt break, kink, or migration, can be evaluated. Disconnections of the shunt tubing can occur at any site but are common at the sites of mobility, such as the neck and at the level of the reservoir.[27] Distal obstruction can occur because of kinking or disconnection of the tubing, migration of catheter, infection, or pseudocyst formation. On an abdominal radiograph, a pseudocyst may be seen is a soft tissue mass at the distal tip of the catheter, which can be confirmed by ultrasound. A low-dose head CT is usually done in conjunction with the shunt survey. Low-dose CT can be used to minimize radiation in children, especially because multiple CTs are usually needed throughout the life span of patients. Three-dimensional (3D) reconstructions of the skull are extremely useful in quickly evaluating for a shunt break, which might not be easily apparent in the axial plane (**Fig. 4**). More recently, a rapid sequence MR imaging, which includes a limited thin-section T2-weighted MR imaging in the axial plane, followed by coronal and sagittal reconstructions, has been adopted in various institutions.[28]

The entire scan lasts for 3 to 4 minutes and is an attractive alternative to CT in children who can lie in the scanner for a few minutes. The scan can be done without sedation, and patients are spared the harmful effects of radiation. On the CT or MR imaging study, the ventricular size is evaluated and compared with prior studies, and an evaluation for periventricular/peri-catheter edema is done. The position of the shunt catheter is evaluated to see if it is intraventricular or not, and the shunt catheter is evaluated for fracture. The imaging study is evaluated for slit ventricle syndrome and for collections around the reservoir, indicating malfunction and extra-axial collections.

Slit ventricle syndrome: This condition is one in which the ventricles appear smaller than normal on the CT or MR study. Various hypotheses have been suggested for slit ventricle syndrome, which include overdrainage of CSF, intermittent shunt malfunction, decreased intracranial compliance, and periventricular fibrosis.[29] Subdural hematomas and hygromas may be associated with low intraventricular pressure and are especially more common when the ventricles are large before shunting.[30]

Third ventriculostomy: In children who have undergone endoscopic third ventriculostomy (ETV), rapid MR imaging is preferred to CT.[31] The surgical defect at the floor of the third ventricle can be nicely depicted. Also, patency of the ETV can be confirmed by the CSF pulsation artifact created through the defect at the floor of the third ventricle (**Fig. 5**).

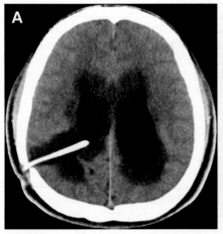
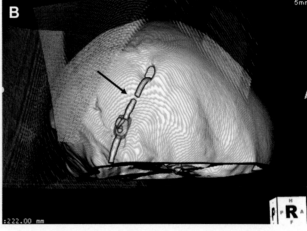

Fig. 4. Shunt malfunction: A 14-year-old boy presenting to the ED with headaches. Axial CT scan of the brain (*A*) demonstrating moderate enlargement of the ventricles, which had increased in size when compared with a prior study 3 months ago. Periventricular hypodensities suggesting transependymal flow of CSF due to acute hydrocephalus are noted bilaterally. The shunt tubing demonstrated a questionable break in the portion close to the reservoir on the axial images. A 3D reformat of the skull (*B*) clearly demonstrates the break (*black arrow*).

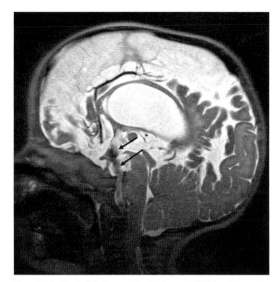

Fig. 5. Patent third ventriculostomy: Child with prior history of Chiari 2 and myelomeningocele and hydrocephalus treated with third ventriculostomy. Thin-section T2-weighted MR image in the midline demonstrating a prominent CSF flow artifact (*arrows*) at the floor of the third ventricle (both above and below the floor) suggestive of a patent third ventriculostomy.

Communicating Hydrocephalus

This condition may be associated with meningitis (bacterial or viral), intraventricular hemorrhage, trauma, or a congenital malformation of the subarachnoid spaces. In communicating hydrocephalus, the lateral, third, and fourth ventricles become enlarged.[24]

Noncommunicating Hydrocephalus

Noncommunicating hydrocephalus is caused by intraventricular obstruction of the flow of CSF. In children, common sites of obstruction include the foramen of Monroe, cerebral aqueduct, the fourth ventricle, and outlet foramina. The most common location of obstruction is at the aqueduct, secondary to congenital aqueductal stenosis. When suspected, a thin-section high-resolution T2-weighted sequence in the sagittal plane is extremely useful in evaluating the patency of the aqueduct. Obstruction can also result because of infection or compression of the aqueduct by a mass, such as a tumor (**Fig. 6**).[24,32] Acute noncommunicating hydrocephalus secondary to masses can be the initial clinical presentation of the child to the ED. Masses causing obstruction can be either intraventricular or in the brain parenchyma near the ventricles. The most common causes of aqueductal obstruction include masses arising in the pineal region or gliomas originating in the tectum, quadrigeminal plate, or thalamus. Posterior fossa tumors, such as medulloblastoma, pilocytic astrocytoma, ependymoma, or atypical rhabdoid teratoma, or metastasis can cause fourth ventricular or aqueductal obstruction either from extrinsic compression or intraventricular extension. These masses are usually first seen on the CT scan done for screening of these children,

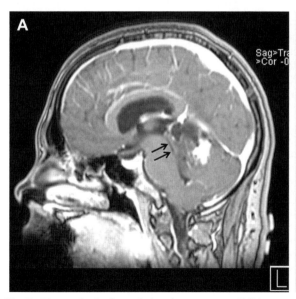
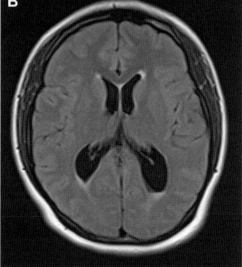

Fig. 6. Obstructive hydrocephalus due to tumor: Child presenting to the ER with nausea, headaches and vomiting. Sagittal postcontrast T1-weighted (*A*) and axial FLAIR (*B*) MR images of the brain demonstrating a heterogeneously enhancing mass centered in the superior vermis causing mass effect and marked narrowing of the aqueduct (*black arrows*) and mild obstructive hydrocephalus of the lateral ventricles. Final path: pilocytic astrocytoma.

but MR imaging is the imaging modality of choice for evaluation. Additional imaging of the spine is often needed in such cases because of the increased incidence of spinal spread of tumor. Congenital malformations, such as a Chiari 1 malformation or arachnoid cysts/webs, may be the cause of the noncommunicating hydrocephalus.[24,32] In addition to conventional MR imaging, a CSF flow study can be used in such cases to determine the degree of obstruction at the level of the foramen magnum for preoperative planning.

What the referring physician needs to know

- The signs and symptoms of obstruction range from mild (eg, headache and nausea) to life-threatening signs of intracranial hypertension.
- In any child presenting to the ED with a CSF shunt, the shunt should be considered as the cause of the problem until proven otherwise.
- A negative result from a CT scan does not rule out a shunt obstruction.

Stroke

Cerebral venous sinus thrombosis

Cerebral venous sinus thrombosis (CVST) is a well-established cause of childhood and neonatal stroke. It is a multifactorial disease that occurs when there is a thrombotic occlusion in the cerebral veins and/or the intracranial dural sinuses. CVST has an incidence of 2.6 per 100,000 newborns per year,[33] with more than 40% of childhood CVST occurring in the neonatal period. Children may present with nausea, vomiting, headache, feeding difficulties, blurry vision, loss of consciousness, seizures, respiratory distress, and coma.[34] The most common predisposing factor is infection, followed by a hypercoagulable/hematological state and dehydration.[35] Other risk factors include perinatal complications, hypoxia, cardiac defects, solid tumors, vascular trauma, oral contraceptive use, and genetic prothrombotic disorders.[36]

Noncontrast CT is usually the first imaging study performed, given the nonspecific clinical presentation, and can detect a cord sign acutely as increased attenuation of the thrombus in the dural sinuses or cortical veins (Fig. 7A, B). As the thrombus becomes less dense, a CT with contrast may reveal an empty delta sign, which is a triangular filling defect in the dural venous sinus.[37,38] Common sites for CVST include the transverse, superior sagittal, sigmoid, and straight sinuses. Anywhere from 33% to 66% of children with CVST will have parenchymal brain lesions, including venous infarction and hemorrhage.[32] CVST involving the internal cerebral veins results in infarction of the thalami and CVST involving the superior sagittal sinus results in

infarction of the parasagittal brain parenchyma, whereas CVST in the vein of Labbe, transverse, and sigmoid sinuses may cause temporal lobe infarction.

On MR imaging, the clot appears isointense on T1 and hypointense on T2, with subacute clots presenting as hyperintense on T1. The T2*-weighted conventional gradient echo sequences are the best method for the detection of cerebral venous thrombosis (Fig. 7C).[39] Contrast MR venography will show an absence of flow in the occluded sinuses. The key to the diagnosis of CVST is a high degree of suspicion in the acute phase and imaging before the venous sinuses recanalize.[35,40,41] Measuring the density of the venous sinuses can help aid in the diagnosis. A threshold of 62 Hounsfield units (HU) on a noncontrast CT can be used, with higher densities indicating CVST (Fig. 7D). In addition, an HU:hematocrit ratio of greater than 1.52 strongly suggests CVST, with an accuracy of 97.5%.[42]

Pearl, pitfalls, and variants

- Examine the periphery of the brain, especially the high frontal regions for cortical vein thrombosis.
- Check the density of the sinuses. A high hematocrit, which is physiologic in neonates, can simulate the appearance of a dense sinus.
- Acute renal failure, causing delayed contrast excretion, can simulate a dense sinus, due to contrast retention, and be confused for sinus thrombosis.[43]
- Acute subdural hemorrhage (SDH), particularly along the tentorium, can be confused for thrombosis within the transverse sinus on the axial images. Therefore, suspected CVST should be evaluated in the other planes as well, which helps differentiate it from true CVST.

What the referring physician needs to know

Because CVST is a rare entity in children, diagnosis is often delayed resulting in high morbidity and mortality. Physicians should maintain a high degree of clinical suspicion, particularly in children with risk factors, because the therapeutic frame for treatment with thrombolytic agents is only 3 to 6 hours.

Hypoxic ischemic encephalopathy

Hypoxic ischemic encephalopathy (HIE) is a type of brain injury due to a hypoxic insult and can occur in various settings, the most common being cardiac arrest, nonaccidental injury (NAI), and infection. Two main patterns of HIE are noted in children. The watershed pattern is seen involving the zones between major vascular territories and is usually present in mild to moderate hypoxic injury. Changes are most prominent in the frontal

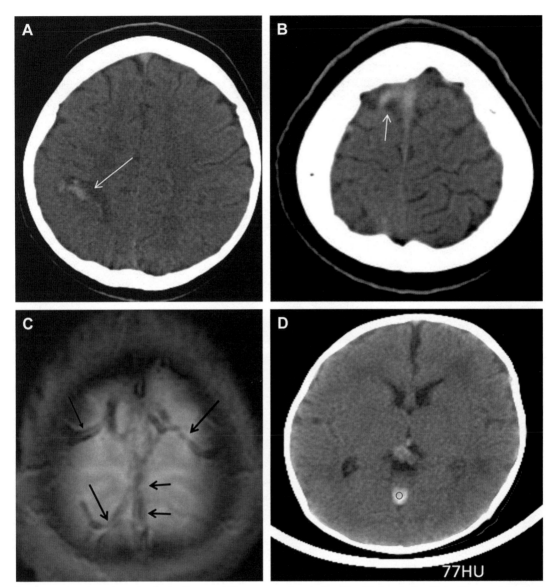

Fig. 7. Venous sinus thrombosis: An 8-year-old boy presenting to the ED with headache. Plain CT scan of the brain (*A, B*) demonstrating linear hyperdense areas in the right parietal lobe due to parenchymal hemorrhage with surrounding hypodensity due to edema (*long white arrow*). Linear increased density along the right frontal convexity consistent with cortical vein thrombosis (cord sign) can be seen (*short white arrow*). Axial gradient echo MR image (*C*) demonstrating the prominent low signal within the cortical veins (*long black arrows*) and the superior sagittal sinus (*short black arrows*) indicating both cortical vein and superior sagittal sinus thrombosis. Axial CT scan of the brain (*D*) in the same patient with region of interest over the vein of Galen (*D*) measures 77 HU, which is consistent with venous sinus thrombosis.

and parietal lobes. The ganglionic pattern is seen in moderate to severe hypoxia, with changes seen involving the basal ganglia, thalami, hippocampi, and corticospinal tracts. In the most severe patterns of injury, the cortex can also be involved.

On CT, normal parenchyma exhibits good gray-white matter differentiation with a distinct appearance of the basal ganglia, which is very important to note, especially in children. Any loss of blood flow or hypoxia can result in diffuse cerebral edema, resulting in loss of gray-white matter differentiation, with sulcal, ventricular, and cisternal effacement. In mild to moderate injury, low attenuation may be seen in watershed zones of vascular territories. Low attenuation of the deep grey nuclei can occur in severe HIE (**Fig. 8A–C**). The least vulnerable regions affected are the midbrain and the cerebellum, which causes a lower attenuation

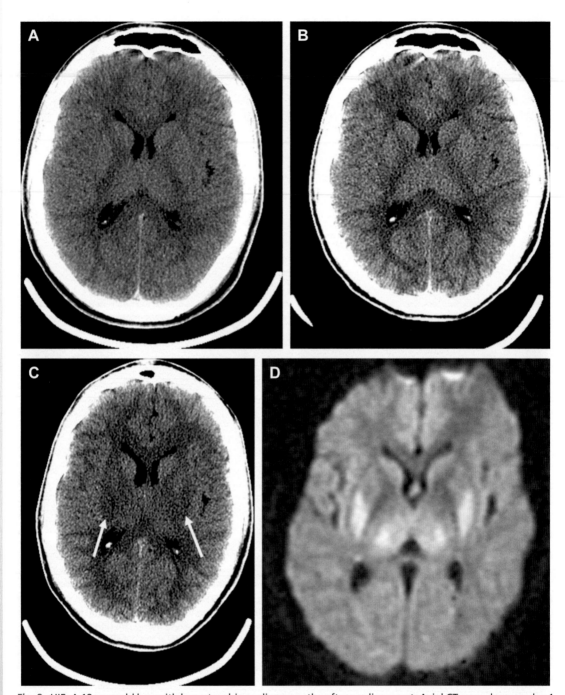

Fig. 8. HIE: A 12-year-old boy with hypertrophic cardiomyopathy after cardiac arrest. Axial CT scans done on day 1 and 2 (*A, B*) appear normal. On day 4 (*C*), using a narrow window, subtle areas of hypodensity can be appreciated in the posterior basal ganglia (*white arrows*). Diffusion image (*D*) from MR imaging done on day 5 shows areas of restricted diffusion in the posterior basal ganglia and thalami, indicating HIE.

in the cerebrum in relation to the cerebellum, resulting in the white cerebellum sign.

MR imaging is known to be more sensitive in the evaluation of HIE. DWI is extremely useful in the first few days when evaluating anoxic injury (**Fig. 8**D). Restricted diffusion is seen from 1 to 7 days, after which point it begins to pseudonormalize. Mild to moderate injury presents as infarcts in watershed zones. In severe HIE, basal ganglia and thalamic involvement are seen as increased T1 hyperintensity, typically of the anterior putamen and posteromedial thalamus. The normal signal of the posterior limb of the internal capsule (hyperintense T1/hypointense T2) is lost. In the most severe forms, increased T1 hyperintensity is noted in the peri-rolandic cortex, insula, and even the cortices.[8,44,45]

Pearls, pitfalls, and variants
- Always look closely at deep gray matter nuclei in children because it is very vulnerable to ischemia.
- The DWI is crucial for diagnosis of HIE; however, it is important to know that it may appear as falsely normalized at 8 to 10 days.

What the referring physician needs to know Interventions are most beneficial if carried out within 2 to 6 hours after the insult to reduce the severity of injury to the brain. Hence, it is crucial for emergency physicians to be able to recognize and diagnose this condition early to decrease the morbidity and mortality in the neonatal period.

Toxic

Methotrexate-induced encephalopathy
Methotrexate (MTX)-induced leukoencephalopathy most often occurs in children undergoing intrathecal or intravenous treatment of acute lymphoblastic leukemia.[46] Patients receiving MTX therapy usually present 2 to 14 days after administration, and clinical features are similar to other encephalopathies.[47] Initial manifestations include headache, confusion, lethargy, seizures, transient paresis, aphasia, and dysarthria. Unlike many other encephalopathies, a notable feature is the waxing and waning of signs and symptoms over the course of the presentation.[46]

MTX toxicity classically presents with diffuse high T2 signal intensity involving the deep white matter of the centrum semiovale on T2-weighted images (**Fig. 9**) and low attenuation on CT. The subcortical U-fibers are characteristically spared. DWI imaging is extremely useful in the evaluation of acute toxicity; high signal can be seen in the involved regions, which eventually resolve once MTX is withdrawn.[46,47]

Cyclosporine-induced posterior reversible encephalopathy syndrome
Posterior reversible encephalopathy syndrome (PRES) is a rare central nervous system (CNS) complication and may manifest with a variable degree of neurologic symptoms, including headaches, seizures, encephalopathy, and visual disturbances.[48] In addition to immunosuppressive or cytotoxic drugs, such as cyclosporine, reported causes of PRES also include acute hypertension, infection, autoimmune disease, eclampsia, and preeclampsia.[49] The pathophysiology of PRES

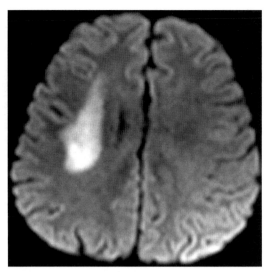

Fig. 9. MTX-induced leukoencephalopathy: An 11 year old with acute lymphocytic leukemia presenting with seizures and altered mental status after intrathecal administration of MTX. Diffusion MR image demonstrating a large area of restricted diffusion (apparent diffusion coefficient map not shown) in the right centrum semiovale. The methotrexate drug administration was stopped and the lesion resolved in the MR imaging done a few days later.

remains unclear, and several mechanisms have been proposed. The cause is thought to be secondary to the inability of the posterior circulation to autoregulate in response to acute changes in blood pressure. Hyperperfusion results in disruption of the blood-brain barrier (BBB).[48] Another theory is that certain drugs (eg, cyclosporine) may have a direct toxic effect on vascular endothelial cells, causing them to release endothelial damaging factors; these may cause microthrombi and also damage the BBB. This damage to the BBB leads to vasogenic edema initially, followed by cytotoxic edema, if the causative cause is not corrected.

Imaging findings initially correlate to vasogenic edema, which is mostly localized to the subcortical white matter of the parietal or occipital lobes (**Fig. 10**).[50] Not infrequently, cortical involvement as well as involvement of other lobes of the brain, including the brainstem, basal ganglia, and cerebellum, can be seen. Lesions appear as ill-defined hypodensities on CT and as T1 hypointense and T2 hyperintense on MR imaging. There is no restricted diffusion noted in the initial stage of vasogenic edema. Later in the disease process, cytotoxic edema might occur, leading to restricted diffusion in 10% to 25% of patients. Because of the breakdown of the BBB, postcontrast enhancement can be seen in the involved regions of the brain. The lesions typically resolve as soon as the offending agent or cause is treated.

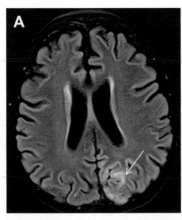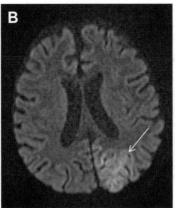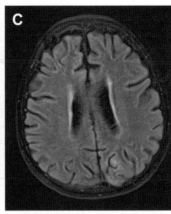

Fig. 10. Posterior reversible encephalopathy syndrome: A 7 year old with acute lymphocytic leukemia on cyclosporine therapy presenting lethargy, change in mental status, and hypertension. Axial FLAIR (*A*) and diffusion (*B*) MR images demonstrating hyperintense signal abnormality and corresponding restricted diffusion involving the left parietal subcortical white matter (*arrows*). FLAIR image (*C*) from repeat MR imaging done 10 days later demonstrates near complete resolution of the FLAIR signal hyperintensity.

Pearls, pitfalls, and variants Classic imaging findings are ill-defined, asymmetric lesions involving the subcortical white matter in the parietal and occipital lobes. Other regions of the brain, including deep gray nuclei, can also be involved.

Resolution of lesions on imaging is noted a few days after treatment of the precipitating cause.

What the referring physician needs to know Rapid diagnosis of this condition is essential, as early treatment and/or withdrawal of the cause can prevent long-term permanent neurologic damage.

Epilepsy

New-onset seizures are the most common neurologic emergency of childhood with approximately 4% to 10% of children and adolescents presenting for the evaluation of a newly occurring seizure disorder every year.[51] A clinical examination, including a detailed neurologic examination and an electroencephalogram, should be performed initially. When imaging is being considered, a plain MR imaging without contrast is usually sufficient and is preferred over CT. Contrast should be considered only if there is a progressive neurologic deficit or if an abnormality is identified on the plain study and needs to be evaluated further.

The most common cause of a seizure in children is a febrile illness. Children with simple febrile seizures do not carry any greater risk for having meningitis than those who have a fever without a seizure, and neuroimaging is not indicated in these children. Children who have a complex febrile seizure, particularly those who present with febrile status epilepticus, have an increased risk of bacterial meningitis or encephalitis; neuroimaging, usually MR imaging with contrast, is indicated in these

children. In children presenting with new-onset seizures without fever, significant findings may be seen in up to 8% of patients, with less than 1% caused by either a tumor or stroke.[52]

An identifiable cause for seizures can be found in up to 90% of full-term newborns, the most common of which is HIE.[53] Other important considerations are infection, hemorrhage, both accidental and nonaccidental, and metabolic abnormalities, such as hypoglycemia (**Fig. 11**). Neonates usually get an ultrasound first, which can show calcifications secondary to a congenital infection or a phakomatosis, such as tuberous sclerosis, among other causes. Ultrasound might also reveal a structural abnormality, which might

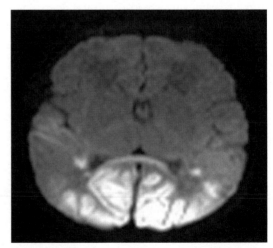

Fig. 11. Hypoglycemia: DWI in a neonate who presented with severe hypoglycemia demonstrating areas of restricted diffusion (apparent diffusion coefficient maps not shown) in the occipital lobes bilaterally.

warrant further investigation with CT or MR imaging. CT is superior at delineating the extent of intracranial hemorrhage, cortical abnormalities, and other emergent conditions. When rapidly available, and in the setting of clinical stability, plain MR imaging of the brain can offer even more detail and can adequately assess the described potential causative entities. It is important to note that transient gyral swelling and enhancement may be seen in patients with status epilepticus, which may be mistaken for other causes of encephalopathy.

What the referring physician needs to know

- Neuroimaging is not indicated in children presenting with simple febrile seizures and should be reserved for complex seizures or new-onset seizures without a febrile illness.
- Neuroimaging should be strongly considered in neonates who present with seizures due to a high incidence of a causative factor associated with seizures in the neonatal period.

Others

Acute disseminated encephalomyelitis

Acute disseminated encephalomyelitis (ADEM) is defined as a monophasic, immune-mediated demyelinating CNS disorder, which causes new-onset poly-focal neurologic symptoms, including encephalopathy, and imaging showing demyelination.[54] Patients usually present 1 to 3 weeks following a viral illness or vaccination. It can also be seen in the absence of an identifiable viral infection. CT may show focal areas of hypodensity (**Fig. 12A**), but the sensitivity is low. The best imaging modality for evaluation is a contrast-enhanced MR of the brain. On MR imaging, patchy, bilateral, often asymmetric areas of hyperintensity are noted on the T2-weighted and FLAIR images in the subcortical and deep white matter of the cerebral hemispheres (**Fig. 12B**).[55] Although it is mainly a white matter disease, gray matter involvement of the cortex and deep nuclei can also be seen. Variable contrast enhancement can be seen (**Fig. 12C**). Cerebellar involvement has also been reported. Thirty percent of cases have spinal cord involvement, so spinal cord imaging may also be indicated in appropriate cases.

The main differential diagnosis that needs to be considered and excluded is multiple sclerosis (MS). MS is less likely to be associated with a prodromal illness. Additionally, the diagnosis of MS is based on evidence of a second demyelinating event involving new areas of the CNS. Patients with MS are generally older (childhood presentation is uncommon), whereas ADEM presents at an earlier age. In MS, the lesion involvement is predominantly in the periventricular white matter and there is a presence of periventricular ovoid lesions perpendicular to the ventricular edge.[56]

Pearls, pitfalls, and variants

- Given that there is no specific diagnostic test, ADEM is typically a diagnosis of exclusion, which makes it very important to rule out mimics, such as infection.
- An ADEM-like first demyelinating event can be the initial involvement by MS.

What the referring physician needs to know Because the symptoms are often nonspecific and may mimic infection, diagnostic difficulty may

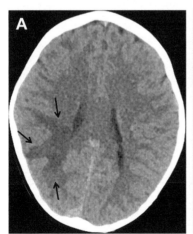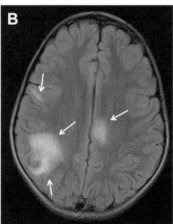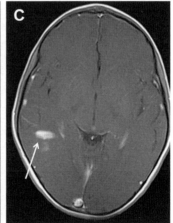

Fig. 12. ADEM: An 8 year old with acute ataxia and diplopia 1 week after a viral infection. Axial plain CT scan of the brain (*A*), demonstrating a large hypodensity in the right parietal lobe (*black arrows*). Axial FLAIR (*B*) and postcontrast (*C*) images demonstrate FLAIR hyperintensities in both cerebral hemispheres (*short white arrows*). Confluent area of underlying enhancement is noted in the right parietal lobe lesion (*long white arrow*).

arise when patients present with headache, fever, meningismus signs, and seizures; infection needs to be excluded in such cases. Once infection is ruled out and ADEM is being considered, treatment with high-dose intravenous steroids followed by oral steroids can be instituted.

TRAUMATIC PEDIATRIC EMERGENCIES

The diagnosis of pediatric head trauma requires a multidisciplinary approach, and the use of neurologic imaging plays a crucial role for diagnosis. The initial imaging study is often a head CT because of its high sensitivity in detecting acute hemorrhages and fractures.[57] However, CT is not always ideal because it requires children to be exposed to radiation.[58] MR imaging has an increased sensitivity and can be performed without radiation; however, it takes a much longer time and may require sedation.[58] The most important goal for anyone reading an imaging study is to be able to recognize the imaging features that may seem benign to the untrained eye but actually are more serious that what they seem to be.

Accidental Injury

Calvarial fractures

Calvarial fractures are a common cause of pediatric emergencies and can be seen in accidental as well as nonaccidental trauma. About 20% of skull fractures occur at the skull base.[59] They are the most fatal, consisting of 80% of fractures at autopsy. About 75% to 90% of depressed fractures are open fractures.

The best imaging modality is a noncontrast CT because it can demonstrate linear, depressed, elevated, skull-base, temporal bone, and growing skull fractures. True acute calvarial fractures demonstrate a linear course with overlying soft tissue swelling.[57] They lack well-defined sclerotic borders and most commonly present unilaterally and asymmetrically. Bilateral fractures are often associated with displacement and/or comminution but will present asymmetrically.[60] If there is a depressed or growing skull fracture, MR imaging is warranted to evaluate for an underlying intracranial injury. In trauma cases, a CT angiography study may be warranted to evaluate for suspected vascular injury. It is important to distinguish normal sutures, accessory sutures, and wormian bones in children from a calvarial fracture (**Fig. 13**). Normal sutures have a zigzag appearance and sclerotic borders and are symmetric. It is crucial for the reader to know the normal sutural anatomy, common accessory sutures, and the timing of typical sutural closure to be able to recognize a true fracture.

Often, a transverse fracture might be present in the same plane as the plane of imaging, which makes visualization of the fracture difficult. Therefore, multi-planar reformats or preferably a 3D imaging of the skull is recommended in all children with skull trauma in order to improve visualization

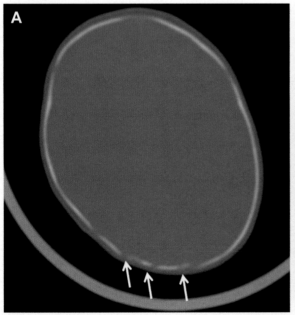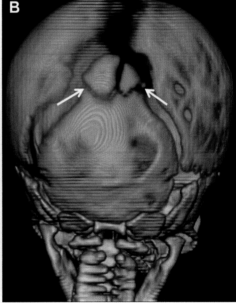

Fig. 13. Wormian bone: Axial CT scan of the brain bone window (*A*) in a newborn demonstrating multiple linear lucencies in the occipital bones (*white arrows*), which could be mistaken for fractures (*short white arrows*). A 3D reconstruction of the skull (*B*) shows these to be large inca (wormian) bones (*white arrows*).

of a fracture. This point becomes particularly more important in cases of suspected NAI whereby an old fracture might be present without overlying soft tissue swelling.[61]

Pearls, pitfalls, and variants

- A child's skull differs from an adult's because of the presence of sutures, accessory sutures, and wormian bones.
- A skull fracture shows a sharp lucency with nonsclerotic edges, can cross adjacent suture lines, widen as it approaches a suture, is often unilateral, and is associated with some soft tissue swelling.
- Accessory sutures, on the other hand, have a zigzag pattern with sclerotic borders, no associated diastasis, merges with the adjacent suture, are often bilateral, fairly symmetric, and do not have overlying soft tissue swelling.

Nonaccidental Injury

NAI is the number one cause of subdural bleeding in children younger than 1 year.[62] The incidence is 17 to 25 per 100,000 children annually, with most children being younger than 2 years at the time of diagnosis. In 80% of cases, the cause of death is cerebral edema, which leads to severe HIE. Retinal hemorrhages are present in about 75% of all child abuse cases with head injury, whereas it is present in only 6% of cases in accidental head injury.[63] Skull fractures are seen in approximately 50% of patients with intracranial injury.[64] Although there is no specific type of fracture indicating child abuse, features favoring NAI include multiple fractures, complex fractures involving both sides of the skull, diastatic fractures, fractures that cross suture lines, fractures of different ages, and depressed skull fractures of the occiput.[65] The

mechanisms of injury include direct injury, strangulation, or shaking. Imaging down to C2 is beneficial to detect associated atlantooccipital injuries.

The best imaging tool for acute trauma is a noncontrast CT to rule out fractures and intracerebral hemorrhage. MR should be done 24 to 48 hours after the injury to evaluate the extent of injury. SDH is a dominant feature in nonaccidental head injury. Subarachnoid hemorrhages are seen in more than 50% of cases, whereas epidural hemorrhages are less common. Neither of these hemorrhages are specific for NAI; however, an interhemispheric SDH, especially when it is the only injury, should raise the suspicion for NAI.[66] An acute SDH is hyperdense on CT. It becomes isodense and finally hypodense as it ages over days to weeks. It is very difficult to time the injury based on the density of blood because blood density is based on several factors and SDHs of the same age can have varying densities.[67] Certain characteristic of SDH may favor NAI, such as SDH with associated retinal hemorrhages, SDH without an associated fracture, isolated interhemispheric SDH, bilateral SDH, or especially SDHs of varying ages. The utility of MR imaging is in differentiating SDHs of various ages (eg, acute vs chronic SDH), detection of associated retinal hemorrhages (**Fig. 14**) or additional injuries, and differentiation from other benign extra-axial collections.

The most common parenchymal injuries in NAI are contusions, shear injuries and cerebral edema.[68] Shear injuries are an acceleration-deceleration pattern of injury which usually result in axonal injuries commonly at the grey-white matter junction. These are frequently hemorrhagic and are seen as focal hyperdensities on CT. On MR, they are T1 hyperintense and T2 hypointense lesions, but are best seen on the more blood-sensitive

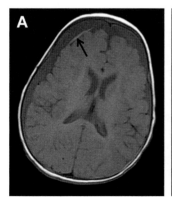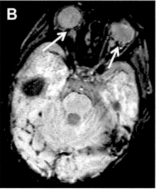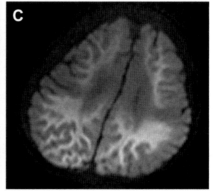

Fig. 14. NAI: Axial T1-weighted (*A*), susceptibility-weighted imaging (*B*), and diffusion (C) MR images in a 2-year-old child with confirmed NAI. Chronic bilateral subdural collections with underlying subacute blood products (*black arrow*), bilateral retinal hemorrhage (*white arrows*), and extensive symmetric supratentorial white matter restricted diffusion. The constellation of these findings is highly suspicious for nonaccidental brain injury.

susceptibility-weighted imaging sequences. Sometimes these lesions may be nonhemorrhagic and seen as focal hypodensities on CT, or T2 hyperintensities on MR, due to edema.

Cerebral edema can be due to direct trauma-related injury or due to secondary causes, such as hypoxia due to strangulation/suffocation or posttraumatic apnea from injury at the craniocervical junction.[69] Imaging findings of edema are described earlier in this article.

Pearls, pitfalls, and variants

- Not all extra-axial collections are due to trauma. It is important to be able to recognize conditions such as subdural empyemas, which can be confused for SDH.
- It is very difficult to find out the exact time intracerebral hemorrhage (ICH) has occurred, which is why it is better to avoid trying to time an ICH. The blood density is based on several different factors (eg, CSF dilution, hematocrit, coagulation studies), and SDHs of the same age can have varying densities.

What the referring physician needs to know

A detailed history is extremely important when suspecting NAI. In the presence of significant intracranial injury, a history of minor trauma is incompatible; NAI should always be suspected whenever there is a discordance between the degree of injury and the clinical history provided. Whenever NAI is suspected, a whole skeletal body survey as well as other imaging tests might be necessary to exclude other associated injuries.

SUMMARY

Physicians not formally trained in radiology play a critical role in the evaluation of children presenting to the ED with neurologic emergencies. Knowledge of the imaging protocol and findings, pearls, pitfalls, and differential diagnosis for some of the common pediatric neurologic emergencies can allow for prompt diagnosis, which can potentially be lifesaving. It is important to keep NAI in mind when dealing with trauma in children, particularly those in whom the clinical and imaging findings are discordant.

REFERENCES

1. Wong J, Quint DJ. Imaging of central nervous system infections. Semin Roentgenol 1999;34:123–43.
2. Kanamalla US, Ibarra RA, Jinkins JR. Imaging of cranial meningitis and ventriculitis. Neuroimaging Clin N Am 2000;10:309–31.
3. van de Beek D, de Gans J, Spanjaard L, et al. Clinical features and prognostic factors in adults with bacterial meningitis. N Engl J Med 2004;351:1849–59.
4. Sze G, Zimmerman RD. The magnetic resonance imaging of infections and inflammatory diseases. Radiol Clin North Am 1988;26:839–59.
5. Mohan S, Jain KK, Arabi M, et al. Imaging of meningitis and ventriculitis. Neuroimaging Clin N Am 2012;22:557–83.
6. Sage MR, Wilson AJ, Scroop R. Contrast media and the brain. The basis of CT and MR imaging enhancement. Neuroimaging Clin N Am 1998;8:695–707.
7. Kastrup O, Wanke I, Maschke M. Neuroimaging of infections of the central nervous system. Semin Neurol 2008;28:511–22.
8. Bano S, Chaudhary V, Garga UC. Neonatal hypoxic-ischemic encephalopathy: a radiological review. J Pediatr neurosciences 2017;12:1–6.
9. AG Osborne. Infections of the brain and its linings. Diagn Neuroradiology 1994;673–715.
10. Karagulle-Kendi AT, Truwit C. Neuroimaging of central nervous system infections. Handb Clin Neurol 2010;96:239–55.
11. Parmar H, Sitoh YY, Anand P, et al. Contrast-enhanced flair imaging in the evaluation of infectious leptomeningeal diseases. Eur J Radiol 2006;58:89–95.
12. Dietemann JL, Correia Bernardo R, Bogorin A, et al. Normal and abnormal meningeal enhancement: MRI features. J Radiol 2005;86:1659–83 [in French].
13. Kioumehr F, Dadsetan MR, Feldman N, et al. Postcontrast MRI of cranial meninges: leptomeningitis versus pachymeningitis. J Comput Assist Tomogr 1995;19:713–20.
14. Hughes DC, Raghavan A, Mordekar SR, et al. Role of imaging in the diagnosis of acute bacterial meningitis and its complications. Postgrad Med J 2010;86:478–85.
15. Kennedy PG. Viral encephalitis: causes, differential diagnosis, and management. J Neurol Neurosurg Psychiatry 2004;75(Suppl 1):i10–5.
16. Cinque P, Cleator GM, Weber T, et al. The role of laboratory investigation in the diagnosis and management of patients with suspected herpes simplex encephalitis: a consensus report. The EU concerted action on virus meningitis and encephalitis. J Neurol Neurosurg Psychiatry 1996;61:339–45.
17. Falcone S, Post MJ. Encephalitis, cerebritis, and brain abscess: pathophysiology and imaging findings. Neuroimaging Clin N Am 2000;10:333–53.
18. Tien R, Dillon WP, Jackler RK. Contrast-enhanced MR imaging of the facial nerve in 11 patients with Bell's palsy. AJR Am J Roentgenol 1990;155:573–9.
19. Noguchi T, Yoshiura T, Hiwatashi A, et al. CT and MRI findings of human herpesvirus 6-associated encephalopathy: comparison with findings of herpes simplex virus encephalitis. AJR Am J Roentgenol 2010;194:754–60.

20. Kuker W, Nagele T, Schmidt F, et al. Diffusion-weighted MRI in herpes simplex encephalitis: a report of three cases. Neuroradiology 2004;46:122–5.

21. Vossough A, Zimmerman RA, Bilaniuk LT, et al. Imaging findings of neonatal herpes simplex virus type 2 encephalitis. Neuroradiology 2008;50:355–66.

22. Bonfield CM, Sharma J, Dobson S. Pediatric intracranial abscesses. J Infect 2015;71(Suppl 1):S42–6.

23. Banerjee AD, Pandey P, Devi BI, et al. Pediatric supratentorial subdural empyemas: a retrospective analysis of 65 cases. Pediatr Neurosurg 2009;45:11–8.

24. Barkovich AJ. Hydrocephalus. New York: Raven Press; 1995.

25. Klein DM. The treatment of shunt infections. Williams and Wilkins; 1990. p. 87–98.

26. Casey AT, Kimmings EJ, Kleinlugtebeld AD, et al. The long-term outlook for hydrocephalus in childhood. A ten-year cohort study of 155 patients. Pediatr Neurosurg 1997;27:63–70.

27. Aldrich EF, Harmann P. Disconnection as a cause of ventriculoperitoneal shunt malfunction in multicomponent shunt systems. Pediatr Neurosurg 1990;16:309–11 [discussion: 312].

28. Patel DM, Tubbs RS, Pate G, et al. Fast-sequence MRI studies for surveillance imaging in pediatric hydrocephalus. J Neurosurg Pediatr 2014;13:440–7.

29. Madsen MA. Emergency department management of ventriculoperitoneal cerebrospinal fluid shunts. Ann Emerg Med 1986;15:1330–43.

30. Zahl SM, Egge A, Helseth E, et al. Benign external hydrocephalus: a review, with emphasis on management. Neurosurg Rev 2011;34:417–32.

31. Robson CD, MacDougall RD, Madsen JR, et al. Neuroimaging of children with surgically treated hydrocephalus: a practical approach. AJR Am J Roentgenol 2017;208:413–9.

32. Kirks DR, Griscom NT. Practical pediatric imaging: diagnostic radiology of infants and children. Lippincott Williams & Wilkins; 1998.

33. Heller C, Heinecke A, Junker R, et al. Cerebral venous thrombosis in children: a multifactorial origin. Circulation 2003;108:1362–7.

34. deVeber G, Andrew M, Adams C, et al. Cerebral sinovenous thrombosis in children. N Engl J Med 2001;345:417–23.

35. Sebire G, Tabarki B, Saunders DE, et al. Cerebral venous sinus thrombosis in children: risk factors, presentation, diagnosis and outcome. Brain 2005;128:477–89.

36. Hashmi M, Wasay M. Caring for cerebral venous sinus thrombosis in children. J Emerg Trauma Shock 2011;4:389–94.

37. Huisman TA, Holzmann D, Martin E, et al. Cerebral venous thrombosis in childhood. Eur Radiol 2001;11:1760–5.

38. Kothare SV, Ebb DH, Rosenberger PB, et al. Acute confusion and mutism as a presentation of thalamic strokes secondary to deep cerebral venous thrombosis. J Child Neurol 1998;13:300–3.

39. Ihn YK, Jung WS, Hwang SS. The value of T2*-weighted gradient-echo MRI for the diagnosis of cerebral venous sinus thrombosis. Clin Imaging 2013;37:446–50.

40. Kenet G, Kirkham F, Niederstadt T, et al. Risk factors for recurrent venous thromboembolism in the European collaborative paediatric database on cerebral venous thrombosis: a multicentre cohort study. Lancet Neurol 2007;6:595–603.

41. Baumgartner RW, Studer A, Arnold M, et al. Recanalisation of cerebral venous thrombosis. J Neurol Neurosurg Psychiatry 2003;74:459–61.

42. Buyck PJ, De Keyzer F, Vanneste D, et al. CT density measurement and H:H ratio are useful in diagnosing acute cerebral venous sinus thrombosis. AJNR Am J Neuroradiol 2013;34:1568–72.

43. O'Neill S, Saigal G. Pseudo empty delta sign due to poor clearance of intravenous contrast in the setting of acute renal failure. Pediatr Radiol 2014;44:761–2.

44. Heinz ER, Provenzale JM. Imaging findings in neonatal hypoxia: a practical review. AJR Am J Roentgenol 2009;192:41–7.

45. Izbudak I, Grant PE. MR imaging of the term and preterm neonate with diffuse brain injury. Magn Reson Imaging Clin N Am 2011;19:709–31, vii.

46. Inaba H, Khan RB, Laningham FH, et al. Clinical and radiological characteristics of methotrexate-induced acute encephalopathy in pediatric patients with cancer. Ann Oncol 2008;19:178–84.

47. Tamrazi B, Almast J. Your brain on drugs: imaging of drug-related changes in the central nervous system. Radiographics 2012;32:701–19.

48. Adams DH, Ponsford S, Gunson B, et al. Neurological complications following liver transplantation. Lancet 1987;1:949–51.

49. Hinchey J, Chaves C, Appignani B, et al. A reversible posterior leukoencephalopathy syndrome. N Engl J Med 1996;334:494–500.

50. Bartynski WS, Boardman JF. Distinct imaging patterns and lesion distribution in posterior reversible encephalopathy syndrome. AJNR Am J Neuroradiol 2007;28:1320–7.

51. Hauser WA. The prevalence and incidence of convulsive disorders in children. Epilepsia 1994;35(Suppl 2):S1–6.

52. Sharma S, Riviello JJ, Harper MB, et al. The role of emergent neuroimaging in children with new-onset afebrile seizures. Pediatrics 2003;111:1–5.

53. Agarwal M, Fox SM. Pediatric seizures. Emerg Med Clin North Am 2013;31:733–54.

54. Pohl D, Alper G, Van Haren K, et al. Acute disseminated encephalomyelitis: updates on an inflammatory CNS syndrome. Neurology 2016;87:S38–45.

55. Tenembaum S, Chamoles N, Fejerman N. Acute disseminated encephalomyelitis: a long-term

follow-up study of 84 pediatric patients. Neurology 2002;59:1224–31.

56. Alper G, Heyman R, Wang L. Multiple sclerosis and acute disseminated encephalomyelitis diagnosed in children after long-term follow-up: comparison of presenting features. Dev Med Child Neurol 2009; 51:480–6.

57. Kralik SF, Finke W, Wu IC, et al. Radiologic head CT interpretation errors in pediatric abusive and non-abusive head trauma patients. Pediatr Radiol 2017; 47:942–51.

58. Ryan ME, Jaju A, Ciolino JD, et al. Rapid MRI evaluation of acute intracranial hemorrhage in pediatric head trauma. Neuroradiology 2016;58: 793–9.

59. Yellinek S, Cohen A, Merkin V, et al. Clinical significance of skull base fracture in patients after traumatic brain injury. J Clin Neurosci 2016;25:111–5.

60. Sanchez T, Stewart D, Walvick M, et al. Skull fracture vs. accessory sutures: how can we tell the difference? Emerg Radiol 2010;17:413–8.

61. Prabhu SP, Newton AW, Perez-Rossello JM, et al. Three-dimensional skull models as a problem-solving tool in suspected child abuse. Pediatr Radiol 2013;43:575–81.

62. Matschke J, Voss J, Obi N, et al. Nonaccidental head injury is the most common cause of subdural bleeding in infants <1 year of age. Pediatrics 2009;124:1587–94.

63. Vinchon M, Defoort-Dhellemmes S, Desurmont M, et al. Accidental and nonaccidental head injuries in infants: a prospective study. J Neurosurg 2005; 102:380–4.

64. Merten DF, Osborne DR, Radkowski MA, et al. Craniocerebral trauma in the child abuse syndrome: radiological observations. Pediatr Radiol 1984;14: 272–7.

65. Rao P, Carty H. Non-accidental injury: review of the radiology. Clin Radiol 1999;54:11–24.

66. Barnes PD. Imaging of nonaccidental injury and the mimics: issues and controversies in the era of evidence-based medicine. Radiol Clin North Am 2011;49:205–29.

67. Park HR, Lee KS, Shim JJ, et al. Multiple densities of the chronic subdural hematoma in CT scans. J Korean Neurosurg Soc 2013;54:38–41.

68. Paul AR, Adamo MA. Non-accidental trauma in pediatric patients: a review of epidemiology, pathophysiology, diagnosis and treatment. Transl Pediatr 2014;3:195–207.

69. Geddes JF, Whitwell HL, Graham DI. Traumatic axonal injury: practical issues for diagnosis in medicolegal cases. Neuropathol Appl Neurobiol 2000;26:105–16.

Head and Neck Injuries
Special Considerations in the Elderly Patient

Claire K. Sandstrom, MD[a],*, Diego B. Nunez, MD, MPH[b]

KEYWORDS

- Geriatric • Elderly • Trauma • Head • Neck • Subdural hematoma • Cervical spine • Fractures

KEY POINTS

- Injury patterns differ in geriatric patients compared with young trauma victims, and the risk of serious complications is higher in the elderly for a given level of trauma.
- Preexisting atrophy of the brain can result in delayed clinical manifestations of increased intracranial pressure from traumatic intracranial hemorrhage. The threshold for computed tomographic imaging of geriatric patients with even minor head trauma should be very low.
- Facial injuries are more likely to involve the orbital floor, lateral orbital wall, and maxilla than in nongeriatric patients.
- Cervical spine fractures are likely to occur between the occiput and C2, most frequently at the dens and C2 body. The presence of underlying diffuse idiopathic skeletal hyperostosis or ankylosis from degeneration increases the likelihood of unstable hyperextension fractures.

INTRODUCTION

Various definitions of elderly exist, but 65 years of age is used most commonly to define the geriatric population, including in the Eastern Association for the Surgery of Trauma practice management guidelines.[1] In coming years, geriatric trauma patients will comprise an increasing percentage of Emergency Department visits as the result of the rapidly growing elderly population in the United States. By 2030, one-fifth of the American population will be aged 65 years or older as the baby boomer generation continues to mature.[2]

Older adults comprise an even larger proportion of the trauma population. Persons aged at least 65 years of age accounted for 30% of patients recorded in the 2015 National Trauma Data Bank.[3] The annual report also shows that falls account for 83% of trauma incidents in those aged 65 years and older, with much of the remainder accounted for by motorized vehicular crashes (MVC) and car-versus-pedestrian accidents.[3] Falls from standing are more likely in the geriatric population for a variety of reasons, including weakness and generalized deconditioning related to chronic diseases, polypharmacy, balance and gait disturbances, vision loss, poor reaction times, and cognitive impairments.[4] Recurrent falls are also more likely in patients who have fallen within the past year.[5]

According to the Centers for Disease Control and Prevention, unintentional injuries, most commonly from falls, were the seventh leading cause of death in those 65 years and older in 2014.[6] Injury patterns differ in geriatric patients compared with their younger counterparts, and the elderly are at higher risk for serious complications. The case fatality rate increases for geriatric

Disclosures: None.
[a] Section of Emergency and Trauma Radiology, Department of Radiology, Harborview Medical Center, Box 359728, 325 Ninth Avenue, Seattle, WA 98104, USA; [b] Emergency Radiology and Neuroradiology Divisions, Department of Radiology, Brigham and Women's Hospital, 75 Francis Street, Boston, MA 02115, USA
* Corresponding author.
E-mail address: cks13@uw.edu

Neuroimag Clin N Am 28 (2018) 471–481
https://doi.org/10.1016/j.nic.2018.03.008

patients, with the mortality for those older than 84 years of age (8.73%) over twice that of all non-geriatric age groups (range 0.97%–4.10%).[3] Mortality is increased in geriatric patients across all injury severity scores, body parts injured, and mechanisms of injury.[3,7,8] Falls in patients 65 years and older resulted in more than 21,000 deaths in 2010, with an estimated $500 million in medical costs and more than $2 billion in work loss costs.[6] Nevertheless, a large proportion of geriatric trauma patients can return to independent living with prompt, appropriate treatment.[9] Elderly patients are also at risk for undertriage because of, among other reasons, normal age-related physiologic differences compared with younger adults, medication effects, and preexisting cognitive deficits.[1] Early diagnosis and aggressive management of injuries in the geriatric trauma patient are imperative, and liberal use of imaging, particularly with computed tomography (CT), plays an essential role in this task. In this article, the authors focus on injuries to the head, face, and cervical spine in geriatric trauma patients and on how they differ from the younger population, based on mechanistic, anatomic, and clinical factors.

HEAD TRAUMA

Head injuries in the elderly are common following trauma and are more likely to be significant, requiring intervention or resulting in a long-term disability or neurologic impairment.[10,11] Although neurosurgical intervention is not usually necessary, it is more likely if focal neurologic deficits are present.[12] Adverse outcomes, including mortality and functional disability, are uniformly higher in geriatric patients when compared with younger patients with similar degree of injury.[11] The most frequent traumatic lesions seen in geriatric trauma patients are contusions and subdural hematomas. Epidural hematoma, intraventricular hemorrhage, skull fractures, and pneumocephalus are seen less commonly in elderly patients.[12]

Frontal and temporal lobe contusions are certainly not unique to older age but are still prevalent in this patient population. Falling backwards from standing or on stairs is frequent in the elderly, and the resulting impact to the occiput can be associated with enough longitudinal deceleration to cause cortical contusions from a coup-contracoup mechanism (**Fig. 1**). Likewise, parasagittal or gliding contusions occur when the paramedian frontoparietal cortex slides against the rigid falx cerebri, as a result of a more lateral traumatic impact (**Fig. 2**).

Subdural hematomas result from tearing of the small bridging veins of the subarachnoid space, which tends to widen with older age secondary to involution of the cerebral cortex. This age-related volume loss partially explains why elderly patients with significant intracranial injury may not display typical neurologic signs of increased intracranial pressure.[13] In geriatric patients, different than younger adults, subdural hematomas frequently present with imaging features of chronicity, and a clear history of trauma is not always elicited on admission to the emergency department. The hematomas can grow gradually over time without significantly increased intracranial pressure. The expansion is likely related to a combination of clot absorption and increased fibrinolytic activity within the hematoma. Recurrent microbleeds from the hematoma capsule also contribute to its growth and are responsible for the mixed density of the collections (**Fig. 3**). The development of membranous adhesions within chronic hematomas is not uncommon in the elderly. They present as relatively hyperdense

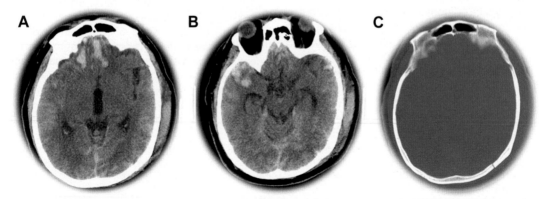

Fig. 1. Contracoup contusions in an 80-year-old patient who fell backwards from standing. Axial CT images show frontal (*A*) and temporal (*B*) hemorrhagic contusions associated with posterior parietal fracture (*C*).

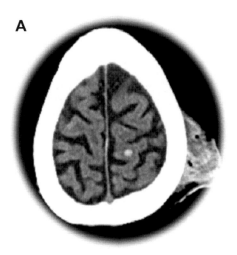

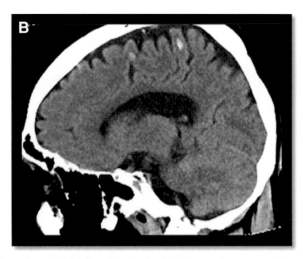

Fig. 2. Paramedian gliding contusions in an elderly patient. Axial (*A*) and sagittal (*B*) CT images demonstrate hemorrhagic foci at the gray/white matter interface with large left parietal soft tissue hematoma.

septations forming pockets of noncommunicating collections that may resemble the configuration of small epidural hematomas (**Fig. 4**A). The dense content and adhesions present in chronic subdural hematomas pose a therapeutic challenge. The evacuation is frequently incomplete (**Fig. 4**B), necessitating additional interventions for drainage and increasing patient morbidity and mortality.

Epidural hematomas are exceedingly rare in geriatric patients, and skull fractures in general are less common than in younger patients.[14,15] The calvarium thickens with age and renders the skull less vulnerable to fractures, particularly in the setting of low-energy trauma. In addition, the periosteal layer of the dura mater becomes very adherent to the inner table and is less prone to strip off from epidural hemorrhage, as seen in younger adults.

Although often used to screen head injury patients, the Glasgow Coma Scale (GCS) may be

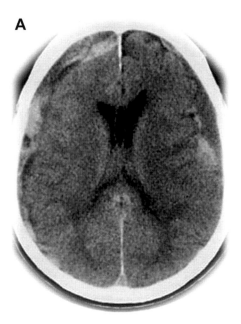

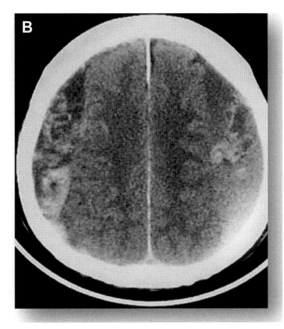

Fig. 3. Mixed density bilateral subdural hematomas in a 76-year-old patient who presented with cognitive decline. Axial CT images (*A*, *B*) show alternating layers of high and low attenuation within bilateral subdural collections. No midline shift is noted.

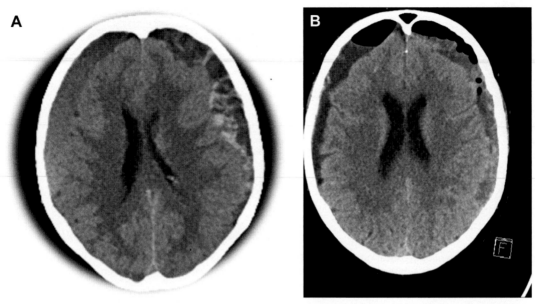

Fig. 4. Bilateral subacute and chronic subdural collections in a 68-year-old patient with a history of remote trivial head trauma. Axial CT images demonstrate (*A*) partially isodense right subdural hematoma and a septated left-sided collection with hyperdense foci consistent with recurrent bleeding. (*B*) Postoperative CT scan shows incomplete evacuation of the hematomas.

unreliable in the elderly trauma patient.[16] The threshold for imaging of the geriatric patient with even minor head trauma (defined as no loss of consciousness, no focal neurologic deficits, and a normal GCS) should therefore be very low. Age older than 65 years is an independent risk factor mandating further assessment with CT following head trauma in both the New Orleans Criteria[17] and the Canadian CT Head Rule.[18] National guidelines currently recommend immediate head CT in all geriatric patients with minor head injury.[19]

Abnormalities of coagulation are common in the elderly and include hematologic disorders, liver disease, and treatment with anticoagulant and antiplatelet medications. Elderly patients who are receiving anticoagulation treatment are at higher risk for intracranial hemorrhage after trauma.[20–22] Hemorrhage progression and complications from or delay in neurosurgical intervention are also higher in anticoagulated patients. Higher mortalities have been seen in elderly patients taking preinjury anticoagulants, including warfarin or antiplatelet agents (clopidogrel, aspirin), than in age-matched controls not on anticoagulants before trauma.[21–24] Ideally, all older adults on anticoagulation with head trauma should be triaged directly to a trauma center.[1,25] Current clinical guidelines recommend head CT immediately after admission for all anticoagulated patients with head trauma.[1,26] Once intracranial injury has been

identified, immediate reversal of coagulopathy is generally warranted despite the potential complications resulting from reversal therapy (including thrombosis and volume overload).[1,27,28] A follow-up CT is performed 6 hours after initial diagnosis to evaluate for stability, unless neurologic deterioration prompts earlier reevaluation (**Fig. 5**). Although rare, delayed intracranial hemorrhage following head trauma may occur in patients receiving warfarin.[20,29–32] Therefore, monitoring for 12 to 24 hours after a head CT negative for intracranial injury is generally appropriate, although whether repeat head CT is routinely needed in this group is still debated.[29,30,32]

CT may on occasion reveal an intracranial cause for the patient's fall, such as hemorrhagic stroke or intracranial mass, as opposed to a complication of the trauma.

FACIAL TRAUMA

As with head injuries, facial trauma most often results from falls in the elderly population, followed by MVC.[33] Most facial injuries in geriatric patients tend to be minimally displaced midfacial fractures that do not require surgical intervention. They are more likely to involve the nose, the orbit, and the zygomaticomaxillary complex resulting from anterior or lateral impacts, whereas nongeriatric adult patients are more prone to suffer fractures of the mandible.[33]

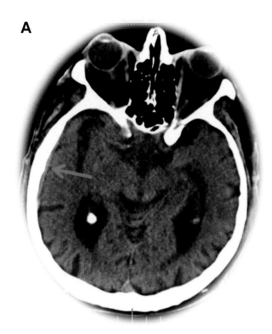
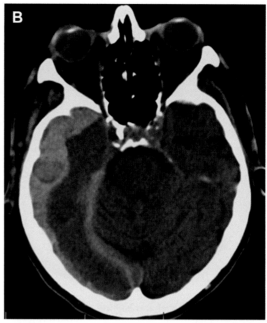

Fig. 5. Rapid progression of acute subdural hematoma in a geriatric patient. Axial CT images demonstrate (*A*) very thin, laminar right temporal subdural collection (*arrow*) that expands in a few hours to a large holohemispheric hematoma (*B*).

Geriatric patients with facial fractures are more likely to have accompanying brain, spine, and extremity injuries than nongeriatric adult patients with facial trauma.[33] Of note, a frequent pattern of combined injuries results from anterior facial or frontal impact associated with hyperextension of the neck and associated injuries of the cervical spine (**Fig. 6**). The population of geriatric patients with facial trauma has also been found to have longer hospitalization, higher in-hospital mortality, and greater need for assistance after discharge.[33]

CERVICAL SPINE TRAUMA

The prevalence of spinal fractures increases with age, regardless of location.[26] In particular, cervical spine injuries differ significantly in geriatric trauma patients compared with their younger adult counterparts. Patients aged 65 years and older are at increased risk for cervical spine injuries for any degree of trauma, with falls again constituting the most common mechanism.[34] In younger adult patients, most cervical spine injuries occur at the most mobile segment, from C4 to C7. Although hyperextension fractures centered at C5-C6 levels occur not infrequently in geriatric trauma patients (**Fig. 7**), cervical spine injuries in the elderly are much more likely to involve the upper cervical spine, from the

occiput to C2.[35,36] This effect is even more pronounced in the very elderly (older than 75 years of age).[35] A combination of age-related factors likely accounts for this increased rate and altered location of cervical spine injuries. These factors include osteoporosis, muscular weakness, and increased rigidity of the lower cervical spine due to degeneration, ankylosing spondylitis (AS), or diffuse idiopathic skeletal hyperostosis (DISH) (**Fig. 8**).[34]

The most common cervical fractures in elderly patients involve the C2 vertebra, most often at the base of the dens (Anderson-D'Alonzo type II) (**Fig. 9**).[37] Fractures involving the C2 vertebral body (Anderson-D'Alonzo type III) are also common, particularly in patients aged 70 years and older.[37] Most C2 odontoid fractures are related to low-energy trauma in the setting of osteoporosis. In contrast, C2 Hangman fractures are usually the result of high-energy trauma, not osteoporosis, and therefore are less prevalent in the geriatric trauma population.[37]

DISH is most commonly found in men and is increasingly widespread because of its association with age, type 2 diabetes mellitus, and obesity. The presence of ankylosis, whether from AS or DISH, creates long lever arms acting on a stiff and brittle spine that results in significantly increased risk for injury, particularly unstable spine

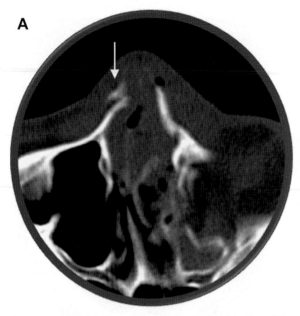
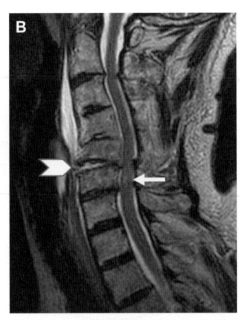

Fig. 6. Combined facial and cervical spine injuries in a 67-year-old female patient who slipped on ice. Axial CT image (*A*) reveals right nasal (*arrow*) and left orbital fractures. Sagittal T2 magnetic resonance (MR) image (*B*) demonstrates hyperintense prevertebral edema/hematoma with interruption of the anterior longitudinal ligament and C5-C6 disc injury (*arrowhead*), and focal cord contusion (*arrow*).

fractures, with even minor trauma.[38] Most fractures in patients with DISH and AS occur as a result of falling from a standing or sitting position and are of a hyperextension type.[38] Although

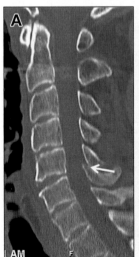
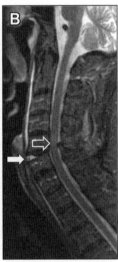

Fig. 7. Hyperextension injury in a 72-year-old patient who fell on a treadmill. Sagittal CT reformation (*A*) shows subtle anterior widening of the C5-C6 intervertebral space and step-off of the interspinous line at the same level (*arrow*). (*B*) Sagittal short T1 inversion recovery (STIR) MR image demonstrates rupture of the anterior longitudinal ligament and intervertebral disc injury (*arrow*) with cord contusion (*open arrow*). Also noted is prevertebral and posterior soft tissue edema.

fractures can occur anywhere in the spine of these patients with ankylosis, the cervical spine is the most common site, particularly at the transition points proximal or distal to a fused segment (**Fig. 10**).[38,39] Delays in diagnosis of fractures in AS and DISH patients are frequent, as a result of failure to request imaging or recognize a fracture on the part of the doctor and as a result of the patient not immediately seeking medical care after a minor traumatic event.[38] Trauma patients with AS and DISH have a very high rate of complications and mortality.[38]

Cervical spine fractures are also more likely to result in spinal cord injuries (SCI) in the elderly, and SCI are associated with a high mortality in geriatric trauma patients.[40] The spinal cord is at increased risk for contusion or transection due to underlying cervical stenosis attributed to degenerative spine disease.[35] As a consequence of cervical spondylosis and stenosis, and probably compounded by smoking or vascular disease,[41] SCI without radiologic evidence of trauma or SCI without CT evidence of trauma is common is the geriatric age group (**Fig. 11**).[42,43] Patients with acute fractures superimposed on AS or DISH have a high rate of neurologic deficits on admission, and secondary neurologic deterioration is also common because of fracture instability.[38]

Any delay in diagnosis of cervical spine fractures should be avoided to prevent secondary neurologic deterioration from unstable injuries.

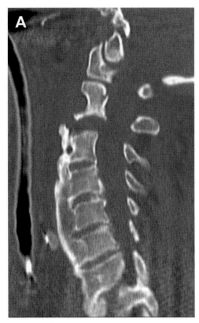

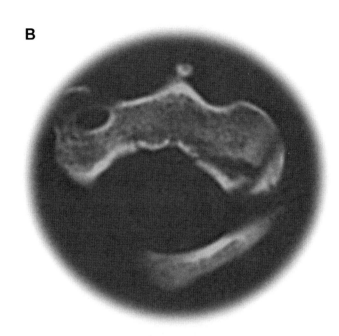

Fig. 8. Distraction injury at the C2-C3 level, proximal to a long fused segment in a patient with DISH. Sagittal CT reformation (A) reveals C2-C3 separation and a coronally oriented fracture of C2 seen in the axial CT image (B).

Cervical spine fractures are much more likely in those elderly trauma patients presenting with new neurologic deficits, with head injuries, or with injuries resulting from moderate- to high-energy trauma, including MVCs and motorcycle crashes, pedestrian struck by vehicle, or fall from height above ground level.[7,44] Depending on the number of these risk factors present, the probability of cervical fracture ranges from 0.4% to 24.2%.[44] All geriatric trauma patients are required to undergo cervical spine imaging following blunt trauma based on the Canadian C-spine Rule.[45] The National Emergency X-Radiography Utilization Study (NEXUS) does not explicitly take age into account.[46,47] Some reports suggest that NEXUS is adequate for screening for significant cervical spine fractures in elderly patients,[36,48] including those at a baseline decreased GCS and those with distracting injuries not related to the head and neck region.[49] However, NEXUS has been criticized by others for having lower sensitivity for detection of cervical spine injuries in geriatric trauma patients.[50–52]

Accurate diagnosis of cervical spine injuries may be more difficult in elderly patients as well.[34] Minimally displaced fractures are more difficult to detect in osteoporotic bone, particularly on radiographs. Morphologic osseous changes associated with degeneration, such as osteophytes and spondylolisthesis, may mask or mimic traumatic

pathologic condition. Also, cervical spine injuries in the elderly tend to be multilevel,[35] sometimes noncontiguous, with missed detection of additional levels due to satisfaction of search (Fig. 12).[34]

Geriatric trauma patients, like younger adult trauma patients, are at risk for blunt cerebrovascular injury (BCVI) as a result of cervical trauma (Fig. 13). The Denver criteria recommend CT angiography (CTA) to screen for BCVI when fractures involve C1 to C3 or the foramen transversarium or are associated with subluxation.[53] Expanded screening criteria have been developed by the Western Trauma Association in 2009 and the Eastern Association for the Surgery of Trauma in 2010 to increase sensitivity of BCVI detection.[54] However, the Denver criteria assume a high-energy mechanism, whereas as discussed, most geriatric cervical spine trauma results from low-energy falls. To that end, in some institutions, a neck CTA may not be mandatory in the setting of an isolated type II dens fracture resulting from a ground-level fall because of a very low risk of BCVI. CTA is performed for type II dens fractures accompanied by C1 ring fractures, type III dens fractures, and fractures from high-energy trauma meeting the expanded Denver criteria. Identification of BCVI usually prompts anticoagulation to prevent the complication of stroke and clinical monitoring for signs of embolic phenomenon.

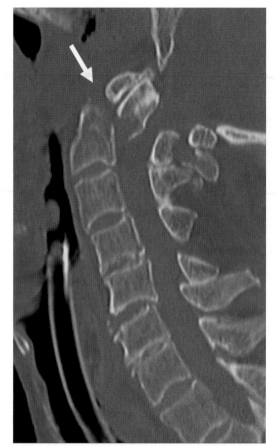

Fig. 9. Severely displaced C2 fracture in an elderly patient. Sagittal CT reformation demonstrates posterior displacement of the fractured dens (*arrow*) and the C1 ring, resulting in significant canal stenosis. Also present is associated hyperextension injury at C5-C6.

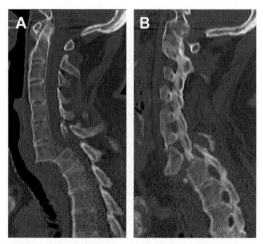

Fig. 10. Severe fracture-dislocation of the cervicothoracic junction in a 66-year-old patient with AS, involved in an MVC. CT sagittal reformations demonstrate anterior displacement of the fused cervical spine on T1 (*A*) with comminuted fracture of the posterior elements (*B*).

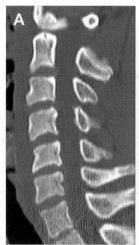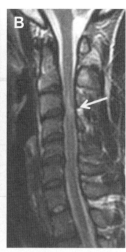

Fig. 11. An elderly patient with mild spinal cervical canal stenosis and cord contusion after whiplash injury. CT sagittal reformation (*A*) shows no fracture or dislocation. Sagittal T2-weighted MR image (*B*) reveals focus of hyperintensity in spinal cord at the C3-C4 level (*arrow*) consistent with contusion, with no injuries noted on CT.

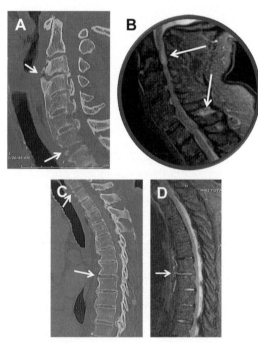

Fig. 12. Multilevel injuries in an elderly patient with a rigid spine secondary to DISH. Sagittal CT reformation of the cervical spine (*A*) shows spinal stenosis and the effect of distraction from hyperextension forces proximal (C3-C4) and distal (C7-T1) to the fused cervical segment (*arrows*). Sagittal STIR MR image (*B*) of the cervical spine reveals associated cord contusion and interspinous soft tissue edema (*arrows*). Sagittal CT reformation of the thoracic spine (*C*) shows the C7-T1 distraction (*short arrow*) and an additional injury at T7-T8 (*long arrow*) with interruption of the generalized anterior fusion. Sagittal STIR MR image (*D*) of the thoracic spine demonstrates the T7-T8 interspace widening and high T2 signal within the disc (*arrow*).

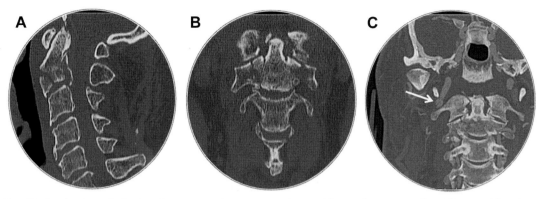

Fig. 13. Proximal cervical spine fractures and posttraumatic carotid pseudoaneurysm in a 72-year-old patient. Sagittal (*A*) and coronal (*B*) CT reformations demonstrate C1 and C2 comminuted fractures with fragment dispersion. (*C*) Maximum intensity projection image of CTA reveals a small carotid pseudoaneurysm (*arrow*) at the segment between fractured fragments and the styloid process.

SUMMARY

Traumatic injuries involving the head and neck region of patients aged 65 years and older are common and will increase in prevalence as the elderly population grows in the coming decades. Injury patterns differ in geriatric patients compared with their younger counterparts, and the elderly are at higher risk for serious complications. Most injuries result from low energy falls, and clinical signs of trauma are less reliable than in younger populations. Liberal use of CT imaging is necessary for prompt diagnosis with even minor trauma. Head injuries most commonly involve cerebral contusions and subdural hemorrhage, and the risk is higher in those with preinjury coagulopathy. Cervical spine fractures are common, and in the geriatric trauma patient, most often involve the upper cervical spine, particularly the odontoid process. Hyperextension fractures in the cervical spine are more likely in elderly with underlying spinal ankylosis and in those with facial fractures from frontal impact. Geriatric patients are also at risk for blunt cerebrovascular injuries and SCI. An understanding of the differing spectrum of head and neck injuries that happen in the elderly population is essential to arriving at a prompt and accurate diagnosis and improving outcomes in this at-risk population.

REFERENCES

1. Calland JF, Ingraham AM, Martin N, et al. Evaluation and management of geriatric trauma: an Eastern Association for the Surgery of Trauma practice management guideline. J Trauma Acute Care Surg 2012;73:S345–50.
2. Vincent GK, Velkoff VA. The next four decades: the older population in the United States: 2010 to 2050, current population reports, P25-1138. Washington, DC: US Census Bureau; 2010.
3. Nance ML, editor. Committee on trauma, American College of Surgeons. Chicago: NTDB Annual/Pediatric Report; 2015.
4. Bonne S, Schuerer DJ. Trauma in the older adult: epidemiology and evolving geriatric trauma principles. Clin Geriatr Med 2013;29:137–50.
5. Ganz DA, Bao Y, Shekelle PG. Will my patient fall? JAMA 2007;297:77–86.
6. Centers for Disease Control and Prevention, National Center for Injury Prevention and Control. Web-based Injury Statistics Query and Reporting System (WISQARS). 2010. Available at: http://www.cdc.gov/injury/wisqars. Accessed April 12, 2017.
7. Brown CVR, Rix K, Klein AL, et al. A comprehensive investigation of comorbidities, mechanisms, injury patterns, and outcomes in geriatric blunt trauma patients. Am Surg 2016;82:1055–62.
8. Finelli FC, Johnsson J, Champion HR, et al. A case-control study for major trauma in geriatric patients. J Trauma 1989;29:541–8.
9. Jacobs DG, Plaisier BR, Barie PS, et al. Practice management guidelines for geriatric trauma: the EAST Practice Management Guidelines Work Group. J Trauma 2003;54:391–416.
10. Nagurney JT, Borczuk P, Thomas SH. Elder patients with closed head trauma: a comparison with non-elder patients. Acad Emerg Med 1998;5:678–84.
11. Rathlev NK, Medzon R, Lowery D, et al. Intracranial pathology in elders with blunt head trauma. Acad Emerg Med 2006;13:302–7.
12. Nagurney JT, Borczuk P, Thomas SH. Elderly patients with closed head trauma after a fall: mechanisms and outcomes. J Emerg Med 1998;16:709–13.
13. Mack LR, Chan SB, Silva JC, et al. The use of head computed tomography in elderly patients sustaining minor head trauma. J Emerg Med 2003;24:157–62.

14. LeRoux AA, Navdi SS. Acute extradural haematoma in the elderly. Br J Neurosurg 2007;21:16–20.

15. Foryoung K, Nautch F, Malhotra A, et al. The patterns of head injury in the elderly. Radiologic Soc North America 2016.

16. Kehoe A, Rennie S, Smith JE. Glasgow Coma Scale is unreliable for the prediction of severe head injury in elderly trauma patients. Emerg Med J 2015;32:613–5.

17. Haydel MJ, Preston CA, Mills TJ, et al. Indications for computed tomography in patients with minor head trauma. N Engl J Med 2000;343:100–5.

18. Stiell IG, Wells GA, Vandemheen K, et al. The Canadian CT head rule for patients with minor head injury. Lancet 2001;357:1391–6.

19. Jagoda AS, Bazarian JJ, Bruns JJ Jr, et al. Clinical policy: neuroimaging and decisionmaking in adult mild traumatic brain injury in the acute setting. Ann Emerg Med 2008;52:714–48.

20. Nishijima DK, Offerman SR, Ballard DW, et al. Immediate and delayed traumatic intracranial hemorrhage in patients with head trauma and preinjury warfarin or clopidogrel use. Ann Emerg Med 2012; 59:460–8.e1-7.

21. Collins CE, Witkowski ER, Flahive JM, et al. Effect of preinjury warfarin use on outcomes after head trauma in Medicare beneficiaries. Am J Surg 2014; 208:544–9.e1.

22. Karni A, Holtzman R, Bass T, et al. Traumatic head injury in the anticoagulated elderly patient: a lethal combination. Am Surg 2001;67:1098–100.

23. Mina AA, Knipfer JF, Park DY, et al. Intracranial complications of preinjury anticoagulation in trauma patients with head injury. J Trauma 2002;53:668–72.

24. Ohm C, Mina A, Howells G, et al. Effects of antiplatelet agents on outcomes for elderly patients with traumatic intracranial hemorrhage. J Trauma 2005;58: 518–22.

25. Nishijima DK, Gaona SD, Waechter T, et al. Out-of-hospital triage of older adults with head injury: a retrospective study of the effect of adding "anticoagulation or antiplatelet medication use" as a criterion. Ann Emerg Med 2017;70(2):127–38.e6.

26. Hu R, Mustard CA, Burns C. Epidemiology of incident spinal fracture in a complete population. Spine (Phila Pa 1976) 1996;21:492–9.

27. Boulis NM, Bobek MP, Schmaier A, et al. Use of factor IX complex in warfarin-related intracranial hemorrhage. Neurosurgery 1999;45:1113–8.

28. Ferrera PC, Bartfield JM. Outcomes of anticoagulated trauma patients. Am J Emerg Med 1999;17: 154–6.

29. Kaen A, Jimenez-Roldan L, Arrese I, et al. The value of sequential computed tomography scanning in anticoagulated patients suffering from minor head injury. J Trauma 2010;68:895–8.

30. Menditto VG, Lucci M, Polonara S, et al. Management of minor head injury in patients receiving oral anticoagulant therapy: a prospective study of a 24-hour observation protocol. Ann Emerg Med 2012; 59:451–5.

31. Miller J, Lieberman L, Nahab B, et al. Delayed intracranial hemorrhage in the anticoagulated patient: a systematic review. J Trauma Acute Care Surg 2015;79:310–3.

32. Peck KA, Sise CB, Shackford SR, et al. Delayed intracranial hemorrhage after blunt trauma: are patients on preinjury anticoagulants and prescription antiplatelet agents at risk? J Trauma 2011;71: 1600–4.

33. Mundinger GS, Bellamy JL, Miller DT, et al. Defining population-specific craniofacial fracture patterns and resource use in geriatric patients: a comparative study of blunt craniofacial fractures in geriatric versus nongeriatric adult patients. Plast Reconstr Surg 2016;137:386e–93e.

34. Mann FA, Kubal WS, Blackmore CC. Improving the imaging diagnosis of cervical spine injury in the very elderly: implications of the epidemiology of injury. Emerg Radiol 2000;7:36–41.

35. Lomoschitz FM, Blackmore CC, Mirza SK, et al. Cervical spine injuries in patients 65 years old and older: epidemiologic analysis regarding the effects of age and injury mechanism on distribution, type, and stability of injuries. AJR Am J Roentgenol 2002;178:573–7.

36. Ngo B, Hoffman JR, Mower WR. Cervical spine injury in the very elderly. Emerg Radiol 2000;7:287–91.

37. Robinson AL, Moller A, Robinson Y, et al. C2 fracture subtypes, incidence, and treatment allocation change with age: a retrospective cohort study of 233 consecutive cases. Biomed Res Int 2017; 2017:8321680.

38. Westerveld LA, Verlaan JJ, Oner FC. Spinal fractures in patients with ankylosing spinal disorders: a systematic review of the literature on treatment, neurological status and complications. Eur Spine J 2009;18:145–56.

39. Hendrix RW, Melany M, Miller F, et al. Fracture of the spine in patients with ankylosis due to diffuse skeletal hyperostosis: clinical and imaging findings. AJR 1994;162:899–904.

40. Keller JM, Sciadini MF, Sinclair E, et al. Geriatric trauma: demographics, injuries, and mortality. J Orthop Trauma 2012;26:e161–5.

41. Kasimatis GB, Panagiotopoulos E, Megas P, et al. The adult spinal cord injury without radiographic abnormalities syndrome: magnetic resonance imaging and clinical findings in adults with spinal cord injuries having normal radiographs and computed tomography studies. J Trauma 2008;65:86–93.

42. Como JJ, Samia H, Nemunaitis GA, et al. The misapplication of the term spinal cord injury without radiographic abnormality (SCIWORA) in adults. J Trauma Acute Care Surg 2012;73:1261–6.

43. Boese CK, Lechler P. Spinal cord injury without radiologic abnormalities in adults: a systematic review. J Trauma Acute Care Surg 2013;75:320–30.

44. Bub LD, Blackmore CC, Mann FA, et al. Cervical spine fractures in patients 65 years and older: a clinical prediction rule for blunt trauma. Radiology 2005; 234:143–9.

45. Stiell IG, Wells GA, Vandemheen KL, et al. The Canadian C-spine rule for radiography in alert and stable trauma patients. JAMA 2001;286:1841–8.

46. Hoffman JR, Wolfson AB, Todd K, et al. Selective cervical spine radiography in blunt trauma: methodology of the National Emergency X-Radiography Utilization Study (NEXUS). Ann Emerg Med 1998;32: 461–9.

47. Hoffman JR, Mower WR, Wolfson AB, et al. Validity of a set of clinical criteria to rule out injury to the cervical spine in patients with blunt trauma. N Engl J Med 2000;343:94–9.

48. Touger M, Gennis P, Nathanson N, et al. Validity of a decision rule to reduce cervical spine radiography in elderly patients with blunt trauma. Ann Emerg Med 2002;40:287–93.

49. Evans D, Vera L, Jeanmonod D, et al. Application of National Emergency X-Ray Utilizations Study low-risk c-spine criteria in high-risk geriatric falls. Am J Emerg Med 2015;33:1184–7.

50. Barry TB, McNamara RM. Clinical decision rules and cervical spine injury in an elderly patient: a word of caution. J Emerg Med 2005;29:433–6.

51. Goode T, Young A, Wilson SP, et al. Evaluation of cervical spine fracture in the elderly: can we trust our physical examination? Am Surg 2014;80: 182–4.

52. Morrison J, Jeanmonod R. Imaging in the NEXUS-negative patient: when we break the rule. Am J Emerg Med 2014;32:67–70.

53. Cothren CC, Moore EE, Ray CE Jr, et al. Cervical spine fracture patterns mandating screening to rule out blunt cerebrovascular injury. Surgery 2007; 141:76–82.

54. Franz RW, Willette PA, Wood MJ, et al. A systematic review and meta-analysis of diagnostic screening criteria for blunt cerebrovascular injuries. J Am Coll Surg 2012;214:313–27.

Current Challenges in the Use of Computed Tomography and MR Imaging in Suspected Cervical Spine Trauma

Frank J. Minja, MD*, Kushal Y. Mehta, MD, Ali Y. Mian, MD

KEYWORDS

- Cervical • Spine • Trauma • Unstable • Ligamentous • Obtunded

KEY POINTS

- Any patient with suspected cervical spine trauma who fails to meet the NEXUS or CCR low risk criteria requires imaging evaluation.
- MDCT is the imaging modality of choice to exclude clinically significant cervical spine injury (CSI).
- There is a small but non-zero rate of clinically significant CSI following a negative CT in obtunded blunt trauma patients.
- The isolated unstable ligamentous CSI is the specific MR imaging target following negative CT.
- MR imaging should specifically evaluate integrity of the discoligamentous complex and document the presence or absence of unstable ligamentous CSI.

OVERVIEW

More than 1 million blunt trauma patients with suspected cervical spine trauma are evaluated in Emergency Departments in the United States each year.[1] The incidence of clinically significant cervical spine injury (CSI) among blunt trauma patients ranges between 1% and 3%.[2–4] The incidence of associated spinal cord injury is fortunately even smaller at 0.07% to 0.26%.[5] The incidence rate of acute traumatic spinal cord injury in the United States has remained relatively stable at 54 cases per million in 2012, compared to 53 cases per million in 1993, with only a modest increase in the estimated absolute number of new cases between 1993 (13,706 cases) and 2012 (16,965 cases), an increase that has been attributed to population growth.[6] Spinal cord injury can result in permanent paraplegia or quadriplegia, and the health care costs associated with spinal cord injury can exceed $1 million per patient in the first 5 years after injury.[5,7] Therefore, although acute traumatic spinal cord injury remains relatively rare among blunt trauma patients in the United States, the devastating neurologic and economic consequences warrant the evaluation for clinically significant CSI.

CLINICALLY SIGNIFICANT CERVICAL SPINE INJURY

Clinically significant CSI are "unstable" bone and/or ligamentous cervical spine injuries that may lead to spinal cord injury, with potentially

Disclosure Statement: The authors have no commercial or financial conflicts of interest to declare. No funding was provided for this work.

Department of Radiology and Biomedical Imaging, Yale University School of Medicine, 333 Cedar Street, New Haven, CT 06510, USA

* Corresponding author.

E-mail address: frank.minja@yale.edu

devastating neurologic consequences. Patients with clinically significant CSI would likely benefit from surgical stabilization or prolonged immobilization in a hard cervical collar to prevent spinal cord injury. Conversely, clinically nonsignificant CSI are unlikely to result in any harm to the patient or require any specific treatment. The National Emergency X-Radiography Utilization Study (NEXUS) and the Canadian C-Spine Rule (CCR) study, both landmark prospective observational studies of patients with suspected cervical spine trauma, clearly defined examples of clinically nonsignificant CSI. In the NEXUS study, clinically nonsignificant CSI included spinous process fractures, simple wedge compression fractures with less than 25% loss of vertebral body height, isolated avulsion without associated ligamentous injury, type I (Anderson-D'Alonzo) odontoid fracture, end plate fracture, osteophyte fracture (not including corner fracture or teardrop fracture), injury to trabecular bone, and transverse process fractures.[3] In the CCR study, clinically nonsignificant (unimportant) CSI included isolated avulsion fracture of an osteophyte, isolated fracture of a transverse process not involving a facet joint, isolated fracture of a spinous process not involving the lamina, or simple compression fracture involving less than 25% of the vertebral body height.[2] These specific examples of clinically nonsignificant CSI may surprise many radiologists who strive to meticulously identify and report each and every CSI on imaging, without any regard to the clinical significance of the reported CSI. The distinction between clinically significant and clinically nonsignificant CSI is critical for subsequent patient management. The remainder of this article focuses on the evaluation for clinically significant CSI in blunt trauma patients.

WHICH PATIENT REQUIRES IMAGING EVALUATION?

In the late 1990s, because of the considerable cost of imaging and the exposure of nearly every blunt trauma patient in the United States and Canada to ionizing radiation, the NEXUS and CCR low-risk criteria were developed to help determine which patients could be safely evaluated in the Emergency Department without any imaging. For the NEXUS low-risk criteria, a blunt trauma patient would need to meet all of the following criteria: no posterior midline tenderness, no evidence of intoxication, a normal level of alertness, no focal neurologic deficit, and no painful distracting injuries.[8] For the CCR, an alert blunt trauma patient would first get screened for the following 3 high-risk criteria: age ≥65 years old, dangerous mechanism, and paresthesias in extremities. If the high-

risk criteria are absent, the patient would be next be screened for the presence of any of the following low-risk factors: simple rear-end motor collision, sitting position in the Emergency Department, ambulatory at any time, delayed onset of neck pain, or absence of midline cervical-spine tenderness. The presence of the low-risk criteria would allow for the safe assessment of range of motion, whether a patient could rotate their neck 45° to the left and right.[8]

The NEXUS low-risk criteria were evaluated in 34,069 blunt trauma patients with sensitivity and negative predictive values of 99.6% and 99.9%, respectively, for clinically significant CSI. Only 2 patients in the entire NEXUS Study cohort were misclassified by the NEXUS low-risk criteria.[3] The CCR rule was evaluated in 8924 blunt trauma patients with a sensitivity of 100% for identifying clinically significant (important) CSI. No blunt trauma patient who met the CCR was subsequently found to have a clinically significant CSI.[2] The NEXUS and CCR low-risk criteria have been compared, with some controversy as to which low-risk criteria is superior.[8] Nevertheless, both the NEXUS and the CCR low-risk criteria are widely used in the United States, and both are endorsed by the American College of Radiology Appropriateness Criteria as the initial step in the evaluation of suspected cervical spine trauma to determine whether any imaging is required.[1] Any blunt trauma patient who fails to meet the NEXUS and/or CCR low-risk criteria requires imaging evaluation to exclude clinically significant CSI.

WHICH IMAGING MODALITY?

The greatest revolution in cervical spine imaging over the past 2 decades has been the near universal adoption of multidetector computed tomography (MDCT) for the evaluation of suspected cervical spine trauma in adult blunt trauma patients. Radiographs are now reserved for patients younger than 14 years of age, or when MDCT images are degraded by patient motion artifact.[1] Furthermore, dynamic flexion and extension radiographs are neither indicated nor recommended in the emergency setting and may have a limited role only at patient follow-up for persistent cervical tenderness.[1]

MULTIDETECTOR COMPUTED TOMOGRAPHY

MDCT is widely available in most Emergency Departments in the United States. Several studies report uniformly high sensitivities, specificities, and negative predictive values of MDCT for clinically significant CSI ranging between 99% and

100%,[1] leading several investigators to recommend MDCT as the primary and only imaging modality for the evaluation of suspected cervical spine trauma. The Western Trauma Association Trial was a large multi-institutional prospective observational trial that enrolled 10,276 blunt trauma patients to evaluate the accuracy of computed tomography (CT) for the detection of clinically significant CSI.[4] One hundred ninety-eight patients were found to have clinically significant CSI, of whom only 3 patients had a negative CT, for a 98.5% sensitivity of CT for the detection of clinically significant CSI. However, all 3 patients with negative CT had neurologic deficits consistent with central cord syndrome on clinical examination, which led the investigators to conclude that CT combined with neurologic examination has 100% sensitivity for detection of clinically significant CSI. Furthermore, none of the 3 patients with negative CT and clinically significant CSI had an unstable bone or ligamentous injury on follow-up MR imaging. Specifically, one patient had a C4-5 disc herniation; one patient had only C4-5 cord contusion, and one patient had both C5-6 degenerative disc disease and C6 spinal cord contusion. In summary, MDCT in the Western Trauma Association Trial revealed 100% of clinically significant CSI from unstable bone or ligamentous injury, whereas MR imaging after negative CT revealed other potential causes for acute cervical myelopathy besides unstable bone or ligamentous injury. Therefore, in awake and alert blunt trauma patients with a reliable neurologic examination, MDCT could serve as the only imaging modality for suspected cervical spine trauma.

OBTUNDED BLUNT TRAUMA PATIENTS

The definition of an "obtunded" patient varies widely in literature, ranging from a Glasgow Coma Scale (GCS) of less than 14 to GCS less than 9.[9] Nevertheless, there is considerable controversy as to whether MDCT could also serve as the only imaging modality in obtunded patients, similar to awake and alert blunt trauma patients. The Eastern Trauma Association systematic review of the literature was an attempt to address this specific question.[9] The final analysis included 11 articles with 1718 obtunded adult blunt trauma patients, in whom following a negative CT, 9% (161 of 1718 patients) were found to have stable CSI and 0% (0 of 1718 patients) were found to have unstable CSI. The additional CSI after negative CT were demonstrated on MR imaging, upright radiographs, flexion-extension CT, and/or clinical follow-up. Despite the zero rate of unstable CSI following a negative CT, the Eastern Trauma Association

systematic review concluded with a conditional recommendation for cervical spine collar removal after a negative high-quality CT in obtunded adult blunt trauma patients. This conditional recommendation was based on the documented nonzero rate of neurologic deterioration following a negative CT in obtunded blunt trauma patients.[9] In other words, although a negative CT is highly reassuring, it does not exclude 100% of clinically significant CSI in every obtunded blunt trauma patient.

MR IMAGING

MR imaging is superior to MDCT for depiction of soft tissue and spinal cord injury. Although MR imaging has a high abnormal rate following negative CT, many of the detected and reported injuries, "edema," "sprain," or "strain," have no clinical significance.[10] Similar to how MDCT reveals most bone CSI regardless of whether they are clinically significant or nonsignificant, many of the soft tissue injuries reported on MR imaging have no clinical significance, yet the reported MR imaging findings often result in prolonged cervical spine immobilization.[10] Isolated unstable ligamentous injury in the cervical spine, without concurrent bony injury, is extremely rare, but may account for the nonzero rate of unstable CSI potentially missed on MDCT. Therefore, the isolated unstable ligamentous CSI is the specific MR imaging target, when screening adult blunt trauma patients for unstable CSI after negative MDCT.

Maung and colleagues,[11] in the reCONECT prospective multicenter observational trial that enrolled 767 adult blunt trauma patients with negative CT who underwent MR imaging for persistent cervicalgia and/or inability to clinically evaluate, found a 23.6% rate of abnormal MR imaging results among this select patient population. This rate of abnormal MR imaging results following negative MDCT is similar to that previously reported in literature, which varies from 8.9% to 21.1%.[12,13] Abnormal MR imaging results in the reCONECT trial included ligamentous injury (16.6%), soft tissue swelling (4.3%), vertebral disc injury (1.4%), and dural hematomas (1.3%). Of the 181 patients with abnormal MR imaging results, 157 patients were kept in a cervical orthotic c-collar, 11 patients underwent surgery, and the remaining 13 patients were presumably managed without cervical immobilization or surgery. The investigators conclude that the clinical significance of the additional injuries identified by MR imaging remains unclear. This recent trial illustrates both the heterogeneity of what constitutes abnormal MR imaging and the varied clinical management following an abnormal MR imaging result.

MR IMAGING FOLLOWING NEGATIVE MULTIDETECTOR COMPUTED TOMOGRAPHY

Studies advocating for MR imaging following negative CT,[12] or against MR imaging following negative CT,[13] are often limited by the heterogeneity of MR imaging findings and the varied clinical management following an abnormal MR imaging result. Furthermore, this literature is complicated by imprecise definitions of clinically significant (unstable) CSI on MR imaging. Some investigators define clinically significant CSI as the need for surgery or prolonged cervical spine immobilization, whereas others deem any injury detected on MR imaging to be clinically significant.[10] Not surprisingly, conclusions in the literature regarding the utility of MR imaging following a negative CT are often diametrically opposed.

The most commonly accepted definition of unstable CSI is a single-level ligamentous injury to 2 or 3 spinal columns, as delineated by Denis in 1983.[14] Malhotra and colleagues[10] recently reported a meta-analysis of 23 studies with a total of 5286 patients seeking to quantify the rate of unstable CSI detected by MR imaging following a negative CT, using the above strict definition of unstable CSI. Malhotra and colleagues found a 15% overall rate for abnormal MR imaging following negative CT; however, the rate of unstable CSI was only 0.3%. Only 16 unstable injuries were reported in 5 of the 23 studies, and when these reported unstable injuries were further critically evaluated, only 11 unstable injuries met the strict definition of unstable CSI for a 0.2% rate of unstable CSI on MR imaging after a negative CT. Therefore, although the overall rate of abnormal MR imaging following negative CT is high, the incidence of unstable CSI not detected on CT is well below 0.3%. The incidence of isolated unstable ligamentous injury is likely less than 0.3%. Isolated unstable ligamentous injury is the specific MR imaging target following negative CT. Therefore, although the incidence of isolated and unstable ligamentous injury is extremely low, it is not zero. This nonzero rate of isolated unstable ligamentous injury following a negative CT must be weighed against the potential for a devastating spinal cord injury.

MR imaging is more expensive compared with MDCT and has a high false positive rate. There is a need to select which patients to image with MR imaging following a negative CT and define clinically significant CSI on MR imaging. In awake and alert blunt trauma patients, MR imaging should be reserved for awake and alert patients with persistent cervicalgia and/or neurologic deficit following a negative CT, to evaluate for both the rare isolated unstable ligamentous injury and other causes for acute cervical myelopathy.[4] Patient selection for MR imaging following negative CT among obtunded blunt trauma patients remains controversial.[1] Reporting the mere presence of any soft tissue injury or edema on MR imaging is similar to reporting every fracture on MDCT without regard for whether the fracture is clinically significant. The imaging target of MR imaging following negative MDCT should be the rare isolated unstable ligamentous injury with potential for devastating spinal cord injury. Adopting the imaging framework of craniocervical junction versus subaxial injury when evaluating the cervical spine on CT and MR imaging could be a first step in critically evaluating the cervical spine for clinically significant CSI. The remainder of this article illustrates this framework using clinical examples of craniocervical junction (CCJ) and subaxial CSI.

CRANIOCERVICAL JUNCTION INJURIES

The craniocervical junction (CCJ) comprises the articulations and ligamentous complexes between the occipital condyles and C1 and C2 vertebral bodies. Evaluating CCJ injuries can be challenging because of the complex anatomy and biomechanics of this region, and whose detailed treatment is beyond the scope of this article.[15–17] The CCJ supports a relatively heavy calvarium, while achieving the dual functions of protecting the spinal cord, cranial nerves, and vessels, and allowing for marked flexibility and range of motion. The CCJ is therefore best evaluated on imaging as a distinct unit of the cervical spine, separate from the subaxial cervical spine, which spans the C3 through C7 vertebral bodies. The focused imaging evaluation of the CCJ will be highlighted using the following examples of CCJ injuries: atlantooccipital dissociation (AOD), occipital condyle fractures, Jefferson C1 ring fractures, C2 odontoid process fractures, and C2 Hangman fractures.

Atlantooccipital dissociation is a devastating injury requiring high-energy trauma. The mechanism for AOD is thought to include simultaneous hyperextension and lateral flexion at the CCJ and more commonly occurs in the pediatric population. High mortality in AOD is likely the result of concurrent brainstem and vascular damage.[16] Three types of AOD have been described.[18] Type 1 is the most common, with anterior translation of the skull with respect to the spinal column. Type 2 involves cephalad distraction of the skull from C1 and is considered the most unstable AOD type. Type 3 is characterized by posterior translation of the occiput relative to the spinal column. All 3 types of AOD involve separation of the

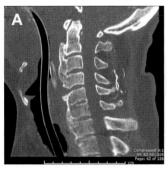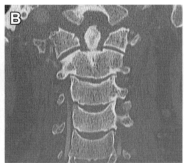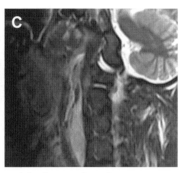

Fig. 1. (*A*) Sagittal CT angiogram image shows a type 2 AOD with widening of the basion-dens distance, greater than 10 mm. (*B*) Coronal CT angiogram image shows widening at the right atlantooccipital joint. (*C*) Sagittal MR imaging STIR image shows fluid signal in the dislocated right atlantooccipital joint.

occipital condyles from the C1 superior articulating facets with disruption of the tectorial membrane and odontoid and cruciate ligaments. A basion-dens distance of greater than 10 mm is highly concerning for AOD.[19] Fisher and colleagues,[20] in a retrospective review of CSI detected on MR imaging after negative CT, included a case of AOD missed on initial CT, but later detected on MR imaging. Review of figure 1 from Fisher and colleagues clearly demonstrates an increased distance between the basion and dens, an observation also pointed out by Plackett and colleagues,[5] which underscores the importance of evaluating the basion-dens distance on sagittal CT images to exclude AOD. **Fig. 1** is an example of type 2 AOD, with cephalad distraction and dislocation of the right atlantooccipital joint.

Occipital condyle fractures have historically been divided by Anderson and Montesano into 3 types.[21] Type 1 are comminuted nondisplaced occipital condyle compression fractures from axial loading; type 2 are skull fractures extending into the occipital condyle from direct blows to the head, and type 3 are avulsion injuries of the alar ligaments from their attachment to the occipital condyles. Tuli and colleagues[22] proposed an updated classification for occipital condyle fractures, which takes into account fracture fragment displacement, stability of the atlantooccipital and atlantoaxial joints, and presence of ligamentous injury. Under the scheme by Tuli and colleagues, type 1 are nondisplaced occipital condyle fractures; type 2A are displaced fractures without ligamentous instability, and type 2B are displaced fractures with ligamentous instability. Surgical management may be indicated for type 2B fractures, whereas type 1 and 2A fractures may only require rigid collar fixation. Note should also be made of osseous fragments in the foramen magnum in the setting of occipital condyle fractures.[16] **Fig. 2** is an example of a type 3 (Anderson and Montesano classification) left occipital condyle fracture, with an avulsed bony fragment.

Jefferson C1 ring fractures are burst-type fractures from axial loading injuries, which often occur at the anterior and posterior arches, where the C1

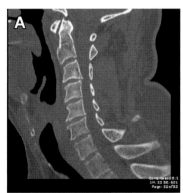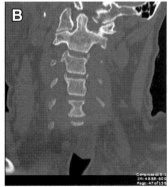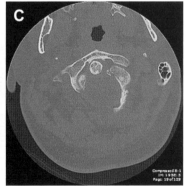

Fig. 2. (*A*) Sagittal CT image shows a normal basion-dens distance and normal atlantodental interval. (*B, C*) Coronal and axial CT images show a type 3 (Anderson and Montesano classification) left occipital condyle fracture, with an avulsed bony fragment and widening of the left C1 lateral mass interval.

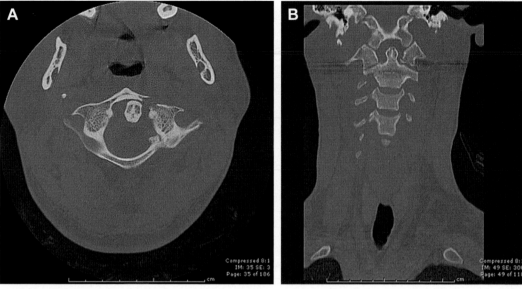

Fig. 3. (*A*) Axial CT image shows Jefferson C1 ring fractures involving the left anterior and posterior C1 arches. (*B*) Coronal CT image shows asymmetric widening of the right C1 lateral mass interval and fracture through the left C1 lateral mass.

vertebral body is narrower. The integrity of the transverse ligament in Jefferson C1 ring fractures should be assessed. Commonly used measurements include the distance between lateral masses of C1 and the atlantodental interval (ADI). A distance of 7 mm or greater between the C1 lateral masses[23] or an ADI of greater than 1.8 mm[24] is concerning for disruption of the transverse ligament. **Fig. 3** is an example of a Jefferson C1 ring fracture, with asymmetric widening of the right C1 lateral mass interval.

C2 odontoid process (dens) fractures have been classified into 3 types by Anderson and D'Alonzo.[25] Type 1 involves a fracture through the tip of the dens; type 2 involves a fracture through the dens neck, and type 3 involves a

fracture through the body of C2. MR imaging short T1 inversion recovery (STIR) sequence is often helpful to distinguish between an acute and a chronic dens fracture, the former showing STIR signal hyperintensity from bone marrow edema. Type 2 dens fractures are unstable and often prone to avascular necrosis and nonunion. Type 3 fractures are typically stable and more likely to heal without avascular necrosis, because of the robust blood supply to the body of C2.[26] **Fig. 4** is an example of a type 2 odontoid fracture with posterior displacement of the superior fracture fragment.

C2 Hangman fractures, also known as axial traumatic C2 spondylolisthesis, usually involve a hyperextension-distraction mechanism and are

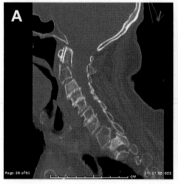
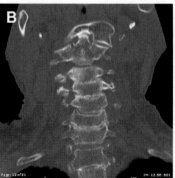
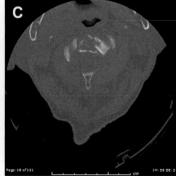

Fig. 4. (*A–C*) Sagittal, coronal, and axial CT images show a type 2 odontoid fracture with posterior displacement of the superior odontoid fracture fragment.

characterized by C2 pedicle fracture and subluxation relative to the C3 vertebral body. Hangman fractures have been classified into 4 basic types by Levine and Edwards.[27] Type 1 are stable fractures with less than 3.5 mm of translational distraction and no angulation, and type 2 fractures have either a significant angular component (type 2a) or significant translational component (type 2b). Type 3 fractures have both large translational and angular components, including C2-3 facet joint dislocation.[27] **Fig. 5** is an example of a type 1 C2 Hangman fracture without significant translational distraction or angulation.

These examples of CCJ injuries illustrate the importance of focused evaluation of the CCJ, as a distinct unit of the cervical spine. The occipital condyle and C1 and C2 vertebral body articulations should be critically evaluated on axial, sagittal, and coronal CT images, with careful attention to the basion-dens distance, atlantodental interval, and C1 lateral mass interval. MR imaging can be helpful to confirm ligamentous or articular involvement; however, the clinical significance of isolated abnormal MR imaging findings in the CCJ following a negative CT remains unclear.

SUBAXIAL CERVICAL SPINE INJURIES

Subaxial injuries of the cervical spine are defined as injuries spanning the C3 through C7 vertebral levels and account for up to 66% of all CSI.[28] Historically, the 3-column model proposed by Denis in 1983[14] has been used to classify subaxial cervical spine and thoracolumbar spine injuries into stable or unstable injuries. In this model, the spine was divided into the anterior, middle, and posterior columns, with spinal stability dependent on at least 2 intact columns. On a lateral radiograph or sagittal CT image of the spine, disruption of at least 2 of 3 spine columns could be determined via the presence of traumatic listhesis, which

would constitute an unstable spinal injury.[14] More recently, the Subaxial Cervical Spine Injury Classification (SLIC) devised by Vaccaro and colleagues[29] has been shown to be more comprehensive and clinically relevant for grading the severity of subaxial CSI.

In the SLIC scheme, 3 major components were determined to be important predictors in clinical outcome, namely, bony morphology, integrity of the discoligamentous complex (DLC), and the neurologic status of the patient.[29] The DLC comprises the intervertebral disc, anterior and posterior longitudinal ligaments, ligamentum flavum, interspinous and supraspinous ligaments, and facet capsules. Each of the 3 major components is given a numeric score, which are subsequently totaled. A total SLIC score greater than or equal to 5 indicates the need for surgical intervention; a score of 3 or less is managed conservatively, and a score of 4 is indeterminate. The bony morphology score is categorized into 5 injury patterns of no injury, compression, burst, distraction, or translation with each receiving a point value of 0, 1, 2, 3, and 4, respectively. If 2 or more patterns are present, the more severe injury will be used in the determination of the SLIC score. Integrity of the DLC is categorized as intact, partially disrupted, or fully disrupted, with a point value of 0, 1, and 2, respectively. The neurologic status is categorized as no injury, root injury, complete cord injury, or incomplete cord injury with a point value of 0, 1, 2, and 3, respectively.[29] The SLIC scheme will be illustrated using the following examples of unstable subaxial CSI: facet fracture-dislocation, hyperflexion teardrop injury, hyperextension teardrop injury, and isolated unstable ligamentous CSI.

Facet fracture-dislocations can be either unilateral or bilateral, and the mechanism of injury usually involves forced hyperflexion with resultant anterior dislocation of the inferior facet of the

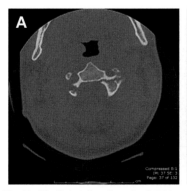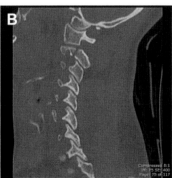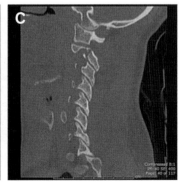

Fig. 5. (*A–C*) Axial and sagittal CT images show a type 1 C2 Hangman fracture involving the bilateral C2 pars interarticularis, without significant translational distraction or angulation.

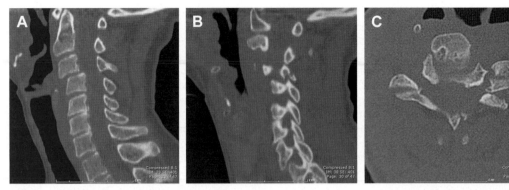

Fig. 6. (*A, B*) Sagittal CT images show grade 1 anterolisthesis at C3-4, and unilateral left C3-4 facture-dislocation. (*C*) Axial CT shows the "reverse hamburger bun" sign, with anterior displacement of the fractured left C3 facet inferior articular process.

superior vertebral body over the superior facet of the inferior vertebral body. The dislocated facet joint is best demonstrated on a sagittal CT image, or on axial CT image as the "reverse hamburger bun sign," in which the inferior articular process of the superior vertebral body lies anterior to the superior articular process of the inferior vertebral body (**Fig. 6**).[30] In **Fig. 6**, the bone morphology score would be 4 because of the facet fracture and grade 1 anterolisthesis; the DLC score would be 2 because the fracture-dislocation implies disruption of the facet capsule. Based on the bone morphology and DLC scores alone, a total SLIC score of 6 would qualify the patient for surgical management of the facet-fracture dislocation.

Hyperflexion teardrop injury is a serious form of subaxial injury resulting from severe flexion and compression forces, such as from diving injuries and motor vehicle collisions. On CT imaging, a flexion teardrop injury demonstrates a triangular-shaped fracture fragment from the anteroinferior aspect of the involved vertebral body. There is also associated posterior displacement of the remainder of the vertebral body into the spinal canal, widening of the interspinous processes and intervertebral disc space (**Fig. 7**).[31] In **Fig. 7**, the bone morphology score would be 3 because of

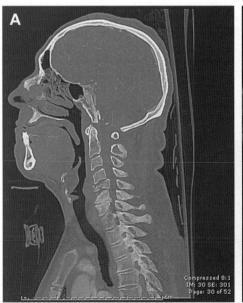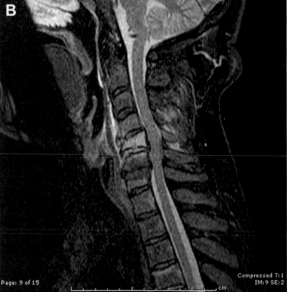

Fig. 7. (*A*) Sagittal CT image shows a hyperflexion teardrop injury at the C5 vertebral body, with posterior displacement of the C5 vertebral body into the spinal canal. (*B*) Sagittal MR imaging STIR image shows disruption of the anterior longitudinal ligament at C4-5 and edema signal in the C4-5 and C5-6 interspinous ligaments.

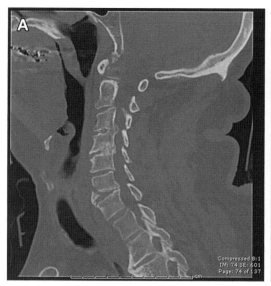
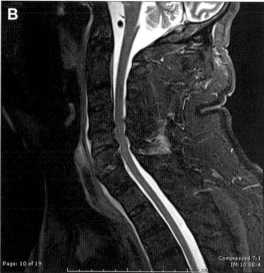

Fig. 8. (*A*) Sagittal CT image shows a classic "teardrop" hyperextension fracture at the anteroinferior aspect of the C6 vertebral body, without posterior vertebral body displacement. (*B*) Sagittal MR imaging STIR image shows complete disruption of the supraspinous ligament at C5-6 and edema signal in the C6-7 interspinous ligament.

the vertebral body fracture and distraction; the DLC score would be 2 because of disruption of the anterior longitudinal ligament. Based on the bone morphology and DLC scores alone, a total SLIC score of 5 would qualify the patient for surgical management of the hyperflexion teardrop injury.

Hyperextension teardrop injuries are considered a less serious form of subaxial injury compared with hyperflexion teardrop injuries but can still

result in significant injury to the cervical spinal cord, with the common mechanism of injury being forced extension of the neck. On CT imaging, hyperextension teardrop injury is usually demonstrated by an anteroinferior avulsion bony fragment by the anterior longitudinal ligament, without any posterior displacement of the vertebral body (**Fig. 8**).[32] Injury to the cervical spinal cord is thought to result from buckling of the

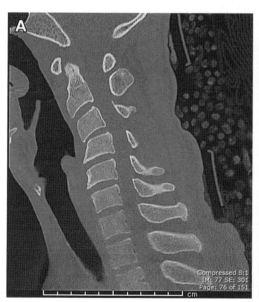
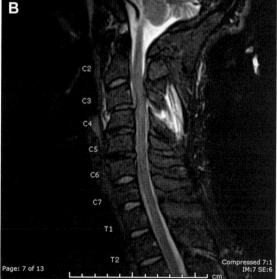

Fig. 9. (*A*) Sagittal CT image shows minimal grade 1 anterolisthesis at C3-4 and subtle widening of the C3-4 interspinous space, without any associated fracture. (*B*) Sagittal MR imaging STIR image shows complete disruption of the posterior longitudinal ligament, ligamentum flavum, and supraspinous ligaments at C3-4, consistent with isolated unstable ligamentous injury.

ligamentum flavum. In **Fig. 8**, the bone morphology score would be 2 because of the vertebral body fracture without distraction; the DLC score would be 2 because of the disruption of interspinous and supraspinous ligaments. Based on the bone morphology and DLC scores alone, with a total SLIC score of 4, the decision for surgical management of this hyperextension teardrop injury would heavily depend on the neurologic status of the patient. Of note, the decision would remain indeterminate for a neurologically intact patient, with a neurologic status score of 0.

Isolated unstable ligamentous CSI are rare subaxial injuries without associated bone injury. The isolated unstable ligamentous CSI may manifest as listhesis, interspinous process, or disc space widening on CT, without any fracture. Isolated unstable ligamentous CSI is the specific imaging target for MR imaging, following a negative CT. MR imaging often demonstrates complete or partial discontinuity of the DLC with associated STIR signal hyperintensity (**Fig. 9**).[33] In **Fig. 9**, the bone morphology score would be 0 because of lack of the any fracture, despite the minimal C3-4 anterolisthesis and subtle widening of the C3-4 interspinous space. The DLC score would be 2 because of disruption of the posterior longitudinal ligament, ligamentum flavum, and supraspinous ligaments at C3-4. Based on the bone morphology and DLC scores alone, with a total SLIC score of 2, the decision for surgical management for this isolated unstable ligamentous CSI would require the patient to also have an incomplete cord injury with a neurologic status score of 3. This example of isolated unstable ligamentous CSI illustrates the application of specific MR imaging findings in the DLC and the patient's neurologic status to determine further management.

SUMMARY

Although several challenges remain regarding the use of CT and MR imaging in suspected cervical spine trauma, some key concepts are now well established. Any patient with suspected cervical spine trauma should be first evaluated using the NEXUS or CCR low-risk criteria, to determine whether any imaging is required to exclude CSI. MDCT is the initial imaging modality of choice to exclude CSI and should be performed in every patient who does not meet the NEXUS or CCR low-risk criteria. Not all CSI detected on imaging are clinically significant. Although the definition of a clinically significant CSI varies widely in literature, the definitions used by the NEXUS and CCR studies are widely accepted. MDCT detects the vast majority of clinically significant CSI, with sensitivity, specificity, and negative predictive values well in excess of 99%. Despite the high accuracy of MDCT, there is a well-documented albeit very small but nonzero rate of CSI missed on MDCT in adult blunt trauma patients.

The key remaining challenges revolve around how to best evaluate for and manage this very small number of CSI missed on MDCT, which includes patients with persistent cervicalgia, persistent neurologic deficits, and those who present with delayed neurologic deficits. MR imaging appears best reserved for alert adult blunt patients following negative CT, if they have persistent cervicalgia and/or neurologic deficits. In non-alert adult blunt trauma patients, there is no consensus as to whether the economic cost and risk of MR imaging for every such patient is justified given the higher expense of MR imaging and the high false positive rate of MR imaging. MR imaging and reports should specifically evaluate the integrity of the DLC and document the presence or absence of an isolated unstable ligamentous CSI, to minimize the false positive rate of MR imaging. The combination of neurologic evaluation, good-quality MDCT, and MR imaging in select patients following negative CT with specific attention to integrity of the DLC should move us closer to 100% detection of CSI and help avoid devastating neurologic consequences in all patients with suspected cervical spine trauma.

REFERENCES

1. Daffner RH, Weissman BN, Wippold FJ, et al. American College of Radiology appropriateness criteria. Reston, VA. 2012. Available at: https://acsearch.acr.org/list. Accessed November 1, 2017.
2. Stiell IG, Wells GA, Vandemheen K, et al. Canadian C-Spine Rule for radiography in alert and stable trauma patients. JAMA 2001;286:1841–8.
3. Hoffman JR, Mower WR, Wolfson AB, et al. Validity of a set of clinical criteria to rule out injury to the cervical spine in patients with blunt trauma. N Engl J Med 2000;343:94–9.
4. Inaba K, Byerly S, Bush LD, et al. Cervical spine clearance: a prospective Western Trauma Association Multi-institutional Trial. J Trauma Acute Care Surg 2016;81:1122–30.
5. Plackett TP, Wright F, Baldea AJ, et al. Cervical spine clearance when unable to be cleared clinically: a pooled analysis of combined computed tomography and magnetic resonance imaging. Am J Surg 2016; 211:115–21.
6. Jain NB, Ayers GD, Peterson EN, et al. Traumatic spinal cord injury in the United States, 1993-2012. JAMA 2015;313:2236–43.

7. Wu X, Malhotra A, Geng B, et al. Cost-effectiveness of magnetic resonance imaging in cervical spine clearance of neurologically intact patients with blunt trauma. Ann Emerg Med 2017. https://doi.org/10.1016/j.annemergmed.2017.07.006.

8. Stiell IG, Clement CM, McKnight RD, et al. The Canadian C-spine Rule versus the NEXUS low-risk criteria in patients with trauma. N Engl J Med 2003;349:2510–8.

9. Patel MB, Humble SS, Cullinane DC, et al. Cervical spine collar clearance in the obtunded adult blunt trauma patient: a systematic review and practice management guideline from the Eastern Association for the Surgery of Trauma. J Trauma Acute Care Surg 2015;78:430–41.

10. Malhotra A, Wu X, Kalra VB, et al. Utility of MRI for cervical spine clearance after blunt traumatic injury: a meta-analysis. Eur Radiol 2017;27:1148–60.

11. Maung AA, Johnson DC, Barre K, et al. Cervical spine MRI in patients with negative CT: a prospective multicenter study of the Research Consortium of New England Centers for Trauma (ReCONECT). J Trauma Acute Care Surg 2017;82:263–9.

12. Menaker J, Philp A, Boswell S, et al. Computed tomography alone for cervical spine clearance in the unreliable patient – are we there yet? J Trauma 2008;64:898–903.

13. Tomycz ND, Chew BG, Chang YF, et al. MRI is unnecessary to clear the cervical spine in obtunded/comatose trauma patients: the four-year experience of a level I trauma center. J Trauma 2008;64:1258–63.

14. Denis F. The three column spine and its significance in the classification of acute thoracolumbar spinal injuries. Spine (Phila Pa 1976) 1983;8:817–31.

15. Siddiqui J, Grover PJ, Grover HL, et al. The spectrum of traumatic injuries at the craniocervical junction: a review of imaging findings and management. Emerg Radiol 2017;24:377–85.

16. Riascos R, Bonfante E, Cotes C, et al. Imaging of atlanto-occipital and atlantoaxial traumatic injuries: what the radiologist needs to know. Radiographics 2015;35:2121–34.

17. Offiah CE, Day E. The craniocervical junction: embryology, anatomy, biomechanics and imaging in blunt trauma. Insights Imaging 2017;8:29–47.

18. Kasliwal MK, Fontes RB, Traynelis VC. Occipitocervical dissociation: incidence, evaluation, and treatment. Curr Rev Musculoskelet Med 2016;9:247–54.

19. Radcliff K, Kepler C, Reitman C, et al. CT and MRI-based diagnosis of craniocervical dislocations: the role of the occipitoatlantal ligament. Clin Orthop Relat Res 2012;470:1602–13.

20. Fisher BM, Cowles S, Matulich JR, et al. Is magnetic resonance imaging in addition to a computed tomographic scan necessary to identify clinically significant cervical spine injuries in obtunded blunt trauma patients? Am J Surg 2013;206:987–94.

21. Anderson PA, Montesano PX. Morphology and treatment of occipital condyle fractures. Spine (Phila Pa 1976) 1988;13:731–6.

22. Tuli S, Tator CH, Fehlings MG, et al. Occipital condyle fractures. Neurosurgery 1997;41:368–76.

23. Marcon RM, Cristante AF, Teixeira WJ, et al. Fractures of the cervical spine. Clinics (Sao Paulo) 2013;68:1455–61.

24. Perez-Orribo L, Snyder LA, Kalb S, et al. Comparison of CT versus MRI measurements of transverse atlantal ligament integrity in craniovertebral junction injuries. Part 1: a clinical study. J Neurosurg Spine 2016;24:897–902.

25. Anderson LD, D'Alonzo RT. Fractures of the odontoid process of the axis. J Bone Joint Surg Am 1974;56:1663–74.

26. Havrda JB, Paterson E. Imaging atlantooccipital and atlantoaxial traumatic injuries. Radiol Technol 2017;89:27–41.

27. Levine AM, Edwards CC. Traumatic lesions of the occipitoatlantoaxial complex. Clin Orthop Relat Res 1989;239:53–68.

28. Patel AA, Hurlbert RJ, Bono CM, et al. Classification and surgical decision making in acute subaxial cervical spine trauma. Spine (Phila PA 1976) 2010;35: S228–34.

29. Vaccaro AR, Hulbert RJ, Patel AA, et al. The subaxial cervical spine injury classification system: a novel approach to recognize the importance of morphology, neurology, and integrity of the disco-ligamentous complex. Spine (Phila PA 1976) 2007; 32:2365–74.

30. Daffner SD, Daffner RH. CT diagnosis of facet dislocations: the "hamburger bun" and "reverse hamburger bun" signs. J Emerg Med 2002;23:387–94.

31. Kim KS, Chen HH, Russell EJ, et al. Flexion teardrop fracture of the cervical spine: radiographic characteristics. AJR Am J Roentgenol 1989;152:319–26.

32. Rao SK, Wasyliw C, Nunez DB Jr. Spectrum of imaging findings in hyperextension injuries of the neck. Radiographics 2005;25:1239–54.

33. Warner J, Shanmuganathan K, Mirvis SE, et al. Magnetic resonance imaging of ligamentous injury of the cervical spine. Emerg Radiol 1996;3:9–15.

Blunt Craniocervical Trauma
Does the Patient Have a Cerebral Vascular Injury?

Aaron Winn, MD[a], Anthony M. Durso, MD[a],
Catalina Restrepo Lopera, MD[b], Felipe Munera, MD[c],*

KEYWORDS

- BCVI • Blunt • Cerebrovascular injury • Carotid injury • Vertebral artery injury • CT angiography
- Trauma

KEY POINTS

- Screening for blunt cerebrovascular injuries in high-risk patients decreases morbidity and may be cost effective (moderate evidence).
- Digital subtraction angiography remains the gold standard for diagnosing vascular injury following blunt trauma (moderate evidence).
- Many institutions have adopted multidetector computed tomography angiography as the primary diagnostic modality for blunt cerebrovascular injury screening.
- Recent evidence supports the potential of multidetector computed tomography angiography as a reference standard in the future.

INTRODUCTION

Blunt cerebrovascular injury (BCVI) involves injury to the carotid and/or vertebral arteries sustained via generalized multitrauma or directed blunt craniocervical trauma, and reflects an increasingly common, potentially catastrophic injury. Stroke remains the most consequential outcome of BCVI, causing 80% of deaths,[1] and is largely responsible for the overall mortality rate of 20% to 30%,[2,3] and permanent neurologic morbidity rate of 37% to 58%.[3]

Motor vehicle collisions contribute to 80% of BCVI; less common causes include a fall from any height, sports related injuries, assault, strangulation, or chiropractic spinal manipulation.[4] Accounting for 5% of all adult trauma,[5] up to 90% of pediatric trauma,[6] and the most common cause of death in young adults,[7] the ubiquitous nature of

blunt trauma impacts health care across all levels. Once thought to account for less than 0.1% of all blunt trauma patients,[8] systematic review of 122,176 patients estimates BCVI to account for 0.18% to 2.70% of blunt trauma admissions.[9] Although estimates continue to vary slightly, most new studies support this trend of increasing incidence.[9–11] Concordantly, a 2017 systematic review demonstrated an incidence increase from 0.33% to 2.00% ($P<.001$) from 1995 to 2015.[12]

This trend seems to be at least partially attributable to a heightened awareness of BCVI, the increasing role of noninvasive imaging strategies,[2,4,13–18] and the expanding implementation of more sensitive screening protocols to identify patients at risk for BCVI.[10,12,14,18–30] Optimum treatment for BCVI is not yet known, although the importance of timely diagnosis and initiation of

Disclosure Statement: The authors have nothing to disclose.
a Department of Radiology, University of Miami Miller School of Medicine, Jackson Memorial Hospital, Ryder Trauma Center, 1611 Northwest 12th Avenue, WW-279, Miami, FL 33136, USA; b CES University, CL 10 A #22-04, Medellin, Antioquia 050021, Colombia; c Department of Radiology, University of Miami Miller School of Medicine, Jackson Memorial Hospital, Ryder Trauma Center, University of Miami Hospital, 1611 Northwest 12th Avenue, WW-279, Miami, FL 33136, USA
* Corresponding author.
E-mail address: fmunera@med.miami.edu

any treatment before the development of neurologic complications has a well-established role in the reduction of morbidity and mortality. Stein and colleagues[31] studied 147 patients with BCVI at R. Adams Cowley Shock Trauma, and reported stroke rates of 25.8% in untreated patients (owing to contraindications) and 3.9% (*P* = .0003) of treated patients, independent of treatment type. Similarly, the recent systematic review by Shahan and colleagues[12] reported BCVI-related stroke mortality to have decreased from 37% to 5% (*P*<.001) over a 30-year duration.

Recent widespread acceptance of multidetector computed tomography (CT) angiography (MDCTA) as an accurate diagnostic modality for BCVI has overcome many of the inherent disadvantages of digital subtraction angiography (DSA); however, disagreement persists for defining the appropriate population to screen via MDCTA. As a noninvasive, rapid, readily accessible, and cost-efficient modality, capable of detecting associated injuries throughout the body, CT now accounts for the greatest source of radiation exposure in trauma patients.[32] Recently, pervasive efforts to keep radiation dose as low as reasonably achievable have shifted, although not supplanted, the essential role of careful clinical examination. This article presents the evidence and controversies surrounding the optimization of diagnostic imaging for patients with suspected BCVI. Discussion centers on the increasing reliance on MDCTA for BCVI screening, also considering the relevant clinical criteria for determining the appropriate patient population to screen.

ANATOMY

An understanding of the anterior and posterior circulation is helpful in evaluating for BCVI. The anterior circulation comprises the bilateral common carotid arteries, from their origins from the brachiocephalic artery (right) or aorta (left) to the carotid bulbs, and the internal carotid arteries (ICA) from the bulbs to their terminus. The ICA most frequently arises at the C3 to C5 vertebral level. The Bouthillier classification[33] divides the ICA into 7 segments: the cervical segment (C1) from the carotid bulb to skull base; the petrous segment (C2), coursing through the skull base in the carotid canal; the lacerum segment (C3), a short segment extending above the petrous apex to the cavernous sinus; the cavernous segment (C4), running through the cavernous sinus; the clinoid segment (C5), ending as the ICA enters the arachnoid space; the supraclinoid segment (C6) extending until the origin of the posterior communicating artery; and the terminal segment (C7) giving rise to the posterior communicating artery, anterior choroidal artery, and finally the anterior and middle cerebral arteries. With the exception of the C7 segment, only the even numbered segments have branches.

The posterior circulation comprises the bilateral vertebral arteries and the basilar artery terminating in the posterior cerebral arteries. The vertebral arteries generally arise from their respective subclavian arteries and are divided into 4 segments: the preforaminal segment (V1), from their origin until they enter the transverse foramen, generally at the C6 level; the foraminal segment (V2), continuing until the C2 level; the Atlantic or extradural segment (V3), extending from the C2 level until the artery passes through the dura; and the intracranial or intradural segment (V4), the intradural extent until they join to form the basilar. Numerous muscular and spinal branches are given off by the vertebral arteries as they ascend the neck, as well as numerous branches originating from the V4 segments and the basilar artery to supply the posterior fossa and the bilateral occipital lobes.

Although BCVI can occur anywhere along the length of the carotid or vertebral arteries, certain anatomic and mechanistic considerations lead to injury more frequently occurring at some sites than others.

ICA are most frequently injured just below the skull base,[34–36] within the cervical segment, and within the petrous and cavernous segments.[34–36] In vertebral artery injury, the V2 segments encompassed by the transverse foramina of C3 to C6 are the most common sites of injury, followed by the V3 segments.[35,36]

PATHOPHYSIOLOGY

Many mechanisms for the pathophysiology of BCVI have been proposed, several sharing the basic theory of disrupting 1 or more layers of the vascular wall through stretching them beyond their physical limits.[36] The pathophysiology of BCVI seems to be a dynamic process, causing grades of injury to change with time, sometimes progressing in a predictable manner. Minimal intimal injury, the least severe form of BCVI described by Biffl and colleagues,[21–24] may result in disruption of the vasa vasorum, commonly progressing to dissection and intramural hematoma. Alternatively, minimal intimal injury may simply expose the underlying thrombogenic subendothelial matrix, causing thrombosis and potential distal embolization.

Blunt carotid artery injury primarily involves a direct cervical blow or cervical hyperextension/hyperflexion complicated by a rotational component,[4,34] resulting in stretching of the carotid vessels over the lateral processes of the upper cervical spine.[37] Blunt vertebral artery injuries, however, most commonly occur in the setting of cervical spine injuries. Mechanism can be a result of direct impingement by a fracture fragment, particularly foramen transversarium fractures, or excessive traction as seen in dislocations and subluxations.[9,14,20–24,26,38,39]

RISK FACTORS

Recently developed screening guidelines for identifying those patients warranting diagnostic screening are mostly derived from research performed by Biffl and colleagues.[21–24] Risk factors were broadly divided into mechanism of injury, clinical findings on initial trauma assessment, or other injuries identified on initial CT evaluation. The Denver Screening Criteria, still the most often cited criteria for identifying those patients for whom screening is appropriate,[15] is presented in **Box 1**.

Several subsequent studies found BCVI present in 20% to 22% of patients not meeting traditional Denver Screening Criteria.[9,25,28,40] In studies performed at R Adams Cowley Shock Trauma Center[25] and the University of Tennessee Health Science Center,[28] 2 of many trauma-heavy institutions that have adopted whole-body CT, retrospective analysis uncovered that 30% and 16% of respective patients diagnosed with BCVI had no standard radiographic or clinical risk factor for BCVI screening. Bonatti and colleagues[41] performed a similar retrospective study, although using the modified Memphis Criteria, reporting that 37.5% of polytrauma patients found to have BCVI on whole-body CT did not show any of the risk factors proposed. It is possible that routine use of whole-body CT to scan severe polytrauma patients would help to identify risk factor negative patients, although this strategy has yet to be proven in a prospective trial.[42]

In 2010, Berne and colleagues[20] developed multivariate logistic regression analysis models to explore the relative roles of several clinical factors in determining which patients should be screened with MDCTA. The factors that were found to be most predictive of the presence of BCVI, and may therefore justify imaging, were cervical spine fracture (odds ratio, 7.46; relative risk, 28.0), mandible fracture (odds ratio, 2.59; relative risk, 2.51), and basilar skull fracture (relative risk, 3.6). On multivariate logistic regression analysis, additional statistically significant predictors of the presence of BCVI include thoracic or lumbar spine

---

> **Box 1**
> **Complete modified Denver screening criteria**
>
> *Signs and symptoms of BCVI*
> - Arterial hemorrhage
> - Focal neurologic deficit
> - Expanding cervical hematoma
> - Cervical bruit
> - Findings on neurologic examination incongruous with head CT
> - Stroke on secondary CT or MR imaging
>
> *Risk factors for BCVI*
> High-energy mechanism with associated
> - LeFort II/III fracture pattern
> - Mandible fracture
> - Cervical spine subluxation, fracture of foramen transversarium, or fracture of C1-C3
> - Complex skull fracture/basilar skull fracture/occipital condyle fracture
> - DAI and GCS of less than 6
> - Cervical Subluxation or ligamentous injury, transverse foramen fracture, any body fracture, any fracture C1-C3
> - Near hanging with anoxic brain injury
> - Clothesline type injury or seatbelt sign with significant pain, swelling, or altered mental status
> - TBI with thoracic injuries
> - Scalp degloving
> - Blunt cardiac rupture
>
> *Abbreviations:* BCVI, blunt cerebrovascular injury; CT, computed tomography; DAI, diffuse axonal injury; GCS, Glasgow Coma Scale; TBI, traumatic brain injury.
> *Data from* Biffl WL, Moore EE, Offner PJ, et al. Optimizing screening for blunt cerebrovascular injuries. Am J Surg 1999;178(6):517–22; and Wu X, Malhotra A, Forman HP, et al. The use of high-risk criteria in screening patients for blunt cerebrovascular injury: a survey. Acad Radiol 2017;24(4):456–61.

---

fracture, any facial injury, or a LeFort fracture. Other clinical parameters did not demonstrate a clear increase risk, including high Injury Severity Score and low Glasgow Coma Scale score.[20]

IMAGING

There are multiple modalities available to assess BCVI: ultrasound examination, CT/CT angiography (CTA), magnetic resonance (MR) imaging/MR angiography, and DSA. Each has its benefits and detractors and are discussed.

Computed Tomography and Computed Tomography Angiography

The performance of CTA in the evaluation of BCVI has been studied by numerous groups. Much of the early data are likely obsolete owing to the advances in CT technology and increased awareness by radiologists for the findings associated with BCVI. Other studies are limited in their design, often not evaluating patients with both CTA and DSA, or only performed DSA after positive findings on CTA. Two recent studies evaluated all patients with both DSA and CTA, reporting 51% sensitivity for 32-channel CTA[43] and 68% sensitivity for 64-channel CTA.[17]

MDCTA offers many practical advantages over DSA for the diagnosis of BCVI. A comprehensive literature review performed by Malhotra and colleagues[44] concluded that selective CTA in high-risk patients is the optimal and cost-effective imaging strategy, even assuming a low CTA sensitivity. Kaye and colleagues[45] evaluated Medicare reimbursement costs for CTA and DSA, reporting costs of $708 and $2674, respectively. If these costs were extrapolated for the 64-channel CTA study by Paulus and colleagues,[17] not performing DSA on the 343 patients with negative CTA would yield a savings of $917,182.

According to a 2011 survey of trauma surgeons, neurosurgeons, and radiologists, 60% of practitioners in North America report using CTA for screening and diagnosis of BCVI, whereas only 15% continue to use DSA despite the low CTA sensitivity at that time.[46] The factors suggest that 64-channel CTA can replace DSA as the primary screening tool for BCVI.

Ultrasound Imaging

Duplex ultrasound imaging is commonly used in the trauma setting, given its noninvasiveness, lack of ionizing radiation, portability, and low cost. Although the specificity is high, the sensitivity of duplex ultrasound imaging for BCVI remains too low to make for an effective screening tool. In a cohort of 1471 patients with a BCVI incidence of 0.9%, Mutze and colleagues[16] reported 38.5% sensitivity of ultrasound imaging for BCVI. An

Table 1
Protocol for multidetector computed tomography (64 detector) whole body computed tomography angiography

Scout	Top of head through feet	
Contrast	150 mL iohexol, 350 mgI/mL	
Contrast bolus	Multiphasic bolus 4 mL/s × 20 s (total 80 mL), then 3.5 mL/s × 20 s (total 70 mL)	
Saline flush	Normal saline 3.5 mL/s × 14 s (total 50 mL)	

Scan Parameters	Arterial Phase	Portal Phase
Scan range	Top of frontal sinus thru pubic symphysis	Diaphragm to iliac crests
Scan delay	20 s after bolus start ≤55 years old 25 s after bolus start >55 years old	20–25 s after arterial phase (70–75 s after contrast bolus start)
Scan mode	Spiral	Spiral
kVp	120	120
Effective mAs	200	200
Rotation time	0.5 s	0.5 s
Slice collimation	0.6 mm	1.2 mm
Pitch	0.7	0.8
Dose modulation	On	On
Slice thickness	3.0 mm	3.0 mm
Kernel	Medium smooth	Medium smooth
Reconstruction interval	3 mm	3 mm
Reconstruction planes	Axial, coronal, sagittal	Axial
Postprocessing	Maximum intensity projection and volume-rendered images reconstructed from arterial phase	

important limitation of duplex ultrasound imaging is the inability to adequately evaluate vessels within bony confines, notably the most commonly injured sites of both the carotid and vertebral arteries.[34–36]

MR Imaging/MR Angiography

The use of MR imaging for the detection of traumatic cerebrovascular injuries has been limited by accessibility and logistical limitations in the acute trauma setting. It is often impossible to assess patients reliably or rapidly for MR imaging contraindications that carry catastrophic potential, such as metallic foreign bodies, incompatible implantable devices, or renal failure. In addition to these prohibitive limitations, there is inadequate evidence to support the adequacy of MR imaging and MR angiography for BCVI screening, with sensitivity and specificity ranging widely from 50% to 100% and 29% to 100%, respectively.[29]

Digital Subtraction Angiography

The high sensitivity, specificity, and ability to provide flow analysis offered by DSA have earned it the role of the traditional reference standard for craniocervical vascular injury since the 1960s. The limited availability of skilled operators and special equipment may lead to delayed time to diagnosis compared with noninvasive modalities.[15] Inherent risks of its invasive nature confer a 1.3% complication rate, including thrombosis or embolization, arterial spasm, arterial dissection, and contrast-induced nephropathy.[29,43,47] In contrast with MDCTA, DSA cannot provide additional information on the vessel itself or extravascular injuries, limiting its usefulness in polytrauma patients.

IMAGING PROTOCOL

Given the widespread use of CTA for evaluating BCVI, a discussion of imaging protocols is warranted. CTA evaluation of the neck can either be performed as a dedicated CTA of the neck, timed to optimize craniocervical vasculature and with arms adducted, or as part of a whole-body CTA (WBCTA), which is performed with arms abducted and includes examinations of the neck, cervical spine, chest, abdomen, pelvis, thoracic spine, and lumbar spine. In 2008, Sliker and colleagues[42] compared patients who underwent both screening CT and DSA, demonstrating similar sensitivities and specificities for carotid and vertebral injuries in an MDCT group that had CT neck as part of a body trauma protocol and a second group that underwent a dedicated CTA neck.

At the authors' institution, a busy level 1 trauma center, dedicated CTA of the neck is performed in

patients with any of the standard clinical criteria for BCVI, and in patients presenting with blunt head or neck trauma who were found to have radiologic criteria for BCVI screening on an initial unenhanced brain and/or cervical spine CT scan. However, in our experience, isolated craniocervical trauma necessitating CTA occurs less commonly than multisystem polytrauma. Therefore, WBCTA is the routine method for screening severe blunt polytrauma patients who have an indication for cervical spine and contrast-enhanced body CT imaging. The dedicated neck and whole body CTA protocols used at our institution can be found in **Tables 1** and **2**, respectively.

We perform dedicated neck CTA on 64-MDCT scanners with 0.6 mm detector configuration. Our region of coverage extends from the aortic arch to the circle of Willis, using an automated triggering device centered on the ascending aorta. The patients receive 50 to 100 mL of iodinated contrast material (350 mg/mL) at 5 mL/s followed

Table 2 Protocol for multidetector computed tomography (64 detector) head and neck computed tomography angiography	
Scout	Top of head through feet
Contrast	100 mL iohexol, 350 mg I/mL
Contrast bolus	4–5 mL/s
Saline flush	Normal saline 4–5 mL/s (total 50 mL)
Scan range	Aortic arch thru top of head
Scan delay	Bolus tracking on descending aorta with trigger set at 40 Hounsfield units
Scan mode	Spiral
kVp	120
Effective mAs	220
Rotation time	0.5 s
Slice collimation	0.6 mm
Pitch	0.8
Dose modulation	On
Slice thickness	2.0 mm
Kernel	Medium smooth
Reconstruction interval	2 mm
Reconstruction planes	Axial, coronal, sagittal
Postprocessing	Maximum intensity projection and volume-rendered images reconstructed from arterial phase

by a 40 mL saline bolus at a similar rate. The images are reconstructed at 0.6 and 1.5 mm slices in axial, coronal, and sagittal planes. Three-dimensional recons are generated by the radiologist at the picture archiving and communication system workstation, using integrated TeraRecon software (TeraRecon, Foster City, CA).

In severe polytrauma patients, WBCTA is performed with 64-MDCT scanners, continuous acquisition with 0.6 mm collimation, and with neck images reconstructed at 1.0 mm slices. Our protocol involves a biphasic injection of 100 mL of iodinated contrast (350 mg/mL) at 4 mL/s for 15 seconds, then at a rate of 3 mL/s, followed by a 40 mL saline bolus at 4 mL/s. Efficiency is improved by using a fixed empiric delay of 20 seconds, or 25 seconds for patients older than 55 years. Separate dedicated coronal and sagittal reformations of the neck in both bone and soft tissue algorithms are generated, with the liberal use of additional postprocessing techniques by the radiologist.

DSA is reserved for definitive diagnosis in equivocal cases or for patients with a negative CTA and persistent clinical concern.

IMAGING FINDINGS AND INJURY GRADING

CTA imaging findings for vascular injury can be divided into both direct and indirect signs,

---

> **Box 2**
> **Signs of vascular injury**
>
> *Direct signs*
> - Abrupt caliber change: can be a sign of dissection
> - Vessel occlusion: abrupt or tapered cut-off
> - Contrast extravasation
> - Intraluminal filling defects: mural thrombi or intimal flaps
> - Abrupt change in vessel contour
> - Pseudoaneurysm: eccentric outpouching of contrast in continuity with the native vessel
> - A fistula: enlarged vein and/or early venous enhancement (equal to the arterial enhancement at the level of injury)
>
> *Indirect signs*
> - Indistinct perivascular fat planes
> - Perivascular hematoma
> - End-organ infarcts (distal emboli from intraluminal thrombus)
>
> *Data from Refs.*[21–24,59,60]

---

summarized in **Box 2**. Detection of these imaging findings aids in diagnosing the severity of injury, and can be used to help grade the BCVI (**Figs. 1–5**).

Biffl and colleagues also devised a classification system for carotid artery injuries (**Box 3**), later adapted for vertebral artery injuries, based on appearance of the vessel, wall, and lumen. Initially devised for use with DSA, the grading system was extrapolated for use with CTA (see **Figs. 1–5**). The importance of injury grading mostly relates to the propensity of higher grade injuries to result in stroke. As reported by Biffl and colleagues, the rates of stroke in blunt carotid artery injury grades 1 to 5 are, respectively, 3%, 11%, 33%, 44%, and 100%. Alternatively, rates of stroke in blunt vertebral artery injuries grades 1 to 4 are 19%, 40%, 13%, and 33%. Grade 5 blunt vertebral artery injuries have not yet been reported.[47]

Scott and colleagues[48,49] found the risk of post-traumatic stroke to be greatest in grade 3 (according to the grading system used by the authors: >50% stenosis of the vessel or the development of a pseudoaneurysm) or grade 4 (complete vessel occlusion) BCVI, at approximately 7%, with follow-up imaging showing progressive worsening without radiographic improvement only in a small number of patients, findings that alone did not correlate with adverse clinical outcome. They reported a stroke rate of only 1% in lower grade BCVI, with a 14% rate of radiographic worsening on follow-up imaging, albeit with no adverse clinical outcomes associated with these radiographic changes.[48,49]

The distinct types of BCVI can occur in combination; for instance, a small, focal intraluminal thrombus may occur on a focal dissection flap, or a thrombosis may occur in the setting of pseudoaneursym formation.

PEARLS, PITFALLS, AND VARIANTS

The diagnosis of BCVI may not always be straightforward and knowledge of various variants and pitfalls will be helpful in accurate diagnosis.

First and foremost, one needs to remember that the anterior and posterior circulation have numerous anatomic variants, both extracranially and intracranially, particularly the posterior circulation. It is beyond the scope of this text to discuss them all owing to the vast number, but variants the authors more commonly encounter are highlighted. One needs to keep in mind that the vertebral arteries are frequently asymmetric in size with 1 vertebral artery being dominant (usually the left), so differences in caliber may

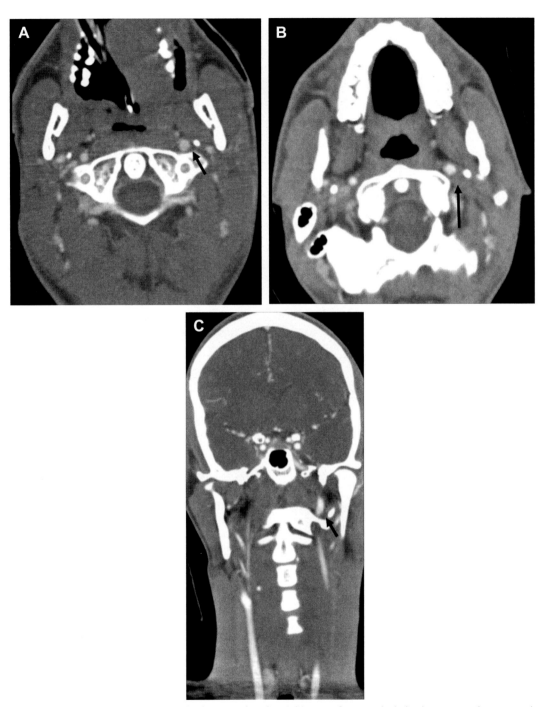

Fig. 1. A 20 year-old male pedestrian hit by a car. (*A, B*) Axial images from a whole body computed tomography angiogram show slight contour irregularity and a small intraluminal filling defect indicating an intimal flap of the left internal carotid artery (*short arrow*). Additionally, note the indistinctness of the perivascular fat planes (*long arrow*), an indirect sign of injury. (*C*) Coronal reformation depicts the intimal flap (*arrow*, grade 1 lesion).

not be a reliable indicator of injury. A left vertebral artery origin directly off the aortic arch is not infrequently seen. Variations in the caliber of the vertebral arteries after the origin of the posterior inferior

cerebellar arteries have been reported as well as vertebral arteries terminating in the posterior inferior cerebellar artery. Vertebral artery fenestrations have a reported prevalence of 0.3% to

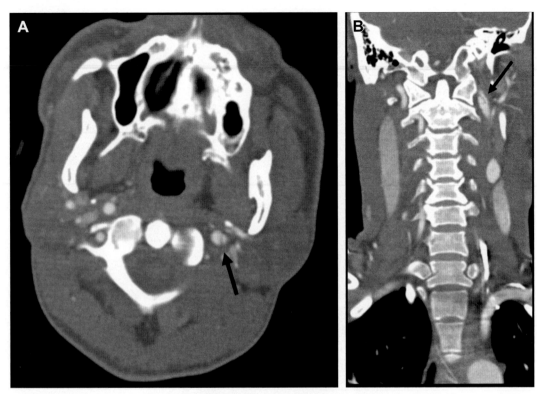

Fig. 2. A 40 year-old male unrestrained driver status post motor vehicle collision. (*A, B*) Axial image and coronal reformation show a raised intimal flap of the left internal carotid artery causing greater than 25% of luminal narrowing (*arrows*, grade 2 lesion).

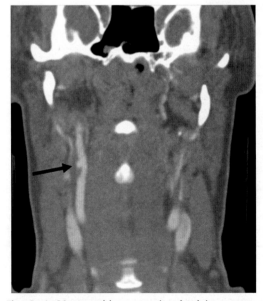

Fig. 3. A 29 year-old woman involved in a motor vehicle collision. Small right internal carotid artery pseudoaneurysm (*arrow*, grade 3 injury) on coronal reformatted image.

2.0%.[50] Last, multiple variants of the circle of Willis are known, to include hypoplastic or aplastic segments of the proximal anterior, middle, and posterior cerebral arteries.

Other pitfalls outside of failure to recognize normal variants include imaging artifacts and pre-existing conditions. Depending on imaging technique, there may be various levels of artifacts that hamper diagnosis. When CTA is performed with the "arms up" technique frequently used with WBCTA, there may be increasing levels of streak artifact that may be confused with intimal flaps. These can usually be differentiated from true vascular flaps by reviewing multiplanar reformatted images. Pulsation artifacts may also simulate intimal or dissection flaps and can be differentiated from true BCVI by their propagation in adjacent veins and anatomy, and by review of multiplanar reformatted images. Subtle patient motion can also cause a diagnostic dilemma that may be alleviated by scrutiny of multiple imaging plans. In some cases, generating oblique multiplanar reformatted images or 3-dimensional postprocessing images may be beneficial. If these additional images are not definitive, repeat dedicated CTA may always be obtained,

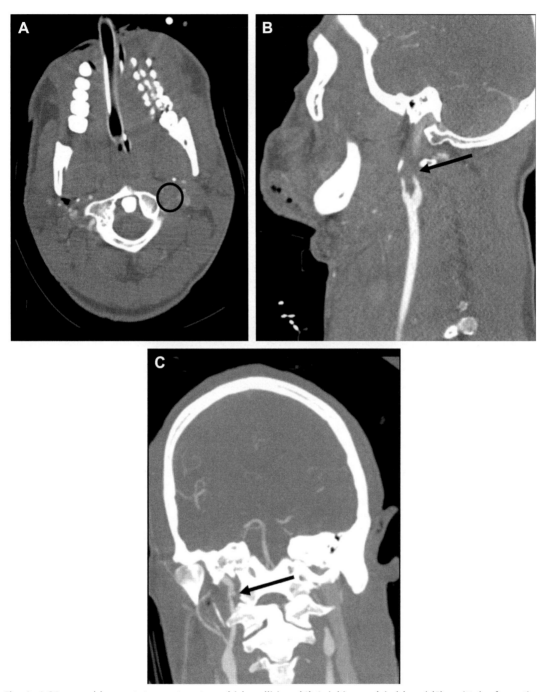

Fig. 4. A 31-year-old man status post motor vehicle collision. (*A*) Axial image (*circle*) and (*B*) sagittal reformation demonstrate left internal carotid artery occlusion (*arrow*, grade 4 injury). Maximum intensity projection images (*C*) on the same patient show a right internal carotid artery pseudoaneurysm (*arrow*, grade 3 lesion).

particularly if the original scan was performed as part of a WBCTA. The most commonly injured segments of the ICAs and vertebral arteries are near the skull base, and streak artifact caused by the dense bone can hamper diagnoses. Again, postprocessing tools allow for various types of reconstructed images including maximum intensity projections, 3-dimensional, and curved planar reformats. Although evaluation for BCVI using nonstandard planes has not been adequately studied, advocation for their liberal use is based on evidence demonstrating

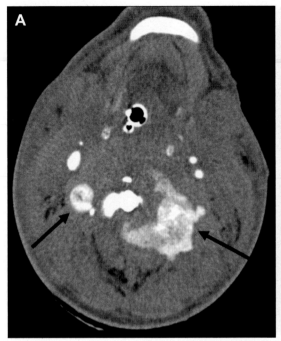
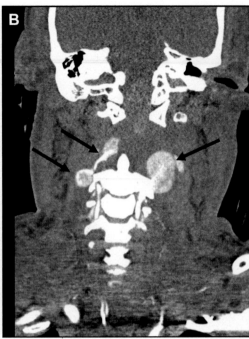

Fig. 5. A 60 year-old male pedestrian hit by a car. (*A*) Axial image from a whole body computed tomography angiogram and coronal reformation (*B*) show severe active arterial extravasation from bilateral vertebral arteries (*arrows*, grade 5 lesions). Note the extreme atlantoaxial dissociation.

improved detection of craniocervical fractures,[51–54] characterization of dislocations and subluxations with rotatory component,[52,53] and detection of cerebral aneurysms.[55]

Preexisting vascular disease, particularly atherosclerotic disease in the older population, or more rarely vasculitides such as fibromuscular dysplasia, may simulate or obscure BCVI, because their appearances may overlap with the direct signs of vascular injury. In our experience, reviewing all imaged vessels and the clinical and imaging presentation can be used as an internal comparison to raise or lower diagnostic suspicion. For instance, an eccentric mural thickening in a young patient without any other vascular disease is more suspicious than a similar finding in an older patient with diffuse vascular disease. Fibromuscular dysplasia is often multifocal and its presence in the contralateral ICA or the renal arteries (if WBCTA was performed) can increase diagnostic confidence.

Vasospasm can result in caliber changes of the vessels and should be considered in the differential of suspected BCVI based solely on the finding.

When BCVI in 1 vessel is diagnosed, a careful review of the remainder of the vasculature should be undertaken. Rather than injury to a single vessel, as classically described, more recent literature suggests that 18% to 32% of patients sustain multivessel injuries (see **Figs. 4** and **5**).[35,42,56] Also, the end-organ effects of BCVI should be evaluated for; cerebral ischemia and infarcts are responsible for the large proportion of morbidity and mortality[1–3] and should be evaluated for.

WHAT THE REFERRING PHYSICIAN NEEDS TO KNOW

- Greater awareness of screening criteria and use of imaging can potentially decrease incidence of stroke in victims of blunt trauma.[57]
- What to order? CTA is the current preferred modality to screen for BCVI at most institutions.[44,46,57]
- How to follow-up? There is no standardized protocol. Follow-up imaging is usually recommended 7 to 10 days after injury or for any change in neurologic status.[21,58]

SUMMARY

MDCTA is increasingly used as the initial screening method in patients suspected of having BCVI. This underscores the need for radiologists to possess significant knowledge about risk factors, pathophysiology, injury patterns and injury grading identified on MDCTA.

ACKNOWLEDGMENTS

The authors thank Catalina Restrepo, MD, for her assistance (Catalina Restrepo, MD, Junior Radiology resident, Universidad CES, Medellín, Colombia, Florida).

REFERENCES

1. Fabian TC, Patton JH Jr, Croce MA, et al. Blunt carotid injury. Importance of early diagnosis and anticoagulant therapy. Ann Surg 1996;223(5):513–22 [discussion: 522–5].
2. Munera F, Foley M, Chokshi FH. Multi-detector row CT angiography of the neck in blunt trauma. Radiol Clin North Am 2012;50(1):59–72.
3. Grabowski G, Robertson RN, Barton BM, et al. Blunt cerebrovascular injury in cervical spine fractures: are more-liberal screening criteria warranted? Global Spine J 2016;6(7):679–85.
4. Chokshi FH, Munera F, Rivas LA, et al. 64-MDCT angiography of blunt vascular injuries of the neck. AJR Am J Roentgenol 2011;196(3):W309–15.
5. Nason RW, Assuras GN, Gray PR, et al. Penetrating neck injuries: analysis of experience from a Canadian trauma centre. Can J Surg 2001;44(2):122–6.
6. Cotton BA, Nance ML. Penetrating trauma in children. Semin Pediatr Surg 2004;13(2):87–97.
7. Mathers CD, Boerma T, Ma Fat D. Global and regional causes of death. Br Med Bull 2009;92:7–32.
8. Schneidereit NP, Simons R, Nicolaou S, et al. Utility of screening for blunt vascular neck injuries with computed tomographic angiography. J Trauma 2006;60(1):209–15 [discussion: 215–6].
9. Franz RW, Willette PA, Wood MJ, et al. A systematic review and meta-analysis of diagnostic screening criteria for blunt cerebrovascular injuries. J Am Coll Surg 2012;214(3):313–27.
10. Harrigan MR, Falola MI, Shannon CN, et al. Incidence and trends in the diagnosis of traumatic extracranial cerebrovascular injury in the nationwide inpatient sample database, 2003-2010. J Neurotrauma 2014; 31(11):1056–62.
11. Esnault P, Cardinale M, Boret H, et al. Blunt cerebrovascular injuries in severe traumatic brain injury: incidence, risk factors, and evolution. J Neurosurg 2017;127(1):16–22.
12. Shahan CP, Croce MA, Fabian TC, et al. Impact of continuous evaluation of technology and therapy: 30 years of research reduces stroke and mortality from blunt cerebrovascular injury. J Am Coll Surg 2017;224(4):595–9.
13. Burlew CC, Biffl WL. Imaging for blunt carotid and vertebral artery injuries. Surg Clin North Am 2011; 91(1):217–31.
14. Geddes AE, Burlew CC, Wagenaar AE, et al. Expanded screening criteria for blunt cerebrovascular injury: a bigger impact than anticipated. Am J Surg 2016;212(6):1167–74.
15. Eastman AL, Chason DP, Perez CL, et al. Computed tomographic angiography for the diagnosis of blunt cervical vascular injury: is it ready for primetime? J Trauma 2006;60(5):925–9 [discussion: 929].
16. Mutze S, Rademacher G, Matthes G, et al. Blunt cerebrovascular injury in patients with blunt multiple trauma: diagnostic accuracy of duplex Doppler US and early CT angiography. Radiology 2005;237(3): 884–92.
17. Paulus EM, Fabian TC, Savage SA, et al. Blunt cerebrovascular injury screening with 64-channel multidetector computed tomography: more slices finally cut it. J Trauma Acute Care Surg 2014;76(2):279–83 [discussion: 284–5].
18. Payabvash S, McKinney AM, McKinney ZJ, et al. Screening and detection of blunt vertebral artery

injury in patients with upper cervical fractures: the role of cervical CT and CT angiography. Eur J Radiol 2014;83(3):571–7.

19. Beliaev AM, Barber PA, Marshall RJ, et al. Denver screening protocol for blunt cerebrovascular injury reduces the use of multi-detector computed tomography angiography. ANZ J Surg 2014;84(6): 429–32.

20. Berne JD, Cook A, Rowe SA, et al. A multivariate logistic regression analysis of risk factors for blunt cerebrovascular injury. J Vasc Surg 2010;51(1):57–64.

21. Biffl WL, Cothren CC, Moore EE, et al. Western Trauma Association critical decisions in trauma: screening for and treatment of blunt cerebrovascular injuries. J Trauma 2009;67(6):1150–3.

22. Biffl WL, Moore EE, Elliott JP, et al. The devastating potential of blunt vertebral arterial injuries. Ann Surg 2000;231(5):672–81.

23. Biffl WL, Moore EE, Offner PJ, et al. Optimizing screening for blunt cerebrovascular injuries. Am J Surg 1999;178(6):517–22.

24. Biffl WL, Moore EE, Ryu RK, et al. The unrecognized epidemic of blunt carotid arterial injuries: early diagnosis improves neurologic outcome. Ann Surg 1998; 228(4):462–70.

25. Bruns BR, Tesoriero R, Kufera J, et al. Blunt cerebrovascular injury screening guidelines: what are we willing to miss? J Trauma Acute Care Surg 2014; 76(3):691–5.

26. Cothren CC, Moore EE, Ray CE Jr, et al. Cervical spine fracture patterns mandating screening to rule out blunt cerebrovascular injury. Surgery 2007; 141(1):76–82.

27. Davis JW, Holbrook TL, Hoyt DB, et al. Blunt carotid artery dissection: incidence, associated injuries, screening, and treatment. J Trauma 1990;30(12): 1514–7.

28. Emmett KP, Fabian TC, DiCocco JM, et al. Improving the screening criteria for blunt cerebrovascular injury: the appropriate role for computed tomography angiography. J Trauma 2011;70(5):1058–63 [discussion: 1063–5].

29. Liang T, Tso DK, Chiu RY, et al. Imaging of blunt vascular neck injuries: a review of screening and imaging modalities. AJR Am J Roentgenol 2013; 201(4):884–92.

30. Tso MK, Lee MM, Ball CG, et al. Clinical utility of a screening protocol for blunt cerebrovascular injury using computed tomography angiography. J Neurosurg 2017;126(4):1033–41.

31. Stein DM, Boswell S, Sliker CW, et al. Blunt cerebrovascular injuries: does treatment always matter? J Trauma 2009;66(1):132–44.

32. Hui CM, MacGregor JH, Tien HC, et al. Radiation dose from initial trauma assessment and resuscitation: review of the literature. Can J Surg 2009; 52(2):147–52.

33. Bouthillier A, van Loveren HR, Keller JT. Segments of the internal carotid artery: a new classification. Neurosurgery 1996;38(3):425–32 [discussion: 432–3].

34. McKevitt EC, Kirkpatrick AW, Vertesi L, et al. Identifying patients at risk for intracranial and extracranial blunt carotid injuries. Am J Surg 2002;183(5): 566–70.

35. Liang T, Tso DK, Chiu RY, et al. Imaging of blunt vascular neck injuries: a clinical perspective. AJR Am J Roentgenol 2013;201(4):893–901.

36. Sliker CW. Blunt cerebrovascular injuries: imaging with multidetector CT angiography. Radiographics 2008;28(6):1689–708 [discussion: 1709–10].

37. Crissey MM, Bernstein EF. Delayed presentation of carotid intimal tear following blunt craniocervical trauma. Surgery 1974;75(4):543–9.

38. Buch K, Nguyen T, Mahoney E, et al. Association between cervical spine and skull-base fractures and blunt cerebrovascular injury. Eur Radiol 2016;26(2): 524–31.

39. Lockwood MM, Smith GA, Tanenbaum J, et al. Screening via CT angiogram after traumatic cervical spine fractures: narrowing imaging to improve cost effectiveness. Experience of a Level I trauma center. J Neurosurg Spine 2016;24(3):490–5.

40. Stein DM, Boswell S, Sliker CW, et al. Blunt cerebrovascular injuries: does treatment always matter? J Trauma 2009;66(1):132–43 [discussion: 143–4].

41. Bonatti M, Vezzali N, Ferro F, et al. Blunt cerebrovascular injury: diagnosis at whole-body MDCT for multi-trauma. Insights Imaging 2013;4(3):347–55.

42. Sliker CW, Shanmuganathan K, Mirvis SE. Diagnosis of blunt cerebrovascular injuries with 16-MDCT: accuracy of whole-body MDCT compared with neck MDCT angiography. AJR Am J Roentgenol 2008; 190(3):790–9.

43. DiCocco JM, Emmett KP, Fabian TC, et al. Blunt cerebrovascular injury screening with 32-channel multidetector computed tomography: more slices still don't cut it. Ann Surg 2011;253(3):444–50.

44. Malhotra A, Wu X, Kalra VB, et al. Evaluation for blunt cerebrovascular injury: review of the literature and a cost-effectiveness analysis. AJNR Am J Neuroradiol 2016;37(2):330–5.

45. Kaye D, Brasel KJ, Neideen T, et al. Screening for blunt cerebrovascular injuries is cost-effective. J Trauma 2011;70(5):1051–6 [discussion: 1056–7].

46. Harrigan MR, Weinberg JA, Peaks YS, et al. Management of blunt extracranial traumatic cerebrovascular injury: a multidisciplinary survey of current practice. World J Emerg Surg 2011;6:11.

47. Willinsky RA, Taylor SM, TerBrugge K, et al. Neurologic complications of cerebral angiography: prospective analysis of 2,899 procedures and review of the literature. Radiology 2003; 227(2):522–8.

48. Scott WW, Sharp S, Figueroa SA, et al. Clinical and radiographic outcomes following traumatic Grade 3 and 4 carotid artery injuries: a 10-year retrospective analysis from a Level 1 trauma center. The Parkland Carotid and Vertebral Artery Injury Survey. J Neurosurg 2015;122(3): 610–5.

49. Scott WW, Sharp S, Figueroa SA, et al. Clinical and radiological outcomes following traumatic Grade 1 and 2 vertebral artery injuries: a 10-year retrospective analysis from a Level 1 trauma center. J Neurosurg 2014;121(2):450–6.

50. Dimmick SJ, Faulder KC. Normal variants of the cerebral circulation at multidetector CT angiography. Radiographics 2009;29(4):1027–43.

51. Chang W, Alexander MT, Mirvis SE. Diagnostic determinants of craniocervical distraction injury in adults. AJR Am J Roentgenol 2009;192(1): 52–8.

52. Deliganis AV, Baxter AB, Hanson JA, et al. Radiologic spectrum of craniocervical distraction injuries. Radiographics 2000;20 Spec No:S237–50.

53. Dreizin D, Letzing M, Sliker CW, et al. Multidetector CT of blunt cervical spine trauma in adults. Radiographics 2014;34(7):1842–65.

54. Junewick JJ. Pediatric craniocervical junction injuries. AJR Am J Roentgenol 2011;196(5): 1003–10.

55. Velthuis BK, van Leeuwen MS, Witkamp TD, et al. CT angiography: source images and postprocessing techniques in the detection of cerebral aneurysms. AJR Am J Roentgenol 1997; 169(5):1411–7.

56. Cothren CC, Moore EE, Biffl WL, et al. Anticoagulation is the gold standard therapy for blunt carotid injuries to reduce stroke rate. Arch Surg 2004;139(5): 540–5 [discussion: 545–6].

57. Wu X, Malhotra A, Forman HP, et al. The use of high-risk criteria in screening patients for blunt cerebrovascular injury: a survey. Acad Radiol 2017;24(4): 456–61.

58. Laser A, Bruns BR, Kufera JA, et al. Long-term follow-up of blunt cerebrovascular injuries: does time heal all wounds? J Trauma Acute Care Surg 2016;81(6):1063–9.

59. Biffl WL, Moore EE, Offner PJ, et al. Blunt carotid and vertebral arterial injuries. World J Surg 2001;25(8): 1036–43.

60. Biffl WL, Moore EE, Offner PJ, et al. Blunt carotid arterial injuries: implications of a new grading scale. J Trauma 1999;47(5):845–53.

The Imaging of Maxillofacial Trauma 2017

Mark P. Bernstein, MD

KEYWORDS

• Maxillofacial trauma • Surgery • Imaging

KEY POINTS

- Multidetector CT is the gold standard for imaging in the setting of suspected maxillofacial trauma.
- Multiplanar reformations and three dimensional reconstructions aid in evaluation of facial fractures.
- Multidetector CT is also the imaging of choice to assess for orbital injuries including ocular injuries.

INTRODUCTION
Epidemiology

Facial fractures account for a large proportion of emergency room visits and 2% of all hospital admissions.[1] Significant facial injuries are clinically occult in more than half of intubated multitrauma patients.[2] Mechanisms include motor vehicle collisions, assaults, falls, sports injuries, and civilian warfare. Together, motor vehicle collisions and assaults account for more than 80% of all injuries and commonly involve young adult men and alcohol use.[3]

By understanding common fracture patterns and the implications for clinical management, radiologists can better construct clinically relevant radiology reports and thus facilitate improved communication with referring clinicians to best serve victims of maxillofacial injuries.

Clinical Issues

The face protects the brain from frontal injury; supports the sensory organs of sight, smell, taste, and hearing; and serves as the point of entry for oxygen, water, and nutrients.

Initial management of any trauma patient begins with life preservation aimed at airway, breathing, and circulation maintenance. In acute facial injury, the presence of fracture fragments, teeth and airway foreign bodies, pharyngeal hemorrhage, and loss of hyomandibular support with posterior displacement of the tongue can all compromise the airway. Stridor and hoarseness are clues to laryngeal injury that may be occult, initially leading to subsequent precipitous airway compromise.

Branches of the external and internal carotid arteries supply circulation to the face. Injuries to these vessels are common and may result in a rapidly expanding hematoma or profuse arterial bleeding. In closed injuries, bleeding is controlled by packing or balloon tamponade using a Foley catheter. When packing fails, angioembolization is necessary to control hemorrhage, often targeting the maxillary and palatine arteries associated with midface fractures and in cases of penetrating arterial injury.

Once patients are stabilized, clinical attention in the setting of facial trauma is directed to restoration of form and function, with attention to facial injury patterns and their impact on sight, smell, taste, speech, and cosmetic deformity.

Biomechanics and Associated Life-threatening Injuries

Injury pattern and severity of maxillofacial fractures are determined by the direction and magnitude of the impacting force and the underlying facial architecture. For example, the prominent positions of the nose, zygoma, and mandible are typically injured in assault with a relatively small amount of energy transfer. Motor vehicle collisions, falls, and other high-velocity injuries result in more complex, midfacial fractures.

The author has no financial support or interests to disclose.
Department of Radiology, New York University Langone Health, Bellevue Hospital and Trauma Center, 550 First Avenue, New York, NY 10016, USA
E-mail address: Mark.Bernstein@nyumc.org

neuroimaging.theclinics.com

A study of major facial fractures in 1020 patients grouped injuries into high G-force and low G-force mechanisms[4]; 21% of patients with low G-force facial trauma had 1 or more associated life-threatening injuries compared with 50% in patients with high G-force mechanisms. Life-threatening injuries included intra-abdominal injury requiring surgery, pneumothorax, chest trauma requiring ventilator support, and severe closed head injury. Mortality in the high G-force group was 12%.

In a study investigating the relationship between facial fractures, cervical spine injuries, and head injuries in 1.3 million trauma patients, 7% of facial fracture patients had concomitant cervical spine injury and 68% had associated head injury.[5] Approximately 8% suffered injuries to all 3 areas.

IMAGING

Imaging in facial trauma aims to define the site and severity of facial fractures and to identify injuries that could compromise the airway, vision, mastication, the lacrimal system, and sinus function. Individual fractures should be listed and associated soft tissue injuries described with attention to these areas. If possible, bony findings should be summarized in one of several typical fracture patterns.

Modalities

Imaging in most emergency departments for significant facial trauma begins with CT scanning. Multidetector CT (MDCT) has supplanted plain radiography and has revolutionized the imaging of the maxillofacial trauma. MDCT, more cost efficient and more rapidly performed than facial radiographs, is considered the optimal imaging modality, particularly in the polytrauma setting. MDCT allows safe and rapid volumetric image data acquisition without patient manipulation and accurately depicts both bony and soft tissue injury. Submillimeter slice thickness permits detailed multiplanar reformations (MPRs) and 3-D reconstructions. Fracture fragment displacement and rotation are easily determined and fracture patterns may be readily classified and assessed for stability. Although 2-D transaxial and coronal images are more accurate and sensitive than 3-D reconstructions for individual fracture detection, 3-D imaging provides a global perspective to help classify fracture pattern types. Additionally, 3-D reconstructions are preferred by surgeons for operative repair planning.[6] Nonetheless, it is important to recognize limitations in 3-D imaging, namely the introduction of artifact during the reconstruction process, decreasing the ability to visualize nondisplaced fractures, and difficulty viewing deep fractures on surface renderings.

MR imaging can be a useful adjunct in patients with cranial nerve deficits not explained or incompletely characterized by CT. Its advantages include multiplanar capabilities, excellent soft tissue contrast, and lack of ionizing radiation. The practical limitations of long scan times, limited patient access, poor evaluation of cortical bone, and contraindication in patients with pacemakers, some aneurysm clips, and ocular metallic foreign bodies prevent its primary application in the emergency setting.

Multidetector CT Technique

At Bellevue Hospital, patients with clinically apparent or suspected maxillofacial fractures are scanned from the top of the frontal sinuses through the hyoid with the field of view from the tip of the nose through the temporomandibular joints to always include the entire face and mandible. Acquisitions using 64-MDCT with 0.625-mm detector width and overlapping sections allow high-quality MPRs to be generated; 2-mm thick images in all 3 planes oriented parallel and perpendicular to the hard palate provide symmetric images for optimal interpretation. Images are produced in bone and soft tissue algorithm for radiologist review. Specialized MPRs may be generated depending on the presence and type of fractures. For example, oblique sagittal reformations along the plane of the optic nerve elegantly characterize orbital floor fractures with respect to depression, orbital depth, and relation to the inferior rectus muscle. Panoramic or oblique sagittal planes optimize evaluation of mandibular angle and ramus fractures. 3-D reconstructions are often acquired in patients with complex injuries for better characterization and surgical planning.

Multitrauma patients often require a comprehensive whole-body CT examination to evaluate multiple body regions in a single visit to the CT suite. With current technology, scanning of the head, face, and cervical spine may be acquired as a rapid single acquisition, without requiring gantry tilt and eliminating overlap of these body sections.

FACIAL FRACTURES

Facial fracture complexes are classified by location and pattern into the following categories: nasal, naso-orbital-ethmoid (NOE), frontal sinus, orbital, zygomatic, maxillary, and mandibular. Manson and colleagues[7] have proposed further categorizing each area by the energy of the injury, namely low energy, moderate energy, and high energy. Low-energy injuries show little or no comminution or displacement. Moderate-energy injuries, the most common, demonstrate mild to moderate displacement, whereas high-energy injuries are characterized by severe fragmentation, displacement, and instability. Impact energy subclassifications dictate management, which range from simple closed reduction to wide exposure open reduction and internal fixation.

Nasal Fractures

Anatomy

The nose is the most prominent facial projection. As such, nasal bone fractures account for approximately 50% of all facial fractures, the majority of which involve the distal third of the nose.[8]

The nasal region consists of bony and cartilaginous portions. The anterior nasal septum is cartilaginous, whereas the remainder of the nasal septum, consisting of the posterior perpendicular plate of the ethmoid, vomer, nasal crest of the maxilla, and nasal crest of the palatine bone, is bony. The upper third of the nasal region is bony, composed of the nasal bones proper, the frontal processes of maxilla, and the nasal process of the frontal bone. Conversely, the middle and lower thirds of the nasal region are composed of the bilateral upper lateral and lower alar cartilages, respectively.

Injuries

The diagnosis of nasal bone fracture is usually made clinically with limited role for dedicated imaging. Imaging directed at identifying other facial fractures or radiology reports from head CTs, however, often bring a nasal bone fracture to the attention of the emergency room staff and facilitate further evaluation. Such evaluation can prevent clinical complications, such as a cosmetic deformity or a septal hematoma, resulting in saddle nose deformity. In these cases, early reduction prevents bony malunion, thereby avoiding osteotomy to anatomically reduce fracture fragments.

Several classification systems exist for nasal and septal fractures, sorting fractures based on laterality (unilateral or bilateral), displacement, comminution, impaction, septal involvement, and soft tissue injury (**Fig. 1**). Generally, nasal trauma with septal fracture or dislocation causing severe alteration of the nasal midline or those with severe soft tissue injury require open repair, whereas most others are treated with closed reduction.

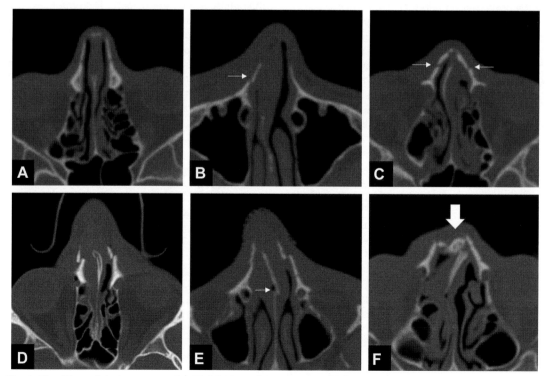

Fig. 1. Nasal bone injuries—transaxial CT. (*A*) Normal appearance of bilateral nasal bones with nasomaxillary sutures visible. (*B*) Unilateral right nasal bone fracture mildly displaced to the left (*arrow*). (*C*) Bilateral undisplaced nasal bone fractures (*arrows*) with overlying soft tissue swelling. (*D*) Bilateral displaced nasal bone fractures. (*E*) Bilateral displaced nasal bone fractures with nasal septal fracture (*arrow*). (*F*) Anterior force (*arrow*) impacting and fracturing bilateral nasal bones and nasal septum.

Naso-Orbital-Ethmoid Fractures

Anatomy

The NOE region refers to the interorbital space—the space between the eyes, representing the bony confluence of the nose, orbit, maxilla, and cranium. The space is defined laterally by the thin medial orbital walls, posteriorly by the sphenoid sinus, superiorly by the cribriform plate, and anteriorly by the bony pillars (composed of the frontal process of the maxilla, nasal process of the frontal bone, and the thick proximal nasal bones). Several key structures lie within this region, including the olfactory nerves, the lacrimal sac, the nasolacrimal duct, the ethmoid vessels, and the medial canthal tendon.

Injuries

An anteriorly directed force sufficient to fracture the nasal bones is likely to progress posteriorly because the ethmoid air cells offer little resistance and are easily fractured with resultant impaction and telescoping. The NOE fracture differs from the simple impacted nasal fracture by additional fractures of the medial orbit, the nasal septum, and the nasofrontal junction (**Fig. 2**A). This pattern results from moderate blunt trauma force directed at the upper nasal bridge.

CT is essential to identifying injury location, type, degree of comminution and displacement, associated facial fractures, and soft tissue injury. CT typically demonstrates hemorrhage within the ethmoid air cells and multiple impacted interorbital fractures. Often, both clinically and on CT, the nose appears pushed back between the eyes (**Fig. 2**B). Left untreated, NOE fractures can result in marked facial deformity with both functional and cosmetic implications, including but not limited to telecanthus, enophthalmos, ptosis, and lacrimal obstruction.[9] These deformities are extremely challenging to correct secondarily and are best addressed immediately.

NOE fractures are commonly associated with Le Fort II and III fractures, and therefore the pterygoid plates should be carefully evaluated. One study showed that 65% of patients with NOE fractures had concomitant facial fractures, most commonly a Le Fort maxillary or frontal sinus fracture. Disruption of the cribriform plate should be assessed because the olfactory nerves can be injured, and more seriously, this fracture can lead to cerebrospinal fluid (CSF) leak, pneumocephalus, or tension pneumocephalus during resuscitation efforts. Also, because NOE fractures are associated with high-impact trauma that involves the midface, ocular injuries, such as lens dislocation, hyphema, vitreous hemorrhage, and globe rupture, should be sought and excluded.

Radiologically, one of the key structures of the NOE fracture to assess and report on is the degree of comminution of medial orbital rim where the medial canthal tendon inserts. The medial canthal tendon anchors the globe medially and maintains eyelid apposition. Disruption of the medial canthal tendon insertion is implied with fracture through the inferomedial orbital rim at the lacrimal fossa (see **Fig. 2**A). Recognizing potential injury is important to ensure appropriate treatment planning and repair. Injury of the medial canthal tendon is closely associated to injury of the lacrimal drainage system, which can lead to obstruction.

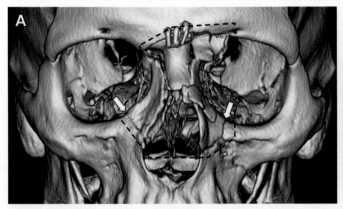
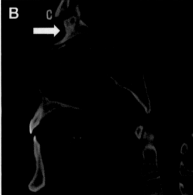

Fig. 2. NOE fractures. 3-D (*A*) and sagittal (*B*) CT reformations of a 35-year-old man after a construction accident. (*A*) 3-D image shows marked comminuted interorbital fractures (*dashed outline*). Note the fractures through the inferomedial orbital rims (*arrows*), implying medial canthal tendon injury. (*B*) Midsagittal CT reformation depicts the posterior displacement of the fractured nasal segment as the nose is pushed back between the eyes (*arrow*).

Many NOE classification algorithms have been proposed in the literature. Markowitz and colleagues[10] system is among the most common, which classifies NOE fractures according to the status of the medial canthal tendon in conjunction with the degree of comminution of the bony fragment to which it attaches.[10] Practically speaking, it is important for the surgeon to know whether a fracture is unilateral or bilateral and whether the fracture is simple (a large single fragment) or comminuted. This, in combination with identifying associated fractures and assessing the internal orbit, determines the degree of surgical exposure required and the type and approach of surgical repair and stabilization necessary. In general, fractures that demonstrate displacement necessitate open reduction and internal fixation. Marked comminution of the medial orbital wall, particularly in the region of the lacrimal fossa, where the medial canthal ligament attaches and the nasofrontal ducts are located, can require transnasal fixation. If the nasofrontal ducts are involved, surgical obliteration is often indicated to prevent mucocele formation. NOE fractures may also extend posteriorly to the optic canal or superiorly to the frontal sinus and intracranial structures, and any such involvement should also be reported.

Frontal Sinus Fractures

Anatomy

Frontal sinus anatomy is highly variable, with 10% of individuals having a unilateral sinus, 5% having a rudimentary sinus, and 4% lacking a frontal sinus. The anterior table of the frontal sinus is thick cortical bone and reportedly can tolerate as much as 1000 kg of force before fracturing, whereas the posterior table is thin and relatively delicate. Just posterior to the posterior table lie the intracranial contents, namely the frontal lobes and overlying dura. Inferiorly, the orbital roofs and nasofrontal ducts are located. The only drainage port from the frontal sinus, the nasofrontal duct, is located at the inferomedial aspect of the sinus and drains into the middle meatus.

Injuries

Frontal sinus fractures result from a direct anterior blow to the forehead driving the head and cervical spine into extension and account for 5% to 12% of all maxillofacial fractures.[11] One-third of injuries are isolated to the anterior table (**Fig. 3**A), whereas two-thirds involve both anterior and posterior tables (**Fig. 3**B). Because of the high-energy G-force necessary for fracture to occur, these injuries result in significant injury including shock, brain injury, coma, and additional facial fractures in 75% of cases.[12]

Displaced posterior table fractures imply disruption of the underlying dura and communication between the frontal sinus and the intracranial contents (see **Fig. 3**B). Prompt and appropriate management is essential, because complications, such as brain abscess, meningitis, encephalitis, mucocele, and mucopyocele, can occur. MDCT should be used as early as possible to exclude injury to the central nervous system and establish the location and extent of injury. Particular attention should be paid to the anterior and posterior tables as well as the nasofrontal duct, because injuries to these 3 structures dictate classification and subsequent treatment.

Injury to the nasofrontal outflow tract is present in 70% of cases and indicated by (1) anatomic outflow tract obstruction, (2) frontal sinus floor fracture, and (3) medial anterior table fracture. Coronal images are particularly helpful for evaluating the base of the frontal sinus at the site of the ostium of the duct. Fracture fragments within the

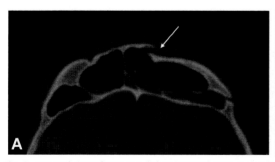
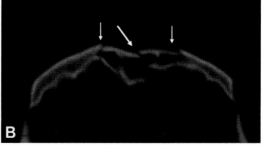

Fig. 3. Frontal sinus fractures. (A) Transaxial CT image of 28-year-old man in a motor vehicle crash with a relatively large frontal sinus and fractures limited to the anterior table (*arrow*). (B) Relatively smaller frontal sinus in a 19-year-old woman after motor vehicle crash with comminuted fractures of both the anterior (*white arrows*) and posterior tables (*black arrows*). Displaced posterior table fracture fragments suggest injury to the dura with risk for intracranial infection and CSF leak.

tract are diagnostic of nasofrontal outflow tract obstruction.[13]

Although treatment goals are similar among surgeons, controversy regarding exact management of frontal sinus fractures exists.[14] As long as the nasofrontal duct remains intact and there is no CSF leakage, nondisplaced fractures of the anterior and posterior walls of the frontal sinus do not usually require surgical treatment. Because of the possibility of delayed infection, however, many facial surgeons recommend long-term CT follow-up.[15]

Nasofrontal duct injury or displaced posterior table injury with a dural tear, often seen on CT as pneumocephalus or with CSF leak, usually requires stripping of the frontal sinus mucosa and obliteration of the cavity (referred to cranialization of the frontal sinus) to prevent mucocele formation.[16] In surgical procedures where the frontal sinus is maintained, serial CT scans in the postoperative period are often performed to ensure adequate sinus drainage. Isolated anterior wall fractures with depression can lead to cosmetic deformities and are treated with anterior wall restoration to obtain aesthetically acceptable contours.

Orbital Fractures

Anatomy
The bony orbit comprises 7 bones: the frontal bone, zygoma, maxilla, lacrimal bone, ethmoid bone, sphenoid bone, and palantine bone. The optic canal, superior orbital fissure, and inferior orbital fissure are the 3 apertures in the posterior orbit. In trauma imaging, fractures of the orbit are usually referenced in relation to the 4 orbital walls: the orbital floor, orbital roof, medial orbital wall, and lateral orbital wall.

Injuries
Orbital fractures may occur in isolation secondary to low-energy injuries or exist as part of a more complex maxillofacial fracture pattern with greater forces, including zygomaticomaxillary complex (ZMC), Le Fort, and NOE fractures. Several typical injury patterns are seen.

The orbital blow-out fracture results from impact to the bony orbital margins by an object larger than the orbit with sufficient force to increase intraorbital pressure and fracture the thin walls of the orbital floor, medial orbital wall, or both.[17] Blow-out fractures are considered pure when the thicker orbital rim remains intact. The free fragment sign on CT denotes an isolated bony fragment within the adjacent sinus reflecting a depressed or displaced orbital floor fracture (**Fig. 4**). With acute fracture, hemorrhage is expected in the adjacent

paranasal sinus. If the sinuses are clear, the injury is almost certainly remote. Fractures through the medial orbital wall that are not simple isolated blow-out fractures should raise suspicion of higher-energy midface fractures, namely NOE, Le Fort II, or Le Fort III fracture patterns.

Complications of orbital blow-out fractures include extraocular muscle herniation, enophthalmos, and orbital emphysema. Although orbital emphysema is usually self-limited, it warrants comment because it can cause mass effect on the adjacent soft tissues and be a rare cause of decreased vision due to either central retinal artery occlusion or optic neuropathy.[18]

The orbital blow-in fracture results from a high-energy impact to the frontal bone with fracture and depression of orbital roof fragments into the orbit (**Fig. 5**A). Blow-in fractures are often associated with intracranial injury (**Fig. 5**B) and decreased orbital volume leading to exophthalmos. Associated ocular injuries are reported in 14% to 29% of cases.[19] If the orbital roof fracture propagates to the orbital apex, the optic nerve can be injured by direct fracture fragment penetration, hemorrhage into the sheath, avulsion from the posterior globe, or ischemia resulting from increased intraorbital pressure. If there is imaging and clinical evidence of optic nerve impingement, emergent surgical treatment is warranted because this can be associated with cavernous carotid artery injury and blindness.

The orbital blow-up fracture is characterized by intracranial displacement of the orbital roof fragment and is strongly indicative of associated intracranial injury (**Fig. 6**).

Isolated lateral orbital wall fractures can occur but are more commonly associated with ZMC fractures.

CT imaging plays a key role not only in diagnosis of these fractures but also in determining management. Although indications for surgical repair are controversial, evidence of mechanical extraocular muscle entrapment or evidence of enophthalmos are well-established criteria mandating urgent repair. Coronal CT is particularly useful for displaying herniation and can suggest entrapment based on kinking of a muscle or isolation of the inferior rectus muscle. The inferior rectus muscle normally appears oval on coronal images; if it appears round, pathology should be suspected. Trapdoor fractures, most common in pediatric patients secondary to more pliable bone, occur when the orbital floor is fractured and displaced inferiorly but then snaps back into place. If the herniated inferior rectus muscle is trapped across the fracture, it is at high risk of ischemia. Extraocular muscle entrapment is a surgical emergency; however, it must be made clear that lack of evidence of

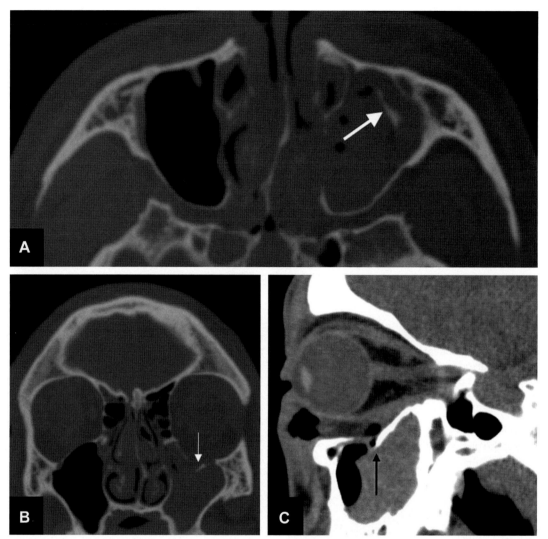

Fig. 4. Orbital blow-out fractures. (*A*) Transaxial CT image of a 34-year-old man after interpersonal assault. There is left malar swelling and opacification of the left maxillary sinus. Within the sinus is a bony free fragment (*arrow*), indicating a displaced or depressed left orbital floor fracture. (*B*) Coronal CT reformation of the same patient shows the left orbital floor fracture displaced into the maxillary sinus (*arrow*). (*C*) Oblique sagittal CT reformation of a different patient with an orbital floor fracture (*arrow*). This projection optimally shows the posterior extent of injury to aid in surgical planning.

entrapment on CT does not exclude the condition and a careful physical examination is critical for diagnosis.

Another parameter in determining the need for surgical intervention is the size of the orbital floor defect. Larger defects increase the risk of future enophthalmos, whereby the globe sinks posteriorly and inferiorly into the underlying maxillary sinus. Many surgeons opt to repair any defect greater than 1 cm^2, whereas others use 50% of the orbital floor involvement. Yet other surgeons estimate the amount of fat or soft tissue displacement to determine the need for surgery.

Some use CT to measure the increase in orbital volume compared with the uninjured side and then use this to determine the risk for postinjury enophthalmos; however, no firm data exist to support this approach. Because criteria vary among surgeons, the size of each orbital floor fracture defect should be estimated in the radiology report.

Surgical repair can consist of either a bone graft from the outer table of the skull or the use of a titanium or resorbable implant. If an implant is used, the patient should be monitored for new-onset diplopia, and, if present, emergent CT scan should

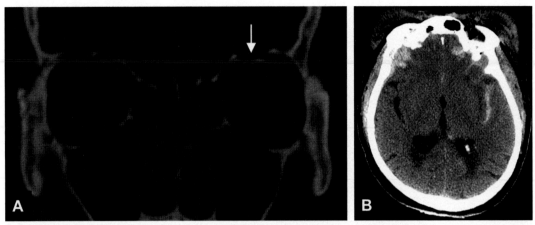

Fig. 5. Orbital blow-in fracture. A 50-year-old man found down. (*A*) Coronal CT reformation through the midorbits demonstrates a left blow-in fracture (*arrow*) of the orbital roof (floor of the anterior cranial fossa) with depressed fragment. (*B*) Transaxial CT head image of the same patient reveals marked bifrontal soft tissue and intracranial injury with extensive subarachnoid hemorrhage and frontal lobe contusions.

be performed to ensure there is no mechanical impedance. When evaluating for placement, care should be taken to ensure that floor implants are properly aligned to simulate the superior incline of the posterior orbital floor.

Globe injury

Injury to the globe or optic nerve or the presence of retrobulbar hematoma is a critical soft tissue

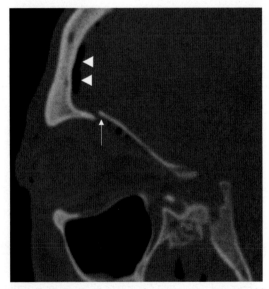

Fig. 6. Orbital blow-up fracture. A 40-year-old man assaulted. Oblique sagittal CT reformation show cranial displacement of orbital roof fracture fragment (*arrow*). Note pneumocephalus (*arrowheads*) implying violation of the dura.

emergency and should be a priority when approaching a facial CT.[20]

Globe rupture is typically the result of a penetrating ocular injury. Higher intraocular pressure and lower infraorbital pressure favor extrusion of the vitreous producing the flat tire sign on CT seen as posterior flattening of the ruptured globe (**Fig. 7A**).[21] Globe hemorrhage can be intravitreous, subscleral, or subretinal (**Fig. 7B**).

Lens dislocation is diagnosed by a lens lying dependently on the retina. Lens subluxation results from a partial tear of the zonular fibers and is seen on CT as an oblique or vertically oriented lens (see **Fig. 7A**). If one lens appears relatively hypodense, acute lens edema should be suspected because this may lead to a traumatic cataract. The difference in attenuation is usually approximately 30 Hounsfield units.[22]

CT scan plays an important role in evaluation of the optic nerve, because clinical examination may be challenging or impossible in the acute setting. Transaxial and oblique sagittal images are particularly helpful in determining the presence of an optic nerve hematoma suggesting injury to the nerve (**Fig. 7C**).

Detectability of intraocular foreign bodies is determined by size and density. Metallic foreign bodies are readily identified; however, plastic and dry wood appear hypodense on CT, similar to fat and air, respectively.[23] Differentiating air from foreign body can be difficult but the presence of geometric margins supports foreign body. In challenging situations for other nonmetallic foreign bodies, MR imaging can be helpful once a

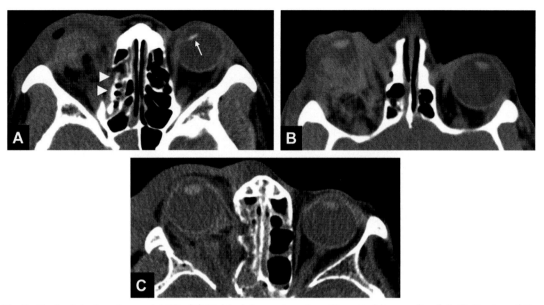

Fig. 7. Ocular injuries—transaxial CTs. (*A*) Right globe rupture in a 42-year-old man after fall. Flattening of the posterior globe is common, referred to as the flat tire sign. Patient also suffered a medial orbital wall fracture (*arrowheads*) and a left ocular lens subluxation (*arrow*). (*B*) Globe hemorrhage on the left seen in a 38-year-old man after penetrating injury. (*C*) Right optic nerve injury in a 77-year-old man after fall seen as ill-defined margins of the optic nerve and its attachment to the posterior globe with retrobulbar hematoma. This patient also suffered a medial orbital wall fracture on the right.

noncontrast head or face CT has excluded a metallic foreign body.

The presence of a carotid-cavernous fistula, although rare, is a condition that requires emergent intervention and must be recognized. This diagnosis is suggested by the presence of a dilated superior ophthalmic vein, a nonspecific finding that mandates confirmation with CT angiography, MR angiography, or conventional catheter angiography.[24]

Zygoma Fractures

Anatomy
The paired zygoma bones form the anterolateral cheek projections and a large portion of the lateral orbital walls and orbital floors. The zygoma is a thick bone and contributes to the buttress system of the midface with 4 principal attachments that are often the site of injury—namely the zygomaticofrontal suture, the zygomaticomaxillary suture, the zygomaticotemporal suture, and the zygomaticosphenoid suture.

Injuries
The prominent position of the zygoma makes it particularly susceptible to traumatic injury and is the second most common isolated facial fracture.[25] A common fracture pattern is the ZMC fracture pattern, resulting from an anterolateral impact

to the cheek that effectively separates the zygoma along its sutural attachments (**Fig. 8**). These fractures can occur from low-energy and high-energy trauma; thus, the ZMC pattern represents a spectrum of fractures varying in the degree of bone loss and displacement. Historically referred to as a tripod fracture, the term is a misnomer and should be avoided, because it overlooks the posterior attachments of the zygoma to the sphenoid bone.

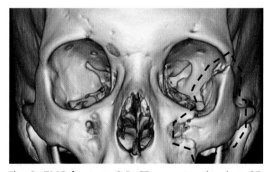

Fig. 8. ZMC fracture. 3-D CT reconstruction in a 25-year-old man after assault shows left ZMC fracture pattern (*dashed outline*). Fracture lines are limited to the zygoma sutural attachments; with higher energy forces, there is often fracture of the zygoma body as well.

Isolated fractures of the zygomatic arch are uncommon and only require operative reduction when there is severe depression causing cosmetic deformity or impingement on the mandibular coronoid process with inability to completely close the jaw (**Fig. 9**).[26] Fractures along the zygomaticomaxillary suture often involve the infraorbital canal injuring the infraorbital nerve (V2), resulting in malar paresthesia.

CT is crucial in determining operative management of zygoma fractures, particularly because acute swelling often precludes accurate clinical assessment of the deformity. 2-D multiplanar and 3-D images are particularly helpful to assess the degree of comminution and displacement, because severe comminution affects the preferred surgical approach for exposing and subsequently aligning the arch.

Zygoma fractures may be isolated or part of other midface fractures. For example, concurrent mandible fractures are seen in 21% of zygomatic arch fractures.[27] The orbital floor and orbital apex are also commonly injured. As discussed with orbital floor fractures, there are multiple criteria for orbital exploration, and CT findings of degree of comminution and displacement should be reported. For orbitozygomatic fractures, the lateral orbital wall in particular should be assessed on the transaxial images. Nondisplaced orbitozygomatic fractures can be managed nonoperatively. With medial displacement of the greater wing of the sphenoid into the orbital apex, however, there is potential danger to the internal carotid artery, cavernous sinus, and cranial nerves.[28] Displaced fractures almost always require operative reduction and internal fixation and should be performed as soon as possible, to avoid malunion and delayed riskier repair.

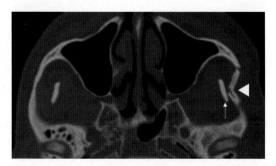

Fig. 9. Depressed zygomatic arch fracture. Transaxial CT image of a 51-year-old man postassault shows a comminuted depressed left zygomatic arch fracture (*arrowhead*). Fragments impinge on the coronoid process of the mandible (*arrow*).

Maxillary Fractures

Anatomy

The central midface is composed of the paired maxillae, which form the upper jaw. The maxillae house the maxillary teeth by way of the alveolus, and attach laterally to the zygomatic bones. The thicker bony margins of the maxillae are major contributors to the facial buttresses. The facial buttress system highlights lines of inherent strength across the midface, with the strongest buttresses being vertically oriented, and the horizontal buttresses providing secondary support (**Fig. 10**).

Injuries

There are 3 classic fracture patterns of the maxilla, the Le Fort I, II, and III, which by definition detach the maxilla from the skull base via fracture through the pterygoid plates (**Fig. 11**).[29] Although Le Fort's descriptions outlined symmetric midface fracture patterns, most midface fractures are asymmetric. Therefore, it is often useful to describe hemi–Le Fort fracture patterns for each side.

The Le Fort I fracture pattern results from direct impact to the upper jaw, creating a free-floating hard palate with consequent malocclusion. This is characterized by a transverse fracture line across the maxilla passing above the tooth roots, crossing the floor of the maxillary sinus and into the anterolateral nasal aperture (also referred to as the piriform aperture), with posterior extension through the pterygoid plates (**Fig. 12**). It does not involve the infraorbital rims.

The Le Fort II fracture pattern results from direct impact to the central midface effectively separating the nasal region from the cranium. This pattern is characterized by a pyramidal fracture line that generally follows the zygomaticomaxillary sutures, fracturing the inferior orbital rims medially, and crossing the nasal bridge. Posteriorly, there is extension of fracture through the pterygoid plates (see **Fig. 11**).

The Le Fort III fracture pattern results from high-energy direct impact to the upper midface causing complete craniofacial disjunction. This pattern is characterized by an essentially transverse fracture crossing the nasal bridge, and the medial and lateral orbital walls, with disruption of the zygomaticofrontal sutures. The fracture continues laterally through zygomatic arches and posteriorly through the pterygoid plates to completely separate the facial skeleton from the calvarium (**Fig. 13**).

Because Le Fort fractures usually result in marked damage to the facial buttresses, they can cause significant functional deficiencies and cosmetic deformities. Often, similar to NOE

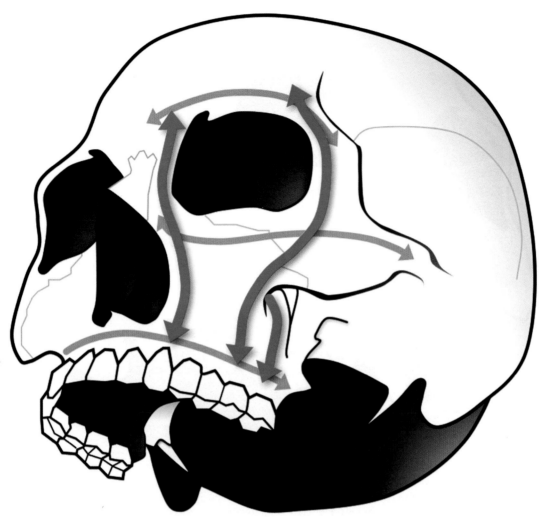

Fig. 10. Facial buttresses. Strong vertical buttresses are shown as curved thick red double arrows. From medial to lateral these are the nasofrontal buttress, zygomatic buttress, and pterygomaxillary buttress. The horizontal buttresses are shown as curved, thinner gray double arrows.

fractures, there is posterior impaction and displacement of the central midface. Additionally, disruption of the vertical buttresses leads of loss of facial height. Given the high incidence of concurrent facial fractures, surgical repair after these injuries is usually complex and surgical planning is aided by high-quality 3-D reconstructions in multiple projections simulating the historic anteroposterior, Water, Towne, lateral, and oblique radiographic views.

Of particular concern are the highly associated concomitant fractures of the hard palate, dentoalveolar units, and mandible, which disrupt the occlusion. Reestablishment of normal occlusion must occur before attempting to surgically anchor the upper midface to the maxilla. Similarly, injury to the supraorbital transverse buttress (frontal bar)

from concurrent NOE, frontal sinus, or ZMC fractures requires correction prior to resuspending and reconstructing the midface from this buttress.

Degree of comminution is another important factor as severe comminution may limit adequate restoration of facial height and projection, thus necessitating bone grafting.

Importantly, many Le Fort III fractures involve the orbital apex with associated injuries to the carotid canal. Because the surgical repair mechanism for Le Fort fractures generally entails the use of significant manual traction on the part of the surgeon, it is important for the surgeon to know preoperatively how close the fracture line extends to the orbital apex and carotid canal so that a more gentle reduction technique can be used.

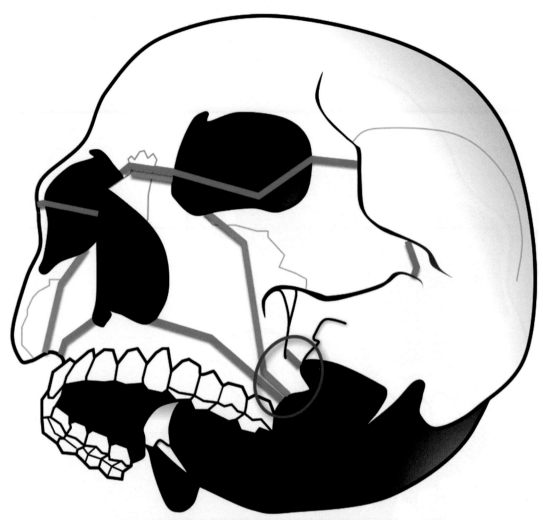

Fig. 11. Le Fort fracture patterns. Le Fort I pattern (*green lines*) traverses the lower maxillae and crosses the nasal aperture and lower nasal septum. Le Fort II pattern (*blue lines*) courses obliquely across the maxillae to the inferior orbital rims and crosses the nasal bridge. Le Fort III pattern (*red lines*) transversely crosses the orbits and nasal bridge, and involves the zygomatic arches. All Le Fort patterns extend posteriorly to fracture the ptyergoid plates (*purple oval*).

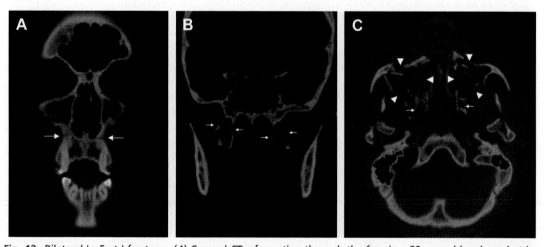

Fig. 12. Bilateral Le Fort I fractures. (*A*) Coronal CT reformation through the face in a 39-year-old male pedestrian struck shows fractures of the anterior maxillary walls extending medially through the nasal aperture bilaterally (*arrows*). (*B*) Coronal CT image of same patient posteriorly shows fractures through the bilateral pterygoid plates (*arrows*), indicative of the Le Fort fracture pattern. (*C*) Transaxial CT image at the level of the maxillae shows multiple fractures of the anterior, medial, and posterolateral maxillary walls bilaterally (*white arrowheads*). There is comminution of the pterygoid plates bilaterally (*white arrows*). Also present are bilateral mandibular condylar fractures (*black arrows*).

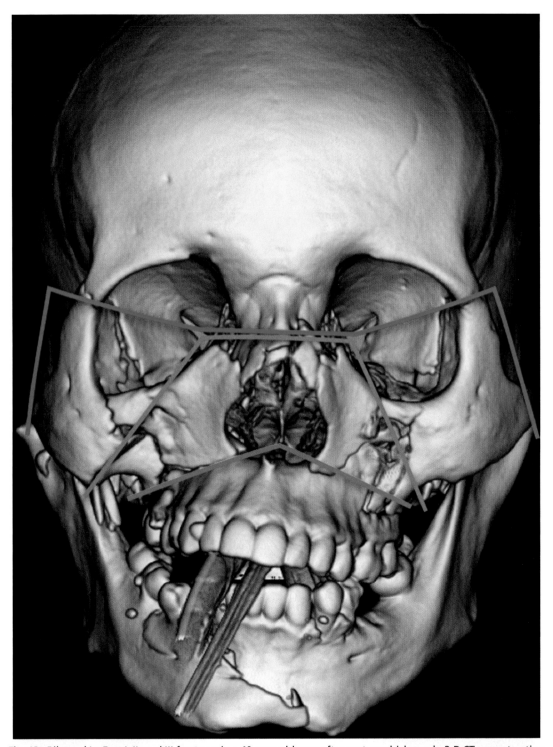

Fig. 13. Bilateral Le Fort I, II, and III fractures in a 40-year-old man after motor vehicle crash. 3-D CT reconstruction shows bilateral Le Fort I pattern (*green line*), bilateral Le Fort II pattern (*blue lines*), and bilateral Le Fort III fracture pattern (*red lines*).

Mandibular Fractures

Anatomy

The mandible forms the lower jaw, holds the mandibular teeth in place, and serves as an attachment for the muscles of mastication. Anatomically, the mandible is a bent horseshoe-shaped bone with a curved anterior symphysis, 2 horizontal mandibular bodies, and 2 perpendicular posterior vertical rami. The junction of the ramus and body is referred to as the mandibular angle. There is a superior anterior projection from each ramus, the coronoid process, which serves as the attachment for the temporalis muscle, as well as a superior posterior projection from each ramus, the condyle, which articulates with the temporal bone at the temporomandibular joint. The temporomandibular joints are the only mobile segments of the facial skeleton and are complex synovial joints that permit hinge, multidirectional translation, and rotational movements. Additionally, the mandible contains the inferior alveolar nerve canal, which houses the inferior alveolar nerve (V3) to provide sensation to the jaw.

Injuries

Mandible fractures are susceptible to low-energy forces and consequently represent a large proportion of facial fractures, typically from interpersonal

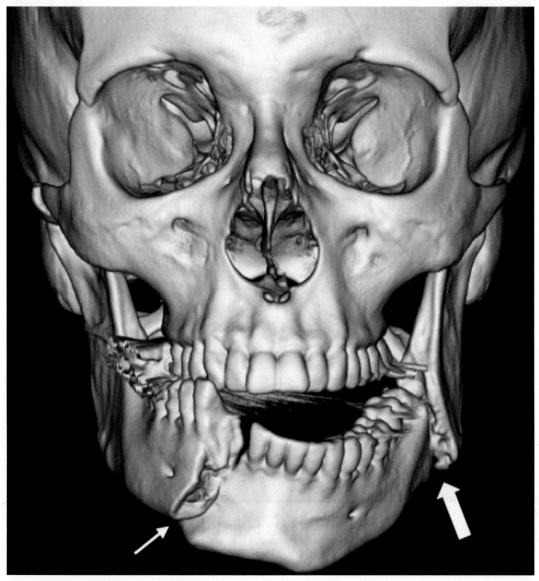

Fig. 14. Mandible fractures. 3-D CT reconstruction in 22 year old postassault shows a right parasymphseal fracture (*thin arrow*) and contralateral angle fracture (*thick arrow*).

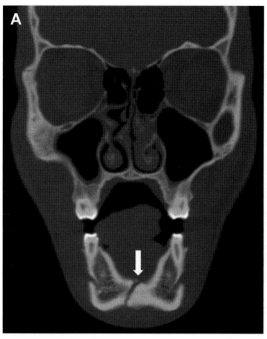
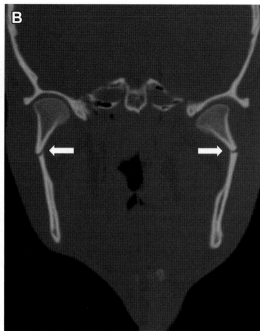

Fig. 15. Flail mandible in 32-year-old man found down intoxicated. Anterior (*A*) and posterior (*B*) coronal CT reformations show a symphyseal fracture (*arrow* [*A*]) and bilateral condylar fractures (*arrows* [*B*]).

assaults.[30] They are classified and described according to anatomic region (symphysis, parasymphysis, body, angle, ramus, coronoid, subcondylar, and condyle). Because the mandible is an incomplete ring a second fracture is present in approximately two-thirds of cases and should always be sought and excluded.[22] Common 2-part fractures include the parasymphyseal fracture with either a contralateral subcondylar or angle fracture (**Fig. 14**). A flail mandible is a symphyseal fracture with bilateral subcondylar fractures that necessitates surgery to restore preinjury facial width and height (**Fig. 15**).

CT with multiplanar reformations is nearly 100% sensitive in detecting fractures of the mandible, which is superior to the 86% sensitivity of curved panoramic (panorex) radiographs. Panoramic CT reformations can be generated and are useful to illustrate bilateral fractures in a single image (**Fig. 16**). CT, however, may be insufficient to evaluate some dental structures and the panorex radiograph can better visualize dental root fractures, particularly when the fracture is located at the angle.[31] The panorex radiograph requires cervical spine clearance and is typically performed in the inpatient or outpatient setting rather than in an emergency department.

Many surgeons consider mandibular fractures through the tooth socket and alveolus as open fractures and, therefore, regard them as contaminated, an indication for antibiotic prophylaxis. Acute tooth loss is implied by a radiolucent socket and should prompt further evaluation for aspirated or ingested tooth fragments. Some surgeons recommend tooth extraction if the fracture contains a tooth or if there is evidence of abscess.

The primary goal in repairing mandible fractures is to restore preinjury occlusion. Management ranges from nonoperative to mandibulomaxillary fixation with arch bars and occlusal wiring, to open reduction and internal fixation, or, in cases of contaminated wound, to external fixation.[32]

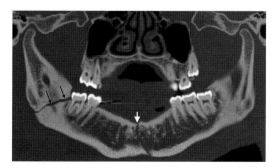

Fig. 16. Mandible fracture in a 37 year old post assault. Panoramic curved CT reformation elegantly shows an angle fracture on the right (*black arrows*) and a midline symphyseal fracture (*white arrow*). The angle fracture extends through the right third molar, thus making this injury an open fracture.

SUMMARY

Maxillofacial fractures and ocular injuries are common. Knowledge of fracture patterns and their implication for management is crucial to facilitating effective and efficient communication between the radiologist and the referring physician to best serve victims of facial trauma.

REFERENCES

1. Pathria MN, Blaser SI. Diagnostic imaging of craniofacial fractures. Radiol Clin North Am 1989;27:839–53.
2. Rehm CG, Ross SE. Diagnosis of unsuspected facial fractures on routine head computed tomographic scans in the unconscious multiply injured patient. J Oral Maxillofac Surg 1995;53:522–4.
3. Rogers LF. The face. In: Rogers LF, editor. Radiology of skeletal trauma. New York: Churchill Livingstone; 1982. p. 229.
4. Luce EA, Tubb TD, Moore AM. Review of 1,000 major facial fractures and associated injuries. Plast Reconstr Surg 1979;63(1):26–30.
5. Mulligan RP, Friedman JA, Mahabir RC. A nationwide review of the associations among cervical spine injuries, head injuries, and facial fractures. J Trauma 2010;68(3):587–92.
6. Levy RA, Edwards WT, Meyer JR, et al. Facial trauma and 3D reconstructive imaging: insufficiencies and correctives. AJNR Am J Neuroradiol 1992;13:885–92.
7. Manson PN, Markowitz B, Mirvis S, et al. Toward CT-based facial fracture treatment. Plast Reconstr Surg 1990;85(2):202–12.
8. Muraoka M, Nakai Y. Twenty years of statistics and observation of facial bone fracture. Acta Otolaryngol Suppl 1998;538:261–5.
9. Leipziger LS, Manson PN. Nasoethmoid orbital fractures: current concepts and management principles. Clin Plast Surg 1992;19:167–93.
10. Markowitz BL, Manson PN, Sargent L, et al. Management of the medial canthal tendon in nasoethmoid orbital fractures: the importance of the central fragment in classification and treatment. Plast Reconstr Surg 1991;87(5):843–53.
11. May M, Ogura JH, Schramm V. Nasofrontal duct in frontal sinus fractures. Arch Otolaryngol 1970;92:534–8.
12. Rohrich RJ, Hollier LH. Management of frontal sinus fractures: changing concepts. Clin Plast Surg 1992;19:219–32.
13. Rodriguez ED, Stanwix MG, Nam AJ, et al. Twenty-six year experience treating frontal sinus fractures: a novel algorithm based on anatomical fracture pattern and failure of conventional techniques. Plast Reconstr Surg 2008;122(6):1850–66.
14. Bell RB. Management of frontal sinus fractures. Oral Maxillofac Surg Clin North Am 2009;21(2):227–42.
15. Tiwari P, Higuera S, Thornton J, et al. The management of frontal sinus fractures. J Oral Maxillofac Surg 2005;63(9):1354–60.
16. Tedaldi M, Ramieri V, Foresta E, et al. Experience in the management of frontal sinus fractures. J Craniofac Surg 2010;21(1):208–10.
17. Pfeifer RL. Traumatic enophthalmos. Trans Am Ophthalmol Soc 1943;41:293–306.
18. Key SJ, Ryba F, Holmes S, et al. Orbital emphysema— the need for surgical intervention. J Craniomaxillofac Surg 2008;36(8):473–6.
19. Lawrason JN, Novelline RA. Diagnostic imaging of facial trauma. In: Mirvis SE, Young JWR, editors. Diagnostic imaging in trauma and critical care. Baltimore (MD): Williams & Wilkins; 1992. p. 243–90.
20. Lee HJ, Jilani M, Frohman L, et al. CT of orbital trauma. Emerg Radiol 2004;10(4):168–72.
21. Sevel D, Krausz H, Ponder T, et al. Value of computed tomography for the diagnosis of a ruptured eye. J Comput Assist Tomogr 1983;7: 870–5.
22. Rhea JT, Rao PM, Novelline RA. Helical CT and three-dimensional CT of facial and orbital injury. Radiol Clin North Am 1999;37:489–513.
23. Myllylä V, Pyhtinen J, Päivänsalo M, et al. CT detection and location of intraorbital foreign bodies: experiments with wood and glass. Rofo 1987;146: 639–43.
24. Anderson K, Collie DA, Capewell A. CT angiographic appearances of carotico-cavernous fistula. Clin Radiol 2001;56(6):514–6.
25. Noyek AM, Kassel EE, Wortzman G, et al. Contemporary radiologic evaluation in maxillofacial trauma. Otolaryngol Clin North Am 1983;16:473–508.
26. Carlin CB, Ruff G, Mansfeld CP, et al. Facial fractures and related injuries: a ten year retrospective analysis. J Craniomaxillofac Trauma 1998;4:44.
27. Obuekwe O, Owotade F, Osaiyuwu O. Etiology and pattern of zygomatic complex fractures: a retrospective study. J Natl Med Assoc 2005;97:992.
28. Linnau KF, Hallam DK, Lomoschitz FM, et al. Orbital apex injury: trauma at the junction between the face and the cranium. Eur J Radiol 2003;48(1):5–16.
29. Le Fort R. Étude experimentale sur les fractures de la machoire supérieure. Rev Chir Paris 1901;23: 208–27, 360–79.
30. Calloway DM, Anton MA, Jacobs JS. Changing concepts and controversies in the management of mandibular fractures. Clin Plast Surg 1992;19:59–69.
31. Wilson IF, Lokeh A, Benjamin CI, et al. Prospective comparison of panoramic tomography (zonography) and helical computed tomography in the diagnosis and operative management of mandibular fractures. Plast Reconstr Surg 2001;107:1369.
32. Stacey DH, Doyle JF, Mount DL, et al. Management of mandible fractures. Plast Reconstr Surg 2006; 117(3):48e–60e.

Radiation Dose Considerations in Emergent Neuroimaging

Walter F. Wiggins, MD, PhD, Aaron D. Sodickson, MD, PhD*

KEYWORDS

- Emergency radiology • Neuroimaging • Radiation dose • Computed tomography • CT angiography
- CT perfusion • Trauma CT

KEY POINTS

- Appropriate computed tomography use with defined imaging algorithms or clinical decision support tools is a crucial step in a patient-centered approach to radiation dose management in emergent neuroimaging.
- Thoughtful computed tomography neuroimaging protocol design reduces radiation exposure by limiting the range and phases of the scan to the minimum necessary to achieve the diagnostic goal.
- Modern scanner and image postprocessing technologies, when properly applied, can synergistically reduce radiation dose while maintaining diagnostic image quality.
- Radiation exposure monitoring on a population level is critical to ensure quality and identify outliers.

INTRODUCTION

Patients presenting with acute problems of the head, neck, spine, and central nervous system frequently require 1 or more diagnostic imaging studies as part of their initial diagnostic evaluation. For many such patients, particularly hospital inpatients and patients presenting to the emergency department (ED), the first imaging test is often a computed tomography (CT) scan of the relevant anatomic region. When appropriate, the benefits of CT typically far outweigh the potential risks. However, for young patients and/or patients with chronic conditions, the cumulative radiation dose from serial diagnostic imaging studies over time raises the concern for possible increased cancer risk as a result of medical imaging.[1,2] Public perception of CT use and radiation dose issues has been heavily influenced by heightened media attention to potential radiation risks in recent years, such as articles published in the *New York Times'* series "Radiation Boom," which have highlighted prominent radiation dose overexposure events[3] as well as the increasing use of CT and concerns regarding the potential cancer risk of the attendant radiation dose.[4,5] As a result, patients are more likely than in the past to have questions about CT radiation dose that prompt a risk–benefit discussion before or after a scan. Referring physicians and physician extenders should have some familiarity with the topic, because they will often be the recipients of such questions. However, radiologists should be prepared to serve as consultants in this regard, and to have these discussions directly with patients. A framework to prepare for such conversations is provided as a reference.[6] Ultimately, the responsibility for managing radiation dose falls on radiologists as the custodians of diagnostic imaging, albeit with considerable collaboration from referring providers, radiologic technologists, medical physicists, and equipment manufacturers.

When considering the risk–benefit calculus of CT radiation dose in emergency neuroimaging, it

Department of Radiology, Brigham and Women's Hospital, Harvard Medical School, 75 Francis Street, Boston, MA 02115, USA
* Corresponding author.
E-mail address: asodickson@bwh.harvard.edu

Neuroimag Clin N Am 28 (2018) 525–536
https://doi.org/10.1016/j.nic.2018.03.010

is critical to remember that CT has become a vital tool for efficiently diagnosing and excluding neurologic conditions that require emergent intervention. To avoid CT or minimize the dose at the expense of adequate diagnostic quality would be folly, because failure to diagnose such conditions in an expedient manner puts patients at far greater risk in the short term, rendering the potential risks associated with radiation exposure irrelevant. However, it is equally important to design CT protocols and monitor the resulting radiation dose to help mitigate both the short-term deterministic effects of a single radiation dose event and the potential long-term, stochastic effects of cumulative radiation dose.

In this article, we explore strategies for a patient-centered approach to managing radiation dose in emergent neuroimaging from the patient's initial presentation to after the scan. This discussion reviews methods for facilitating the appropriate use of diagnostic CT in emergent neuroimaging, taking full advantage of commonly available scanner and image postprocessing technologies in the design and modification of CT examination protocols, and tracking data from these examinations at a population level to inform future iterations of these processes. We conclude with a brief discussion of emerging CT technologies that may facilitate further decreases in radiation exposure from CT in the future. Detailed discussions of more general strategies for reducing CT radiation dose and the concerns regarding cumulative radiation exposure are beyond the scope of this article, although examples from the literature are provided as references.[1,2,7,8]

BEFORE THE SCAN: THE APPROPRIATE USE OF COMPUTED TOMOGRAPHY IMAGING

The most important consideration in patient-centered management before the patient arrives in the CT scanner suite is the determination of the most appropriate imaging study for a given phase of a patient's care. This is no longer simply part of best practices in patient care, but a legal requirement for reimbursement when providing diagnostic imaging services to Medicare patients. In 2014, the US Congress passed bill H.R. 4302, or the Protecting Access to Medicare Act of 2014 (PAMA), which will require medical providers to consult appropriate use criteria (AUC) using an approved clinical decision support (CDS) mechanism before ordering advanced diagnostic imaging for Medicare patients in the outpatient setting, including the ED.[9] As of January 1, 2017, this rule is in effect and any diagnostic imaging services provided to a Medicare patient will be reimbursed by CMS only if documentation indicating the CDS mechanism consulted and supporting whether (a) the service provided adheres or does not adhere to the available AUC or (b) if no applicable AUC were available. It is pertinent to note that there are exceptions defined for patients with "emergency medical conditions" and for providers exempted on a case-by-case basis owing to "significant hardship" in consulting a CDS mechanism. It is also pertinent to note that Sec. 218(a) of PAMA, in which these requirements for AUC and CDS are defined, is titled "Quality Incentives to Promote Patient Safety and Public Health in Computed Tomography Diagnostic Imaging," suggesting that the lawmakers involved in writing PAMA were motivated by concerns for potential overuse of CT imaging and its attendant radiation exposure to patients.

The Medicare Appropriate Use Criteria Program maintains a list[10] of qualified "provider-led entities" that have been approved for the development and endorsement of AUC. For example, the American College of Radiology has been named by the Centers for Medicare & Medicaid Services as a provider-led entity, which means that the American College of Radiology Appropriateness Criteria,[11] a freely available, searchable online database of evidence-based guidelines for both diagnostic and interventional radiology, meet the requirements for AUC as defined in PAMA. For each topic in the Appropriateness Criteria database, "Narrative & Rating Table" and "Evidence Table" documents are provided. Examples of common indications for neuroimaging that can be found in the Appropriateness Criteria database include focal neurologic deficit, head trauma, headache, and low back pain. The Medicare AUC Program also maintains a list of qualified CDS mechanisms, including commercially available software packages that can be integrated into an electronic health record or computerized physician order entry (CPOE) systems.

The authors of this article advocate for the use of CPOE-integrated CDS, given the support in the literature for its role in facilitating appropriate CT use. In a recent study of interphysician variability in head CT ordering among emergency physicians, the authors identified 2-fold variability for all indications, increasing to nearly 3-fold for patients diagnosed with atraumatic headaches.[12] A subsequent study from another institution found that head CT was ordered for minor head injuries with an excess of 37% in comparison with the number of scans expected by application of the Canadian CT Head Rule.[13,14] This observation was particularly pronounced in younger patients. In their analysis of ordering patterns, the authors identified physician specialty and mechanism of injury as significant contributors to the overuse of head CT scans, suggesting that CPOE-integrated CDS might help to reduce the incidence of nonindicated CT by encouraging more careful consideration of the indications, citing 1 of 2 recent studies from another institution.[15,16] In the first of these 2 studies, the authors found a 56% relative increase in adherence to evidence-based guidelines after the implementation of CDS for head CT ordering in the context of mild traumatic brain injury in the institution's CPOE system.[15] A follow-up study demonstrated an absolute decrease of 8% in the number of ED visits for mild traumatic brain injury resulting in a head CT scan.[16] These data suggest that one might expect some positive effect of similar interventions for ordering of other CT neuroimaging studies as well.

Given the legal requirements from the Centers for Medicare & Medicaid Services for the consultation of AUC in the ordering of CT imaging and complementary data in the literature supporting the use of CPOE-integrated CDS systems, a key point to consider is the implementation of such a system. An interdisciplinary approach to the implementation of a CPOE-integrated CDS system is critical to ensure the success of such a system. Collaboration with clinicians on the ordering end of the system should help to identify potential barriers to implementation and appropriate use, as well as preemptive solutions that may be implemented before the institutional launch of the new system. Not only should this help to mitigate some of the initial problems that may arise for the end-users, but it may also help to increase compliance and perceived usefulness by involving representatives on both ends of the system. The inclusion of structured indications into such a system may provide additional benefit and increase efficiency on both ends by presenting referring clinicians with a "pick list" of structured indications deemed appropriate for a given study, while providing the individuals protocolling and interpreting the studies with succinct, relevant clinical history for each patient. For example, the implementation of a structured CPOE for trauma CT imaging studies was shown to significantly increase the percentage of requisitions containing relevant, specific clinical history, as well as the billing efficiency and reimbursement success of examinations submitted to insurance providers, which can be interpreted as a "soft" indicator for the appropriateness of the indications.[17]

Although CT is often the first-line imaging test for acute neurologic syndromes, MR imaging can perform as well or better than CT for certain indications without concern for ionizing radiation. Rapid acquisition brain MR imaging protocols have been suggested and evaluated for certain indications.[18,19] The potential for radiation dose savings are particularly pronounced for young individuals and/or individuals undergoing frequent imaging evaluation, as is the case for many patients with ventricular shunt with suspected shunt malfunction.[20] Ultrafast brain MR imaging in the setting of suspected acute ischemic stroke has been studied and shown to be safe,[20] with potential for improved selection of candidates who might benefit from intraarterial thrombolytic therapies.[21–23]

DURING THE SCAN: TECHNICAL CONSIDERATIONS
Patient-Centered Protocol Optimization

Once the requisition for CT examination has been submitted, the next step in a patient-centered approach to emergent neuroimaging is to consider the extent of imaging required to achieve the diagnostic goal. This is of importance when planning neurovascular CT imaging, including CT angiography (CTA) and CT brain perfusion, and for CT examinations of multiple anatomic regions along the neuroaxis, including CT neuroimaging in the setting of trauma. Multiple approaches to protocolling emergent CT neuroimaging can be considered, ranging from active monitoring and live protocolling of certain scans by a radiologist to the selection of standardized protocols for specific indications by a radiologist or CT technologist. The preferred approach at any given institution will depend on the availability and training of staff, as well as the impact of different approaches on the clinical workflow from the perspectives of the radiology department and the management of individual patients. The approach may also differ depending on the specific indication for the study. In this section, we focus on considerations affecting radiation dose in the general design of neuroimaging protocols for the evaluation of suspected acute stroke/intracranial hemorrhage and in the setting of trauma.

Per the most recent guidelines from the American Heart Association and American Stroke Association for the early management of patients with acute ischemic stroke, the preferred initial diagnostic imaging study is unenhanced (or noncontrast) CT imaging of the brain to assess for the presence of hemorrhage and determine eligibility for treatment with intravenous administration of tissue plasminogen activator.[24] The guidelines further recommend noninvasive intracranial vascular imaging if endovascular therapy is considered. Neurovascular CTA is preferred over

MR angiography, given its rapid acquisition time, slightly higher sensitivity/specificity, and high interobserver agreement for such lesions.[25,26] Although the American Heart Association/American Stroke Association guidelines focus on the management of patients with acute ischemic stroke, other recommendations emphasize the usefulness of neurovascular CTA to evaluate for underlying lesions in the assessment of intracranial hemorrhage.[27]

Neurovascular computed tomography imaging protocols in suspected stroke

Apart from image acquisition technique (discussed elsewhere in this article), the principal considerations when designing protocols for neurovascular CT imaging include the anatomic range of the scan, which phase(s) of contrast will be imaged, and whether CT perfusion (CTP) imaging will be performed, if available. Regarding the anatomic range of the scan, the American Heart Association/American Stroke Association guidelines for acute ischemic stroke only explicitly recommend intracranial vascular imaging; however, a common practice with modern scanner technology is to image from the aortic arch to the vertex of the skull to evaluate the anatomy of the aortic arch and assess for lesions of the neck vessels. A retrospective study of ED neurovascular CTA examinations questioned the value of this practice, the low incidence of clinically significant findings in the mediastinum (1% of cases studied), and the relatively high proportion of the overall radiation dose to the patient (50% in this study) derived from scanning the upper chest.[28] However, this study did find that 31% of patients had clinically significant findings in the neck vessels, leading the authors to conclude that there is likely sufficient benefit to justify the inclusion of the neck in the neurovascular CTA protocol. The authors further identified an important limitation of their study, which was that the retrospective nature of their study and its reliance on review of radiologic reports for identification of significant findings may have excluded important discussions between radiologists and members of the neurology and neurointervention teams at the time of interpretation and, thus, potentially underestimated the percentage of cases with clinically significant findings in the upper chest that were not ultimately included in the final report. Nevertheless, this study raises the possibility that excluding the upper chest from the neurovascular CTA protocol may afford radiation dose reduction without significant loss of important diagnostic information. However, it is our opinion that such a decision should not be made without first having an interdisciplinary discussion with representatives from all specialties involved in the management of patients with suspected acute stroke and/or intracranial hemorrhage.

Different choices for the imaged phases of contrast enhancement have specific advantages in the evaluation of suspected stroke or intracranial hemorrhage. Although neurovascular CTA imaging is typically timed to optimize arterial enhancement, minimize motion artifacts, and reduce venous "contamination," the inclusion of images obtained in a delayed phase of contrast may decrease the number of false positives and increase localization accuracy in the detection of large vessel occlusions.[29] Imaging in more than 1 phase of contrast may also increase the sensitivity and specificity of CTA for detection of the "spot sign" or active contrast extravasation within an intraparenchymal hematoma, a strong prognostic indicator of continued hemorrhage.[30]

CTP imaging of the brain is a somewhat more controversial topic in patient-centered radiation dose management given concerns over the uncertain clinical benefit of CTP from early studies,[31,32] as well as the medical errors in CT brain perfusion imaging in the late 2000s that drew lay media attention to rising medical radiation use in diagnostic imaging[3] and resulted in a US Food and Drug Administration Safety Investigation.[33] At the time, CT brain perfusion imaging was limited by available multidetector CT scanner technology to a 2- to 4-cm volume of the brain.[34,35] The advent of new multidetector CT scanner technologies allowing volumetric CTP of the entire brain has renewed interest in this tool for evaluation of cerebrovascular pathology and treatment planning.[35–37] For example, properly used, volumetric CTP on a 320-detector array CT scanner can produce thin section axial images in arterial and/or delayed phases of contrast enhancement that are comparable with conventional CTA, with the added benefits of reduced radiation dose and additional temporal information.[35] With these advances in technology, research interest has renewed to use CTP in the evaluation of acute stroke patients, particularly in the context of evaluation for mechanical thrombectomy for large vessel occlusions, or to better inform risk–benefit decisions for patients outside traditional treatment windows.[37,38]

Neurovascular imaging in trauma computed tomography protocols

Another potential opportunity for radiation dose reduction in emergent neuroimaging is in the planning of CT protocols for imaging of blunt trauma patients. Many institutions have adopted standard protocols for whole-body trauma CT examinations, commonly referred to as "panscans," which are used in patients who have sustained significant blunt trauma to screen for injuries in multiple anatomic regions of the body.[39] Studies have shown this practice to be an efficient and effective means of expediting treatment and reducing mortality in severe trauma.[40–42] Although there is variability between institutions in the implementation details of a panscan protocol, these scans generally examine the head, neck, chest, abdomen, and pelvis, along with the entire spine. When designing a panscan protocol, one must consider whether each anatomic region will be acquired separately in segmented acquisition, combined with other anatomic regions, or acquired all together in a single pass through the scanner, as well as how many phases of contrast will be imaged. An important part of this process is deciding how screening for blunt cerebrovascular trauma will be incorporated into the protocol.

Overlap between adjacent anatomic regions is a necessary component of segmented acquisition panscan protocols and results in increased total radiation dose. Single pass, contrast-enhanced, whole body CT protocols can significantly reduce total radiation dose,[43] reportedly without substantial loss of diagnostic information.[39] In practice, many scanner consoles limit the number of reconstructions that can be built into a protocol for a single pass. As a result, single pass acquisition of multiple anatomic regions requires additional postprocessing by the CT technologists to achieve the reconstructions required for diagnostic evaluation of the included anatomic regions, which may impede the workflow in the CT scanner suite. More important, such a protocol may rely on the technologist's memory of numerous reformations, which can be problematic in a high-pressure trauma setting.

The desired phases of contrast often differ between anatomic regions, providing an additional argument for separate acquisition of body regions. For example, a separate noncontrast head acquisition is considered vital to differentiate intracranial hemorrhage from contrast enhancement.[44–46] When screening for blunt cerebrovascular and other arterial injuries, including active arterial bleeding within injured organs, CTA with arterial-timed bolus tracking is generally preferred to standard contrast-enhanced CT protocols with fixed timing,[39,47–49] although 2 studies have shown the 2 techniques to be similar in the detection of high-grade blunt cerebrovascular[50] and aortic injuries.[51] In an attempt to decrease the radiation dose, some groups have evaluated split bolus protocols for contrast administration in trauma CT

imaging, in which the total contrast volume is divided over 2 phases of intravenous administration to achieve both arterial and venous enhancement during a single pass image acquisition.[7,8,52,53] The diagnostic performance of split bolus protocols compared with conventional approaches has yet to be established, particularly with respect to cerebrovascular injury (and abdominal solid organ injury), but initial studies have reported similar quality of arterial and venous enhancement.[54,55]

Although a single, standardized trauma CT protocol may increase the efficiency of patient care and scanner throughput to some degree, it is worth considering whether a one-scan-fits-all approach to trauma CT is the optimal solution for any given patient, particularly if a single pass, whole body trauma CT protocol will not be used. A patient-centered, radiation dose-conscious approach may involve expanding on a base trauma CT protocol with a simple algorithm for determining whether certain components of the scan, such as neurovascular CTA, are indicated for a given patient. The Biffl Screening Criteria for blunt cerebrovascular injury were initially proposed in 1999 to assist in screening patients for further evaluation with diagnostic cerebrovascular angiography.[56,57] These criteria have been more recently modified to account for the increasing use of noninvasive imaging and renamed the Denver Criteria,[58] which represent a high-yield subset of clinical and imaging findings that significantly raise the likelihood of blunt cerebrovascular injury and, thus, provide an indication for further screening with neurovascular CTA (**Table 1**). Use of the Denver Criteria substantially decreases the use of neurovascular CTA in the setting of blunt trauma.[59]

In our institution, we use a radiologist-driven protocol to determine the need for neurovascular CTA for nearly all blunt trauma patients. Initially, the head and cervical spine (including the face, if specifically requested by the trauma team) are scanned before the administration of intravenous contrast. The unenhanced images are rapidly reviewed by a radiologist at the CT scanner console to screen for the imaging findings in the Denver Criteria with a preference toward the inclusion of neurovascular CTA if there is any uncertainty, so as not to further delay the remainder of the trauma CT protocol. This approach eliminates additional radiation for patients at low risk for cerebrovascular injury, while preserving the remainder of the base trauma CT protocol. In our experience, this approach is worth the trade-off for a slight increase in time spent in the CT scanner room with the added benefit of improving our relationship

Table 1
Denver screening criteria for blunt cerebrovascular injury

Mechanism	Clinical Findings	Imaging Findings
• Near hanging • High-energy transfer mechanism	• Cervical bruit • Expanding cervical hematoma • Focal neurologic deficit • Neurologic examination incongruous with head CT scan findings	• Arterial hemorrhage • Stroke on secondary CT scan • LeForte II or III fracture • Cervical spine subluxation • C1-C3 fractures • Fracture extending into a vessel foramen • Diffuse axonal injury

Abbreviation: CT, computed tomography.

From Burlew CC, Biffl WL, Moore EE, et al. Blunt cerebrovascular injuries: redefining screening criteria in the era of noninvasive diagnosis. J Trauma Acute Care Surg 2012;72(2):330–7. doi:10.1097/TA.0b013e31823de8a0; with permission.

with the trauma team by providing them with a real-time interpretation of the scan. However, for many institutions where real-time review of images at the scanner console is not feasible, it may be more practical to devise an algorithm for assessing risk for cerebrovascular injury before the scan.

Using Available Scanner and Image Postprocessing Technologies

State-of-the-art CT scanner technology allows the incorporation of many advanced image acquisition and reconstruction techniques into protocol design, resulting in improved image quality at lower radiation doses than ever before.[7,8,53] Taking advantage of these features, as available, is a key component of a patient-centered approach to radiation dose management in emergent neuroimaging. A more detailed, general discussion of strategies for reducing radiation dose in the acute care setting is provided as a reference.[8]

Measures of x-ray tube output: volume computed tomography dose index and dose–length product

The most commonly used measures of x-ray tube output in CT are the volume CT dose index (CTDI-vol) and dose–length product, typically included in a screenshot of the radiation report provided for each CT examination. The CTDI$_{vol}$ is derived from calibrated, standardized measurements of ionization events in a cylindrical, acrylic phantom (either a 16-cm "head" or 32-cm "body" model) at a given point during the scan. It depends heavily on selected scan parameters such as peak tube kilovoltage (kVp), tube current–time product (mAs), rotation time, and pitch. CTDI$_{vol}$ is typically reported as the average value over the scan region. The dose–length product is simply the average CTDI$_{vol}$ over the whole scan multiplied by the exposed length of the patient along the

z-axis. These values are best thought of as measures of x-ray tube output rather than radiation dose to the patient, because true radiation dose estimation (organ doses and overall effective dose) requires more involved calculations accounting for additional patient- and scan-specific parameters.

Tailoring the computed tomography technique: adjusting the tube current–time product and peak tube kilovoltage

Automated tube current modulation (TCM) is one of the most robust approaches to adjust CT imaging technique to body composition, such as the differential anatomy, shape, and thickness of the body in each imaged slice. With information about the patient's body composition obtained via CT projection radiographs acquired before the scan (and in some cases supplemented by data from the previous gantry rotation acquired in real time), TCM software can modulate the tube current (mAs) along both the z-axis and within the axial plane to maintain the desired level of image quality between patients of widely varying sizes, and throughout an entire CT scan between portions of a patient's anatomy that can vary greatly in their x-ray attenuation. Along with maintaining desired image quality, this protocol typically results in substantial reductions in CTDI$_{vol}$ and dose–length product for smaller patient anatomy, while increasing x-ray tube output as needed to maintain image quality in areas of greater x-ray attenuation. Specific to emergent neuroimaging, the ovoid contour of the head lends itself to radiation dose savings with the use of TCM (TCM would have insignificant impact in a uniform cylinder), which typically reduced mAs through the vertex and neck. In contrast, shoulder elevation within the scan range drives dose higher with TCM, as does increased skull thickness; however, the latter is appropriate to maintain desired image quality. These factors are among the contributors to the variability in tube current output observed between patients scanned with the same scanner protocol in **Fig. 1**. Proper use requires a detailed understanding of the available vendor approach, including the relevant adjustable parameters: Inappropriate configuration of TCM is thought to have contributed to the medical errors resulting in excessive CTP doses that resulted in hair loss and were investigated by the US Food and Drug Administration.[33]

Along with the dynamic mAs adjustments achieved with TCM, one can also consider decreasing the baseline mAs used in certain types of CT examinations. For inherently high-contrast examinations, such as spine imaging, neurovascular CTA, and CT brain perfusion imaging, one can tolerate more image noise without significant loss of diagnostic information. Additionally, owing to the intrinsic attenuation properties of iodine, scanning at a lower kVp for CTA and CTP examinations results in increased image contrast and vascular contrast-to-noise ratio for the same concentration of iodine. As a result, low kVp vascular imaging is commonly performed to accomplish improved image quality at a reduced radiation dose[60,61] (**Fig. 2**). For neurovascular CTA, these improvements can generally be performed in patients of all sizes, because it is typically possible to achieve adequate x-ray penetration through the neck and head, although image quality may degrade through the great vessel origins owing to photon starvation through the region of the shoulders.

Postprocessing: iterative reconstruction
Use of iterative reconstruction (IR) algorithms for image postprocessing, as opposed to traditional filtered back projection algorithms, can allow for even greater decreases in tube output, resulting in further radiation exposure savings. In theory, IR reduces reconstructed image noise through successive applications of a procedure that begins with filtered back projection of raw CT data into the image domain and then iterates on the following steps: (1) models of image noise and other factors are used to refine an estimate of the actual image data, (2) forward projection of the image estimate into the raw data domain, where the estimate is compared with the actual raw data and further refined, and (3) filtered back projection of the refined raw data estimate back into the image domain with filtered back projection, where the process is repeated. In practice, this procedure would require a prohibitive amount of computer processing speed and time to implement, so vendors have developed complex algorithms that approximate the theoretic IR procedure, while remaining computationally tractable in the context of clinical workflow. These algorithms can often be applied at incremental "strengths" to afford greater reductions in image noise. A caveat is that higher strengths of IR may result in an undesirable image texture. **Fig. 3** illustrates how image texture changes and image

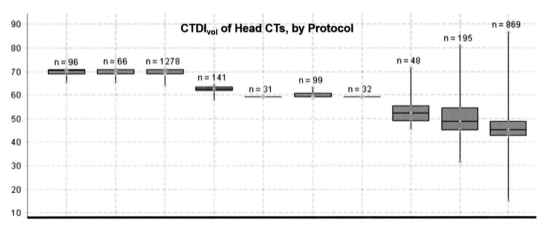

Fig. 1. Historical comparison of mean volume computed tomography (CT) dose index (CTDI$_{vol}$) among different head CT protocols across multiple scanners. The CTDI$_{vol}$ varies considerably between protocols largely owing to differences in selected scan parameters (such as the quality reference tube current–time product [mAs]), and in technique options (such as iterative reconstruction) available on the scanner platforms of different ages. CTDI$_{vol}$ for most scans falls well below the American College of Radiology Diagnostic Reference Level of 75 mGy. The protocols to left with narrow CTDI$_{vol}$ ranges use fixed technique without tube current modulation (TCM), while the 3 to the right use TCM with reduced quality reference mAs level enabled by iterative reconstruction. High outliers result from TCM increasing mAs to compensate for elevated shoulders or unusually thick calvaria. Low outliers result from rescans through the topmost portion of the vertex.

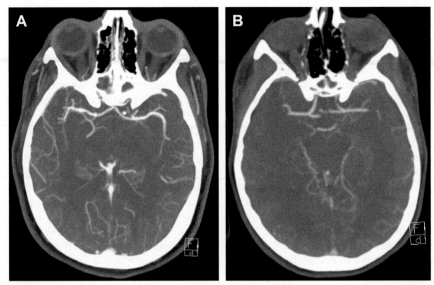

Fig. 2. Maximum intensity projection images through the proximal middle cerebral arteries (MCAs) from head computed tomography angiography obtained at 100 kVp (*A*) versus 120 kVp (*B*). Images were obtained with reference tube current–time products of 250 and 175, respectively, reconstructed at the same image thickness and displayed with the same window width and level. Note the improved visualization of proximal and distal MCA branches in (*A*), partly owing to increased contrast resolution at 100 kVp. Despite this improved image quality, the 100 kVp scan was obtained with approximately 10% lower CTDI$_{vol}$ than the comparison 120 kVp scan.

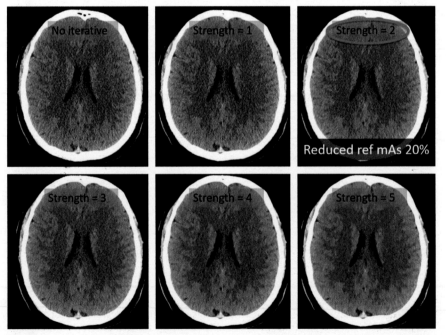

Fig. 3. Images from the same unenhanced head computed tomography scan obtained at 120 kVp and reconstructed using different strengths of iterative reconstruction (IR). Note the reduced noise at higher IR strengths. Some radiologists find the higher strengths to have an unusually "plastic" appearance raising concerns about masking fine detail. After internal "taste testing" among radiologists within our institution, a modest IR strength of 2 was selected for clinical use, along with a modest 20% radiation dose reduction accomplished by reducing the quality reference tube current–time products from 450 to 360.

noise progressively decreases at higher strengths of IR. At our institution, a modest strength of IR was implemented on noncontrast head CT scans with a corresponding modest 20% dose reduction. At another institution, radiation dose for neurovascular CTA was reduced by 50% with a combination of scanning at 80 kVp (as compared with 120 kVp) and postprocessing with IR.[61]

AFTER THE SCAN: MONITORING RADIATION EXPOSURE FROM COMPUTED TOMOGRAPHY IMAGING

Monitoring of patient radiation exposure from CT imaging is an important part of ensuring the success of the broader strategy for radiation exposure management. It should involve a multitiered approach spanning individual CT examinations up to the institutional patient population.[62] The first tier should involve a review by the interpreting radiologist of the CT radiation report attached to each study on Picture archiving & communication system (PACS) to ensure the $CTDI_{vol}$ does not deviate significantly from institutional norms or the American College of Radiology Diagnostic Reference Level for a given study (eg, 75 mGy for an unenhanced head CT reported on a 16-cm CTDI phantom). This practice can help to identify outliers at the high end of radiation exposure, potentially triggering further review of the dose event to identify any modifiable contributors. Periodic review of protocols must be performed by the CT operations team, ideally including a physician, medical physicist, and technologist collaborators. Institutional CT dose monitoring software permits comparison of performed scan doses with external benchmarks, and allows for the real-time investigation of outliers to prevent any protocol deviations from propagating to other patients.[63] An example of radiation dose variability across different CT scanners and neuroimaging protocols is shown in **Fig. 1**.

EMERGING COMPUTED TOMOGRAPHY TECHNOLOGIES: DUAL ENERGY AND MULTIENERGY SPECTRAL COMPUTED TOMOGRAPHY

Dual energy and multienergy CT has yet to achieve widespread adoption, but ongoing research in this area has exposed significant opportunities for improved diagnostic capabilities in emergent CT neuroimaging. A review of potential applications for dual energy CT neuroimaging is provided as a reference.[64] Briefly, the diagnostic value of dual energy and multienergy spectral CT lies in the ability to differentiate materials based on their varied x-ray attenuation behavior as a function of x-ray energy.

For example, dual energy CT can differentiate intracranial hemorrhage from calcium[65] or iodinated contrast.[45] This property may enable radiation dose reduction by reducing the number of needed scan phases, or by eliminating the need for subsequent follow-up scans. For example, in the setting of trauma, accurate differentiation of preexisting calcium from posttraumatic hemorrhage may obviate the need for follow-up imaging, thereby reducing radiation dose and duration of stay. After intraarterial thrombolysis for stroke, iodine maps may differentiate postprocedural iodine staining from new hemorrhage, reducing the need for subsequent scans to make the differentiation. In other specific situations, virtual noncontrast scans in which the iodine has been subtracted from the images may be used in place of a true noncontrast scan, enabling dose reducing in certain multiphase scan protocols. Dual energy CT also offers improvements on existing bone subtraction and metal artifact reduction methods, which may provide better assessment of vessels within cranial or vertebral foramina and may in some cases improve the diagnostic quality of neurovascular CTA for patients with metallic implants, respectively.

SUMMARY

Although the benefits of obtaining and/or excluding a diagnosis often outweighs any theoretic risk of radiation exposure in the setting of acute, emergent neurologic conditions, radiation dose from medical imaging remains an important concern. The first step in a patient-centered approach to radiation dose management in emergent neuroimaging is to promote the appropriate use of emergent CT neuroimaging studies through CDS tools. Before the patient arrives in the scanner, a thoughtful approach to protocol design will ensure a given CT neuroimaging examination is limited to the minimum necessary to achieve the diagnostic goal. During the scan, modern scanner technologies and image postprocessing techniques can synergistically reduce radiation exposure while preserving diagnostic imaging quality. After the scan, population-level monitoring of radiation exposure will help to identify outliers, as well as factors that may contribute to increased radiation dose for certain examinations. Emerging technologies such as dual energy and multienergy spectral CT may result in additional opportunities for radiation dose savings.

REFERENCES

1. Griffey RT, Sodickson A. Cumulative radiation exposure and cancer risk estimates in emergency

department patients undergoing repeat or multiple CT. Am J Roentgenol 2009;192(4):887–92.

2. Sodickson A, Baeyens PF, Andriole KP, et al. Recurrent CT, cumulative radiation exposure, and associated radiation-induced cancer risks from CT of adults. Radiology 2009;251(1):175–84.

3. Bogdanich W. After stroke scans, patients face serious health risks. New York Times 2010;2–7. Available at: http://www.nytimes.com/2010/08/01/health/01radiation.html?_r=2&scp=1&sq=perfusion&st=cse.

4. Bogdanich W. Radiation offers new cures, and ways to do harm. New York Times 2010;1–12. Available at: www.nytimes.com/2010/01/24/health/24radiation.html?pagewanted=all.

5. Bogdanich W, McGinty JC. Medicare claims show overuse for CT scanning. New York Times 2011;4–7. Available at: http://www.nytimes.com/2011/06/18/health/18radiation.html%5Cnpapers2://publication/uuid/1DC22A0D-C241-47C9-9720-94BD6D0E10A4.

6. Shyu JY, Sodickson AD. Communicating radiation risk to patients and referring physicians in the emergency department setting. Br J Radiol 2016;89(1061). https://doi.org/10.1259/bjr.20150868.

7. Sodickson A. Strategies for reducing radiation exposure in multi-detector row CT. Radiol Clin North Am 2012;50(1):1–14.

8. Sodickson A. Strategies for reducing radiation exposure from multidetector computed tomography in the acute care setting. Can Assoc Radiol J 2013;64(2):119–29.

9. Protecting Access to Medicare Act of 2014 (H.R. 4302). 113th United States Congress, Washington, DC. 2nd Session. April 1, 2014.

10. Appropriate Use Criteria. Centers for Medicare & Medicaid Services website. 2017. Available at: https://www.cms.gov/Medicare/Quality-Initiatives-Patient-Assessment-Instruments/Appropriate-Use-Criteria-Program/index.html. Accessed October 4, 2017.

11. ACR Appropriateness Criteria. American College of Radiology website. 2017. Available at: https://www.acr.org/Quality-Safety/Appropriateness-Criteria. Accessed October 4, 2017.

12. Prevedello LM, Raja AS, Zane RD, et al. Variation in use of head computed tomography by emergency physicians. Am J Med 2012;125(4):356–64.

13. Stiell IG, Wells GA, Vandemheen K, et al. The Canadian CT Head Rule for patients with minor head injury. Lancet 2001;357(9266):1391–6.

14. Klang E, Beytelman A, Greenberg D, et al. Overuse of head CT examinations for the investigation of minor head trauma: analysis of contributing factors. J Am Coll Radiol 2017;171–6. https://doi.org/10.1016/j.jacr.2016.08.032.

15. Gupta A, Ip IK, Raja AS, et al. Effect of clinical decision support on documented guideline adherence for head CT in emergency department patients with mild traumatic brain injury. J Am Med Inform Assoc 2014;21(e2):e347–51.

16. Ip IK, Raja AS, Gupta A, et al. Impact of clinical decision support on head computed tomography use in patients with mild traumatic brain injury in the ED. Am J Emerg Med 2015;33(3):320–5.

17. Wortman JR, Goud A, Raja AS, et al. Structured physician order entry for trauma CT: value in improving clinical information transfer and billing efficiency. Am J Roentgenol 2014;203(6):1242–8.

18. U-King-Im JM, Trivedi RA, Graves MJ, et al. Utility of an ultrafast magnetic resonance imaging protocol in recent and semi-recent strokes. J Neurol Neurosurg Psychiatry 2005;76(7):1002–5.

19. Prakkamakul S, Witzel T, Huang S, et al. Ultrafast brain MRI: clinical deployment and comparison to conventional brain MRI at 3T. J Neuroimaging 2016;26(5):503–10.

20. Boyle TP, Paldino MJ, Kimia AA, et al. Comparison of rapid cranial MRI to CT for ventricular shunt malfunction. Pediatrics 2014;134(1):e47–54.

21. Köhrmann M, Jüttler E, Fiebach JB, et al. MRI versus CT-based thrombolysis treatment within and beyond the 3 h time window after stroke onset: a cohort study. Lancet Neurol 2006;5(8):661–7.

22. Li Y-H, Li M-H, Zhao J-G, et al. MRI-based ultrafast protocol thrombolysis with rt-PA for acute ischemia stroke in 12-hour time window. J Neuroimaging 2011;21(4):332–9.

23. Gerischer LM, Fiebach JB, Scheitz JF, et al. Magnetic resonance imaging-based versus computed tomography-based thrombolysis in acute ischemic stroke: comparison of safety and efficacy within a cohort study. Cerebrovasc Dis 2013;35(3):250–6.

24. Powers WJ, Derdeyn CP, Biller J, et al. 2015 American Heart Association/American stroke association focused update of the 2013 guidelines for the early management of patients with acute ischemic stroke regarding endovascular treatment: a guideline for healthcare professionals from the American Heart Association/American stroke. Stroke 2015;46(10):3020–35.

25. Mair G, von Kummer R, Adami A, et al. Observer reliability of CT angiography in the assessment of acute ischaemic stroke: data from the Third International Stroke Trial. Neuroradiology 2015;57(1):1–9.

26. Vachha BA, Schaefer PW. Imaging patterns and management algorithms in acute stroke: an update for the emergency radiologist. Radiol Clin North Am 2015;53(4):801–26.

27. Wintermark M, Sanelli PC, Albers GW, et al. Imaging recommendations for acute stroke and transient ischemic attack patients: a joint statement by the American Society of Neuroradiology, the American College of Radiology and the Society of

NeuroInterventional Surgery. J Am Coll Radiol 2013; 828–32. https://doi.org/10.1016/j.jacr.2013.06.019.

28. Deipolyi A, Hmaberg L, Gonzaléz RG, et al. Diagnostic yield of emergency department arch-to-vertex CT angiography in patients with suspected acute stroke. AJNR Am J Neuroradiol 2015;36(2): 265–8.

29. Chung HJ, Lee BH, Hwang YJ, et al. Delayed-phase CT angiography is superior to arterial-phase CT angiography at localizing occlusion sites in acute stroke patients eligible for intra-arterial reperfusion therapy. J Clin Neurosci 2014;21(4):596–600.

30. Peng W-J, Reis C, Reis H, et al. Predictive value of CTA spot sign on hematoma expansion in intracerebral hemorrhage patients. Biomed Res Int 2017; 2017:1–9. Figure 1.

31. Goyal M, Menon BK, Derdeyn CP. Perfusion imaging in acute ischemic stroke: let us improve the science before changing clinical practice. Radiology 2013; 266(1):16–21.

32. Lev MH. Perfusion imaging of acute stroke: its role in current and future clinical practice. Radiology 2013; 266(1):22–7.

33. US Food and Drug Administration (FDA). Safety investigation of CT brain perfusion scans. Silver Spring (MD): Center for Devices and Radiological Health; 2010. Available at: http://www.fda.gov/MedicalDevices/Safety/AlertsandNotices/ucm185898.htm. Accessed September 10, 2017.

34. Klotz E, König M. Perfusion measurements of the brain: using dynamic CT for the quantitative assessment of cerebral ischemia in acute stroke. Eur J Radiol 1999; 30(3):170–84. Available at: http://www.ncbi.nlm.nih.gov/pubmed/10452715. Accessed September 10, 2017.

35. Saake M, Goelitz P, Struffert T, et al. Comparison of conventional CTA and volume perfusion CTA in evaluation of cerebral arterial vasculature in acute stroke. AJNR Am J Neuroradiol 2012;33(11): 2068–73.

36. Orrison WW, Snyder KV, Hopkins LN, et al. Whole-brain dynamic CT angiography and perfusion imaging. Clin Radiol 2011;66(6):566–74.

37. Van Seeters T, Biessels GJ, Kappelle LJ, et al. The prognostic value of CT angiography and CT perfusion in acute ischemic stroke. Cerebrovasc Dis 2015;40(5–6):258–69.

38. Haussen DC, Dehkharghani S, Rangaraju S, et al. Automated CT perfusion ischemic core volume and noncontrast CT ASPECTS (Alberta Stroke Program Early CT Score): correlation and clinical outcome prediction in large vessel stroke. Stroke 2016;47(9):2318–22.

39. Fanucci E, Fiaschetti V, Rotili A, et al. Whole body 16-row multislice CT in emergency room: effects of different protocols on scanning time, image quality and radiation exposure. Emerg Radiol 2007;13(5): 251–7.

40. Huber-Wagner S, Lefering R, Qvick LM, et al. Effect of whole-body CT during trauma resuscitation on survival: a retrospective, multicentre study. Lancet 2009;373(9673):1455–61.

41. Yeguiayan J-M, Yap A, Freysz M, et al. Impact of whole-body computed tomography on mortality and surgical management of severe blunt trauma. Crit Care 2012;16(3):R101.

42. Kimura A, Tanaka N. Whole-body computed tomography is associated with decreased mortality in blunt trauma patients with moderate-to-severe consciousness disturbance: a multicenter, retrospective study. J Trauma Acute Care Surg 2013;75(2):202–6.

43. Ptak T, Rhea JT, Novelline RA. Radiation dose is reduced with a single-pass whole-body multi-detector row CT trauma protocol compared with a conventional segmented method: initial experience. Radiology 2003;229(3):902–5.

44. Ferda J, Novák M, Mírka H, et al. The assessment of intracranial bleeding with virtual unenhanced imaging by means of dual-energy CT angiography. Eur Radiol 2009;19(10):2518–22.

45. Phan CM, Yoo AJ, Hirsch JA, et al. Differentiation of hemorrhage from iodinated contrast in different intracranial compartments using dual-energy head CT. AJNR Am J Neuroradiol 2012;33(6):1088–94.

46. Bonatti M, Lombardo F, Zamboni GA, et al. Dual-energy CT of the brain: comparison between DECT angiography-derived virtual unenhanced images and true unenhanced images in the detection of intracranial haemorrhage. Eur Radiol 2017;27(7): 2690–7.

47. Dreizin D, Munera F. Blunt polytrauma: evaluation with 64-section whole-body CT angiography. Radiographics 2012;32(3):609–31.

48. Bruns BR, Tesoriero R, Kufera J, et al. Blunt cerebrovascular injury screening guidelines. J Trauma Acute Care Surg 2014;76(3):691–5.

49. Uyeda JW, LeBedis CA, Penn DR, et al. Active hemorrhage and vascular injuries in splenic trauma: utility of the arterial phase in multidetector CT. Radiology 2014;270(1):99–106.

50. Laser A, Kufera JA, Bruns BR, et al. Initial screening test for blunt cerebrovascular injury: validity assessment of whole-body computed tomography. Surgery 2015;158(3):627–35.

51. Zaw AA, Stewart D, Murry JS, et al. CT chest with IV contrast compared with CT angiography after blunt trauma. Am Surg 2015;81(10):1080–3. Available at: http://www.ncbi.nlm.nih.gov/pubmed/26463312. Accessed September 10, 2017.

52. Mayo-Smith WW, Hara AK, Mahesh M, et al. How I do it: managing radiation dose in CT. Radiology 2014;273(3):657–72.

53. Kalra MK, Sodickson AD, Mayo-Smith WW. CT radiation: key concepts for gentle and wise use. Radiographics 2015;35(6):1706–21.

54. Leung V, Sastry A, Woo TD, et al. Implementation of a split-bolus single-pass CT protocol at a UK major trauma centre to reduce excess radiation dose in trauma pan-CT. Clin Radiol 2015;70(10):1110–5.

55. Beenen LF, Sierink JC, Kolkman S, et al. Split bolus technique in polytrauma: a prospective study on scan protocols for trauma analysis. Acta Radiol 2015;56(7):873–80.

56. Biffl WL, Moore EE, Offner PJ, et al. Blunt carotid arterial injuries: implications of a new grading scale. J Trauma 1999;47(5):845–53. Available at: http://www.ncbi.nlm.nih.gov/pubmed/10568710. Accessed October 5, 2017.

57. Biffl WL, Moore EE, Offner PJ, et al. Optimizing screening for blunt cerebrovascular injuries. Am J Surg 1999;178(6):517–22.

58. Burlew CC, Biffl WL, Moore EE, et al. Blunt cerebrovascular injuries: redefining screening criteria in the era of noninvasive diagnosis. J Trauma Acute Care Surg 2012;72(2):330–7.

59. Beliaev AM, Barber PA, Marshall RJ, et al. Denver screening protocol for blunt cerebrovascular injury reduces the use of multi-detector computed tomography angiography. ANZ J Surg 2014;84(6):429–32.

60. Sodickson A, Weiss M. Effects of patient size on radiation dose reduction and image quality in low-kVp CT pulmonary angiography performed with reduced IV contrast dose. Emerg Radiol 2012; 19(5):437–45.

61. Zhang W, Li M, Zhang B, et al. CT angiography of the head-and-neck vessels acquired with low tube voltage, low iodine, and iterative image reconstruction: clinical evaluation of radiation dose and image quality. PLoS One 2013;8(12):e81486. Zuffi A, editor.

62. Sodickson A, Khorasani R. Patient-centric radiation dose monitoring in the electronic health record: what are some of the barriers and key next steps? J Am Coll Radiol 2010;7(10):752–3.

63. Sodickson A, Warden GI, Farkas CE, et al. Exposing exposure: automated anatomy-specific CT radiation exposure extraction for quality assurance and radiation monitoring. Radiology 2012; 264(2):397–405.

64. Potter C, Sodickson A. Dual-energy CT in emergency neuroimaging: added value and novel applications. Radiographics 2016;36(7):2186–98.

65. Hu R, Daftari Besheli L, Young J, et al. Dual-energy head CT enables accurate distinction of intraparenchymal hemorrhage from calcification in emergency department patients. Radiology 2016; 280(1):177–83.

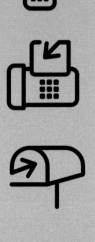